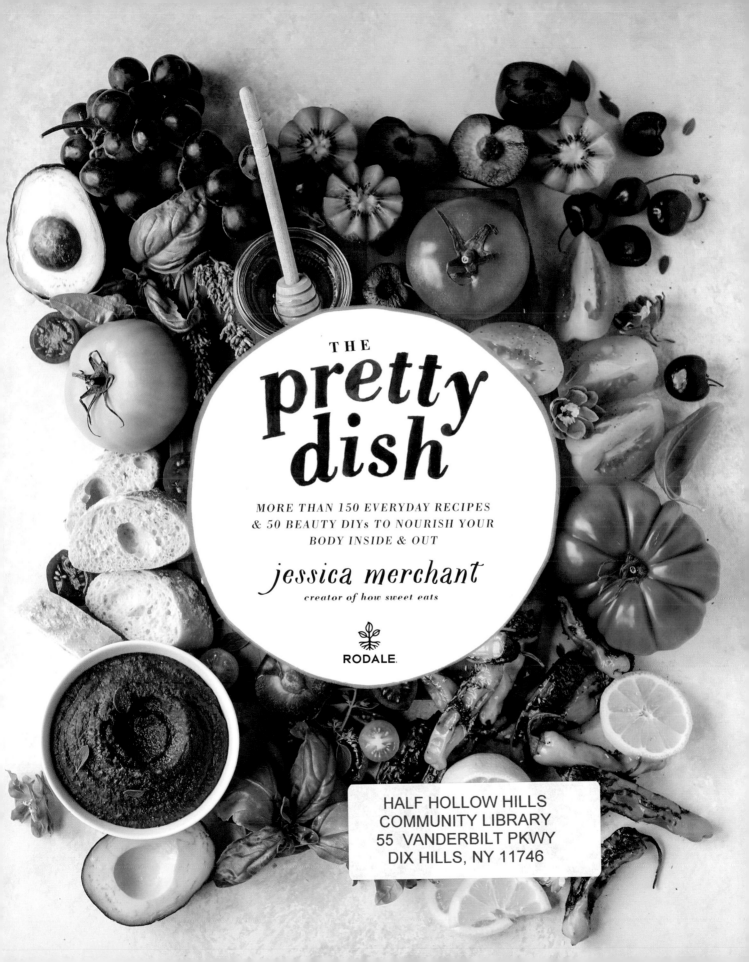

THE
pretty dish

MORE THAN 150 EVERYDAY RECIPES
& 50 BEAUTY DIYs TO NOURISH YOUR
BODY INSIDE & OUT

jessica merchant
creator of how sweet eats

RODALE.

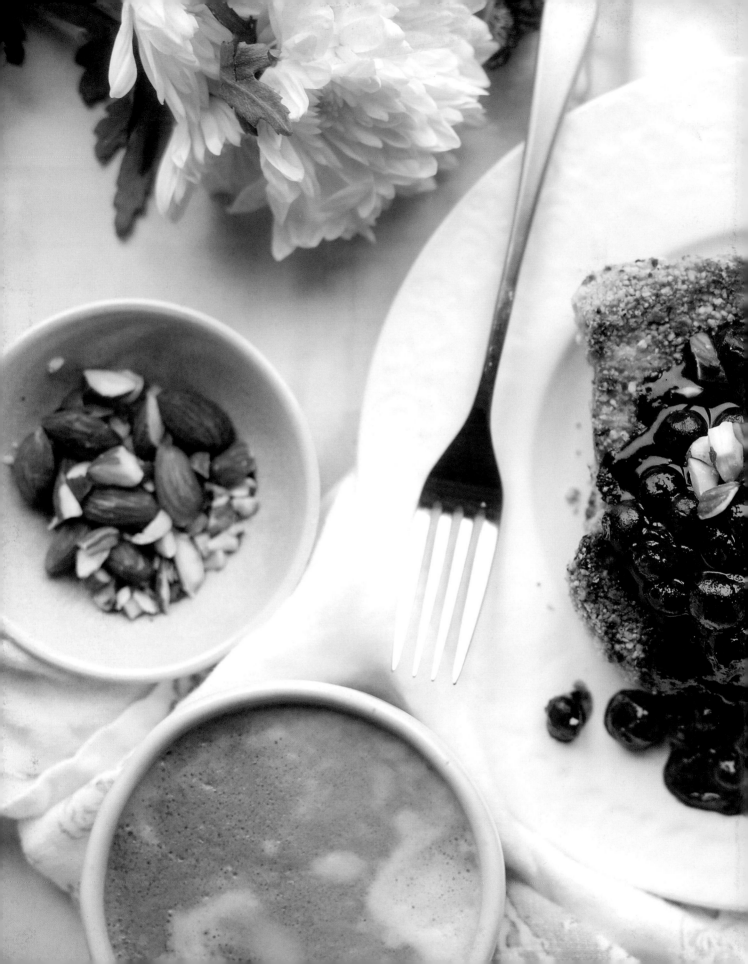

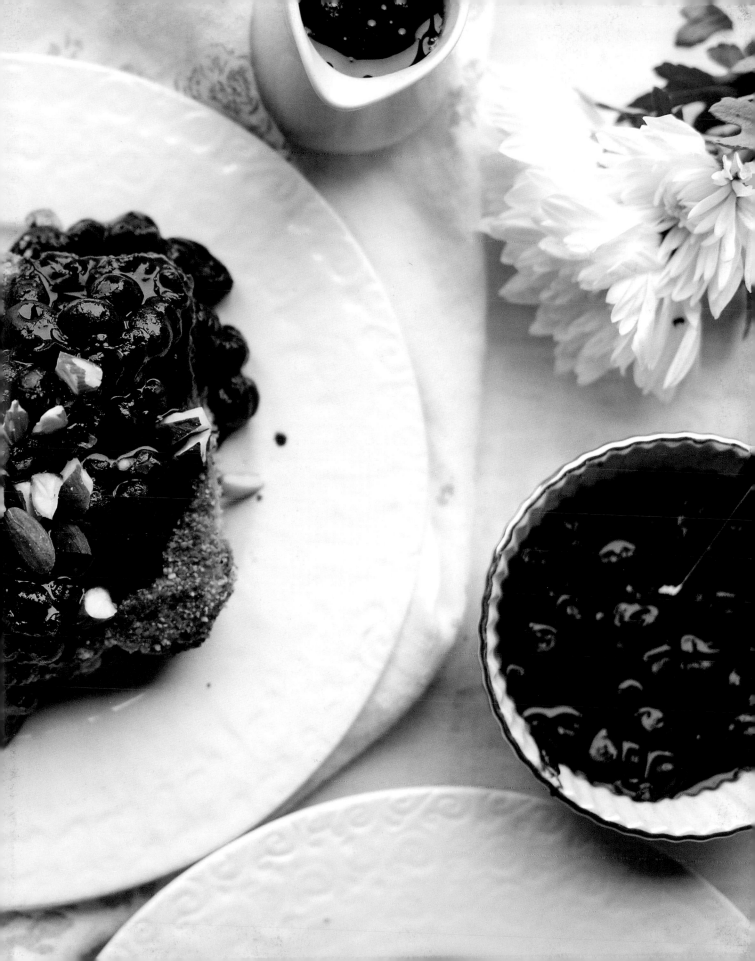

RODALE *wellness*

Live happy. Be healthy. Get inspired.

Sign up today to get exclusive access to our authors, exclusive bonuses, and the most authoritative, useful, and cutting-edge information on health, wellness, fitness, and living your life to the fullest.

Visit us online at RodaleWellness.com
Join us at RodaleWellness.com/Join

Rodale books may be purchased for business or promotional use or for special sales. For information, please e-mail: BookMarketing@Rodale.com.

Printed in China

Rodale Inc. makes every effort to use acid-free ∞, recycled paper ♻.

Book design by Yeon Kim

Library of Congress Cataloging-in-Publication Data is on file with the publisher.

ISBN 978-1-62336-969-9

Distributed to the trade by Macmillan

2 4 6 8 10 9 7 5 3 1 hardcover

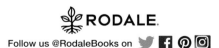

Follow us @RodaleBooks on 🐦 📘 📌 📷

We inspire health, healing, happiness, and love in the world.
Starting with you.

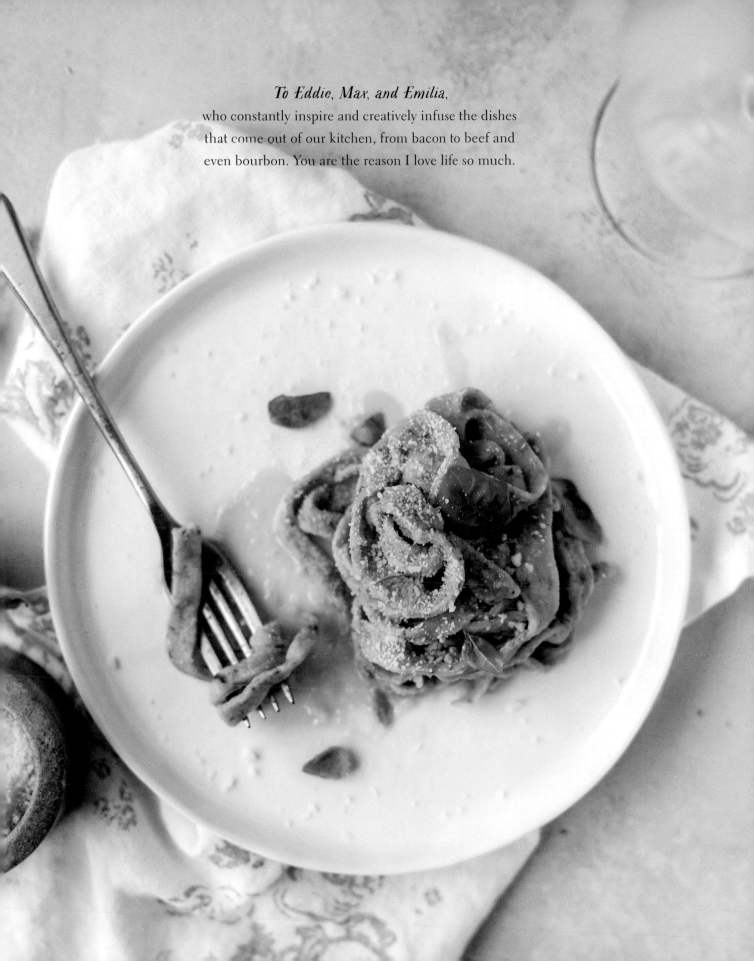

To Eddie, Max, and Emilia,
who constantly inspire and creatively infuse the dishes
that come out of our kitchen, from bacon to beef and
even bourbon. You are the reason I love life so much.

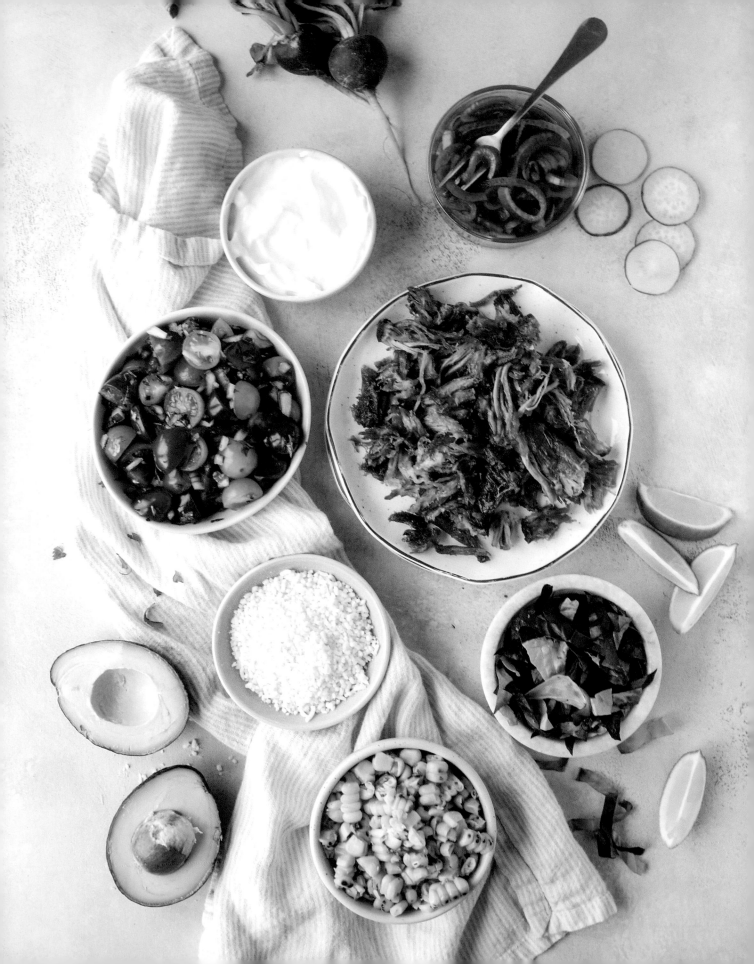

contents

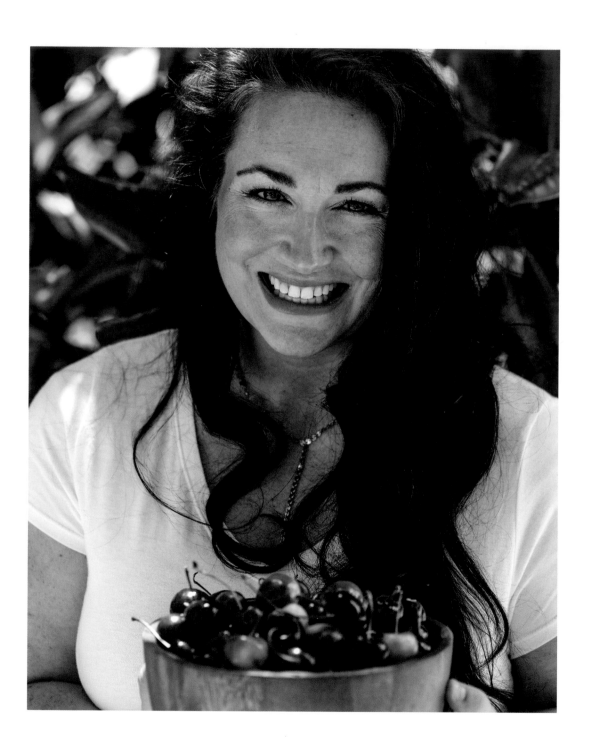

introduction

IT'S 6:47 A.M. WHEN MY ALARM GOES off, and as I peek at my phone screen with one eye open, I see that I have six texts from last night at 1:32 a.m. from my cousin Lacy. It's a group text—one of my least favorite things in the universe—but it includes food, so that softens the blow a bit. Plus, the notifications all went off while I was sleeping and not doing something important like scrolling through Instagram and falling into the vortex of my brother's ex-girlfriend's sister who just got married to a guy I "went together with" in fourth grade, so it's cool.

Speaking of Instagram, that's what the group text was all about. Lacy sent a screenshot of a crazy dessert that she thinks we have to try out together, and she must have been scroll happy, because what follows are screenshots of things that are equally delicious and increasing in calories. A pizza supreme fondue, a peanut butter truffle doughnut, a quinoa salad that would utilize everything we could get at the farmers' market on Saturday morn-

ing, and because life doesn't exist without cocktails: a blueberry mojito punch.

Thanks to her, at 7 a.m. on a Monday morning I am now starving for *anything* but the bowl of overnight oats that sits in my fridge, waiting for a sprinkling of chia seeds and dried raspberries.

There is nothing worse than the dreaded Monday breakfast, when you're still in a food coma from the weekend and craving all sorts of crispy, crunchy tacos with white Cheddar queso and an endless pitcher of margaritas.

Gosh. This just keeps getting worse.

Food is one of the things that tie Lacy and I together; it's one of the ways that we honor our grandmother and one of the activities that we enjoy doing together. Eating *and* cooking, that is. It seems like in the last 4 years, time has both sped up and slowed down. When I was pregnant with my son, Max, everyone told me over and over again how it would be life-changing, and boy were they right. The thing was, though, that I didn't quite feel like *I* had changed. My life and circumstances changed, and it took a lot of adjusting to the "new normal" to feel like things were back in place.

Which is totally a joke, because I think I'm still adjusting to the "new normal"! Two-and-a-half years later, here I am secretly pregnant (only Eddie knows!) with my second child as I write this book, preparing to enter the next new normal that will come with the pitter-patter of multiple baby toes under my own feet.

Of course, there were times in my son's newborn stage when I didn't think I could even manage to make it into the kitchen. Nights when we ate egg sandwiches for dinner, and certainly not ones that you would see on the cover of *Food & Wine*. I had running lists of recipes that sounded *so* fantastic, but days that were rather exhausting and led me to make quick chicken quesadillas for dinner instead.

One thing that has remained constant is my complete and utter adoration for sharing food with people I love. It's funny, because I often tell others how I really have no desire to be a chef in a restaurant and cook for strangers—my true passion lies in cooking and sharing food with people I know and love.

That totally includes *you*. Writing a blog on the Internet has been world-altering for me, even if my parents (and occa-sionally even my husband, Eddie) ask, "Wait, *what* is it that you actually do? Is this really . . . work?"

Writing the blog has been such gratifying work that it has changed my life. While I've never claimed to be a professional chef or culinary expert—and I relish the fact that I'm mom-taught, grandma-taught, and, let's be real, Internet-taught—sharing the experiences that I've had making thousands of recipes over the last 8 years has been so much fun. I have met some of my closest friends this way and feel an incredible connection with the community on my website.

Because of all that, I find that my love for sharing food is twofold. Sharing recipes with readers of my blog, new readers of my cookbooks, and general invisible Internet friends (I know you're real!) has bridged the gap with so many people that I would have never been able to connect with otherwise. It's an easier way to find others who share the same tastebuds that I do, who have a passion for home cooking, and who possibly even enjoy reading the ridiculous rambles that find their way onto the pages of my little corner on the Internet.

However, the other part of this love is that this entire experience has broadened my expertise in being able to share food with family and friends. One of Eddie's and my favorite things to do is host a

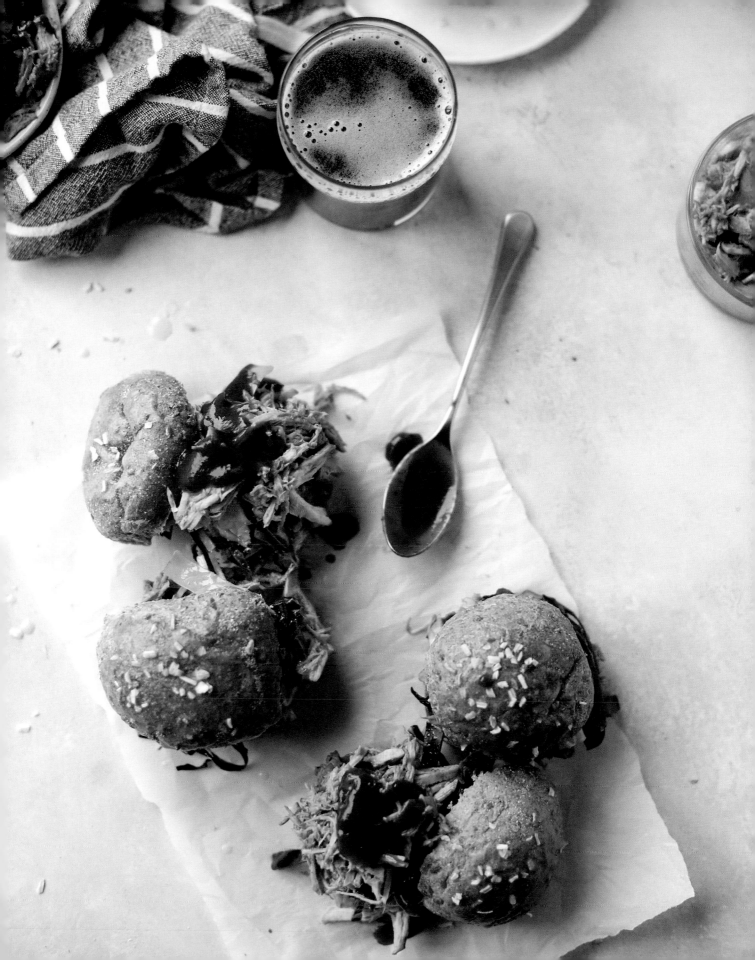

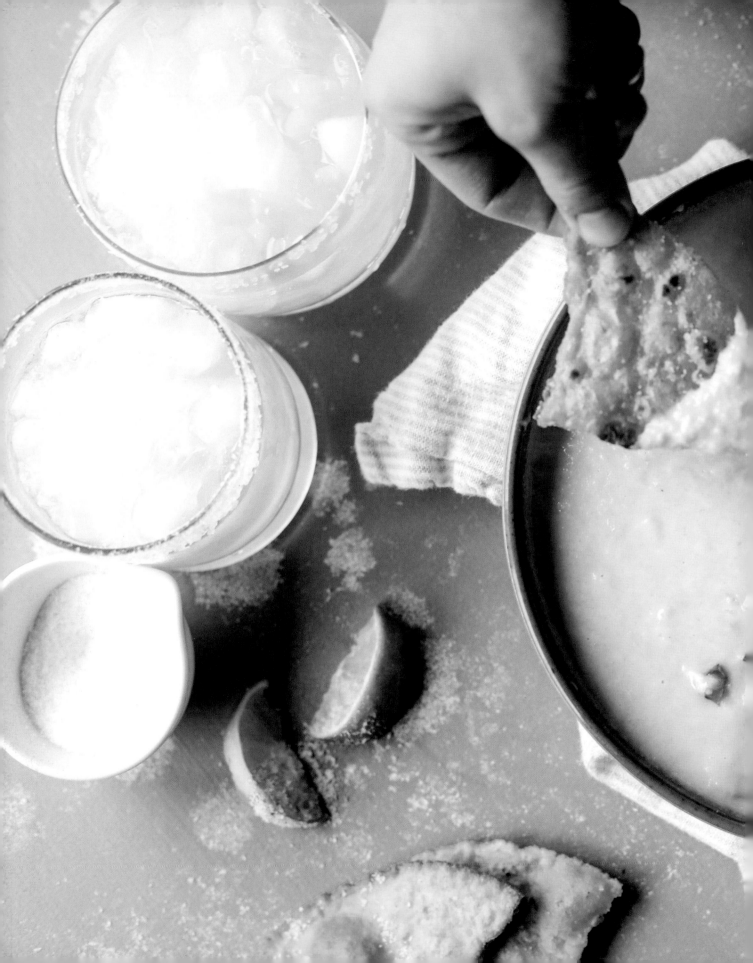

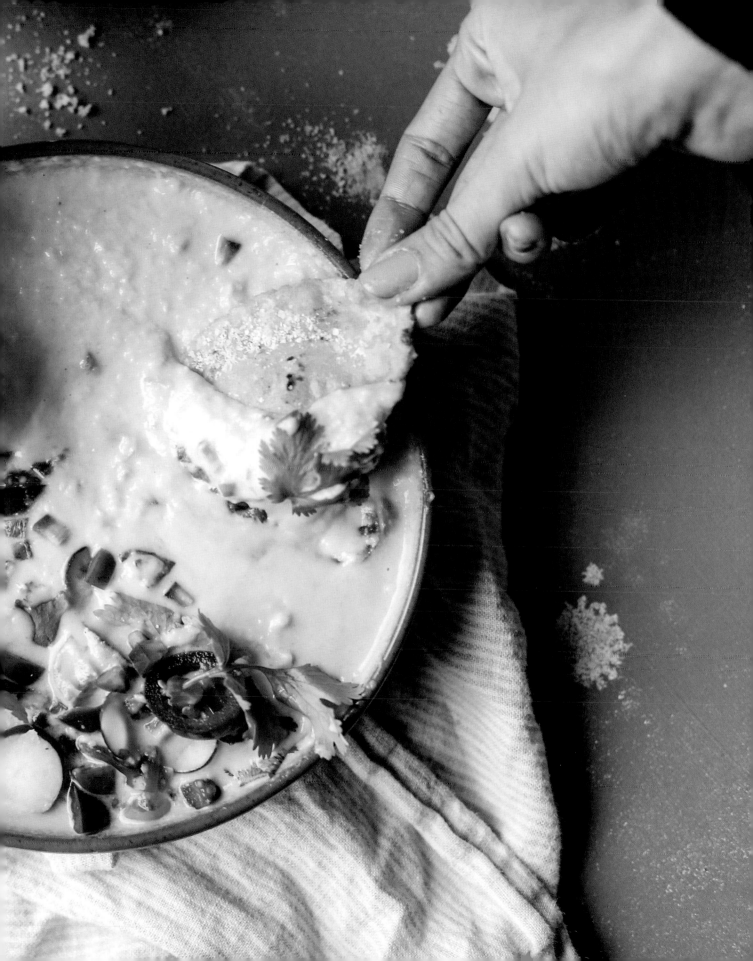

homemade pizza night, which includes grilled pizzas in the summer or baked pizzas in the winter, and I've learned to let go of the stress of cleaning up the mess while we entertain others.

The meals in our home are not always picture-perfect. There are many nights (occasionally, even once a week) when I will eat cereal for dinner or Eddie will make pancakes and eggs. Cooking and sharing food does not have to be glamorous or even Instagram-worthy, though of course I do love a great social media–inspired cheese plate. We have our days (and weeks!) that include plain peanut butter toast, bagged salad, and more cups of yogurt than I can count. But what I like to emphasize most in our house is feeding our family and friends with love and joy, even if it isn't perfect.

With all of this in mind, there is a big constant in these recipes: Almost all of them can be made in 60 minutes or less! 98 percent of them, to be exact. I bent the rules when it came to a few recipes, mainly ones that include use of the slow cooker, because sometimes that is just more convenient. And while those recipes may technically take 6 to 8 hours to cook, the prep and hands-on time is still well under an hour.

I want our food to taste amazing, but I want it to be made in an amount of time that doesn't make my head hurt. I'm a true member of the Internet generation, and I want our time with family, friends, siblings, children, girlfriends—everyone!—to be taken up with good conversation and lots of ice-cold rosé (okay, not for the kids), and not while I'm slaving away to make sure a three-course meal will fit the bill.

Self-care is a trendy term these days, and I find that cooking and sharing a delicious meal with people is my own form of self-care. And, perhaps, self-indulgence! In the best way possible, that is what I hope you take from this book that is so full with recipes from my own head and heart. I want you to take care of yourself and your loved ones. I want you to read the pages of this cookbook like a novel and feel like you are cooking with your BFF. These recipes, from the food that goes in your belly to the food that goes on your face, are ones that you can make with your best group of girlfriends or your family on a Monday night at the start of a busy week. I want these recipes to feel like *you*.

See, there's a whole other section to this book that I haven't even touched on yet, and while it does include "recipes," they aren't so much ones that you will want to put in your mouth. Well, technically, some of them sound and smell so delicious that you might be tempted, but these recipes come with one very specific thing in mind: your skin! It's food for your face *and* your body, if you will.

The truth is that I've been a beauty junkie my entire life. I'm convinced that some of us are born with this love for products, while others are not. Of course, that's ridiculous, and I'm sure it has to do with nature versus nurture or whatever, but really, I'm almost positive that I left the womb with one arm out grabbing for my mom's lipstick.

Some of my earliest memories include sitting on the floor with my mom while she did her makeup, getting ready to go out for a night on the town with my dad. I can still remember the smell of her perfume (Calvin Klein Obsession at the time . . . *Hello '80s!*), the scent of her shampoo mixing with the electric smell of our hair dryer in 1987, the smell of powder bouncing off her brushes, and that classic lipstick taste that you either grow to love or hate.

Beauty love was all around me. My maternal grandmother (whom I refer to lovingly on my blog as Mother Lovett) would sit on one of those stunning plush velvet cushions in front of a gorgeous vanity from the '50s to apply her makeup. (My cousin Lacy has it in her bedroom now, by the way.) She did this for as long as I can remember—even in her late eighties before she died, when it was much more common for her to draw in her eyebrows with mauve lip liner instead of an eyebrow pencil. Being legally deaf and blind made

makeup application a bit harder, but somehow, she still looked classy in her heels, with her snow-white hair and purplish pink eyebrows on at the age of 87.

I would often sneak into my mom's room and go through her stash of makeup samples, presumably from all the "free gifts" that you would get with a purchase back in the '80s and '90s. The gifts in those days were fairly generous, and I'd take the eyeshadow and lipstick that did nothing for my skin and sit in front of my own light-up makeup mirror (one of the best Christmas presents *ever!*) and experiment. My paternal grandmother only heightened my love because she would give me the free gift makeup samples each time I saw her, and by the age of 11 or 12, I'd say that I had quite the "collection" of samples—albeit nothing I technically purchased (aside from 20 flavors of Bonne Bell Lip Smackers) and all full of shades that were anything but complementary to my skin.

These ladies, my grandmothers especially, were truly the epitome of grace and elegance in a way that came across as anything but pretentious. If they were alive today, they'd never be the women going through the drive-thru for iced coffee or wearing glitter on their faces. In fact, they'd make simple sandwich lunches for road trips, pull off on the side of the road where a picnic table just happened to be placed under a tree, and enjoy a patient, non-rushed lunch without worrying about reaching their destination. I'm still aiming for that grace!

I've never had artistic talent in the form of drawing, painting, or sculpting, but in a weird way, I loved that makeup was like art for the face. I was never interested in using makeup to cover up my freckles or make my eyes appear larger. But I was totally interested in using the brightest, boldest shades and wacky, glittery shimmers to make my eyelids look like a splatter painting.

This love for makeup and beauty products has never, ever left me. But by no means do I think it's a crime to leave the house without makeup—heck, I will go anywhere and everywhere right after I leave the gym, something neither of my grandmothers would *ever* do. These days, I get just as excited about an awesome skincare regimen as I always have about colorful eyeshadow.

The minute I found out that I was pregnant with Max, I read up on things to avoid, which basically included . . . everything. I pared down a lot of the skincare products and makeup I use, because as a first-time mom, I flipped out about everything. After he was born, I slowly allowed a few beloved products back into my life. But it did beg the question of "If it isn't safe while I'm pregnant, isn't it sort of hyp-ocritical to use it even when I'm not?"

I will forever be a beauty junkie, and I doubt that I'll ever stop purchasing products to try. But creating the "recipes" for these beauty DIY products has been such an awesome experience. I've found a sugar scrub consistency that I completely adore, to the point where I'm not sure I will ever purchase another sugar scrub unless the consistency matches this exactly. I love my homemade lip balm as much as the ones I buy from Sephora or the drugstore. I even put together a homemade coconut sea salt spray to make those beachy waves in my hair that I have craved every June since I turned 12 years old.

You'll find that most of my recipes use sugar instead of salt. This is a personal preference I developed after the multiple times I used a salt scrub after shaving my legs or got a bit of salt scrub in a cut on my finger. That is *no* fun.

You'll find a lot of projects here use coconut oil. I'm always super late to trends, but I like to think that I was using coconut oil waaaaay before coconut oil was cool. It's been a staple in my home for years. Coconut oil itself makes a great moisturizer, cuticle cream, or makeup remover, but I also like to mix it with a few other ingredients to create something amazing.

And finally, you'll also find a lot of projects with essential oils! Essential oils are a part of our daily life. One of the biggest ways I love to use them is to eliminate cooking odors from my home. You'll feel my pain if you ever cook bacon or fish, caramelize onions, or make homemade taco beef with tons of spices. The scent can linger for *days*. I've found that diffusing essential oils removes odors from my kitchen so much better than a candle can, and trust me, I am one crazy candle lady!

A few drops of the oils into my favorite at-home body products give them a spa-like scent, and mixing essential oils with the aforementioned coconut oil is another one of my favorite ways to use them.

Long story made longer—all the recipes in here have a place in our home and in my heart. I hope they can find one in yours, too!

Don't forget! If you make a recipe from the book, be sure to post it on Instagram with the hashtag #theprettydish.

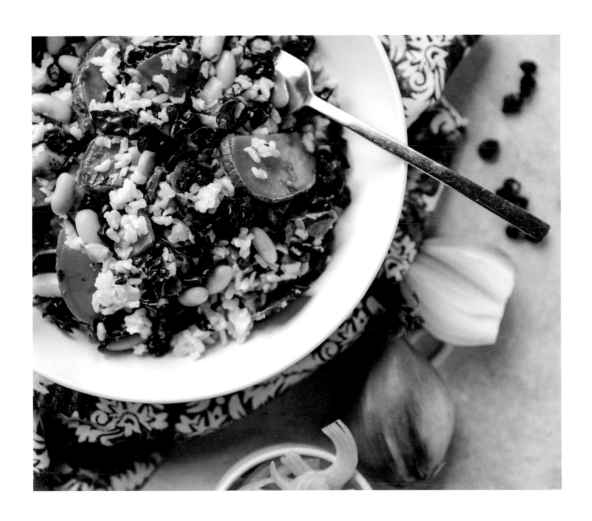

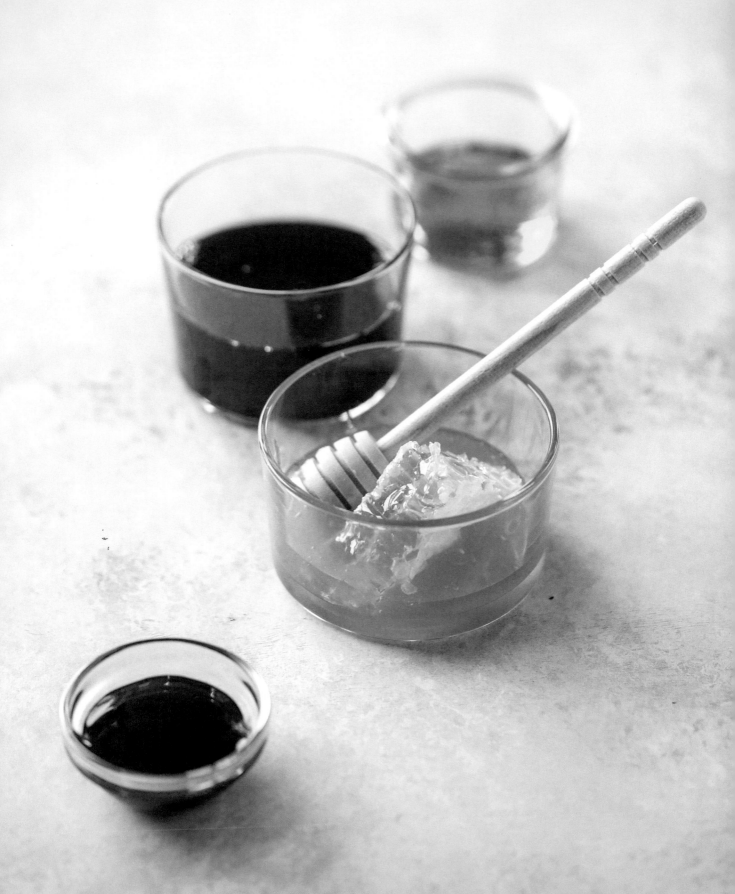

MY FAVORITE PANTRY STAPLES

As somebody who develops recipes for a living, I've found that my pantry can often turn into one gigantic mess. It occasionally looks like a natural disaster came through. And while I'd love to have every single staple available all the time, like my own personal market in my home, it's not practical, nor is it economical!

I could wax poetic for hours on all the pantry staples I need to do my job, but the truth is that for our daily life, daily meals, and general living purposes, those listed below are the ones that are a bit out of the norm (but still worth a mention!) that I just can't live without.

Cannellini beans
(and most other beans, too).
I would love to tell you that I am the person who soaks dry beans every week. I agree that they make the most delicious hummus, and I do keep some on hand for soups. But ever since Max came into the picture, there are a few staples that I have on hand out of convenience, and canned beans are one of them. I try to buy the ones with the lowest sodium, and I always rinse them under cold water before using.

Whole wheat pasta.
Any and all versions!

Vanilla bean paste.
This is the middle ground between vanilla extract and vanilla beans. It provides so much flavor, and those little bean flecks are perfection in desserts. My favorite brand is Rodelle.

Honey.
This is my go-to sweetener for desserts and breakfasts. Also, I use it in salad dressings! I try my best to use local honey that I can find at farmers' markets and farms near my home.

Pure maple syrup.
Same as honey, plus . . . pancakes! Need I say more? Make sure you are getting 100 percent pure maple syrup and nothing with artificial colors or flavors!

Unsweetened flaked coconut.
I love this so much more than the traditional sweetened coconut that I

grew up with. Plus, if you know anyone who can't take the squeak-beneath-your-teeth texture of shredded coconut, this is what they need to try.

Balsamic glaze.
I live for balsamic glaze on vegetables. It's also fabulous on pizza and even great on fresh strawberries!

Unfiltered apple cider vinegar.
Aside from taking a shot of this every morning when I wake up, it's my go-to for any and all salad dressings.

Chia seeds.
Chia seeds are a must-have for things like granola, granola bars, plain yogurt, smoothies, and chia pudding. They are a nutrition powerhouse.

Hemp hearts.
These little seeds are so packed with protein that I find adding them to smoothies, salads, or toast is such an easy way to amp up my daily meals. Plus, they add a nice little crunch, and I'm all about the texture.

Nut butters.
I might have a slight nut butter obsession that goes much further than peanut and almond butter. I love keeping cashew, macadamia, pistachio, and walnut butters on hand—or better yet, making my own. To make my own, I simply grind the nuts in my food processor until they are blended and smooth. Delicious!

Grapeseed oil.
Grapeseed oil is my go-to oil for roasted veggies. It works great at high heat and is mostly flavorless.

Canned fire-roasted tomatoes.
I love having diced fire-roasted tomatoes on hand for Bolognese, soups, chili, and sauces. They add a touch of smoky flavor that takes meals to another level.

Canned coconut milk.
I use coconut milk in many of my recipes, and the canned full-fat version is so rich and luxurious. I love having a few cans in the pantry, as well as a few cans in the fridge to make coconut whipped cream! To make coconut whipped cream, the milk must be refrigerated for about 12 hours so it whips into a fluffy consistency.

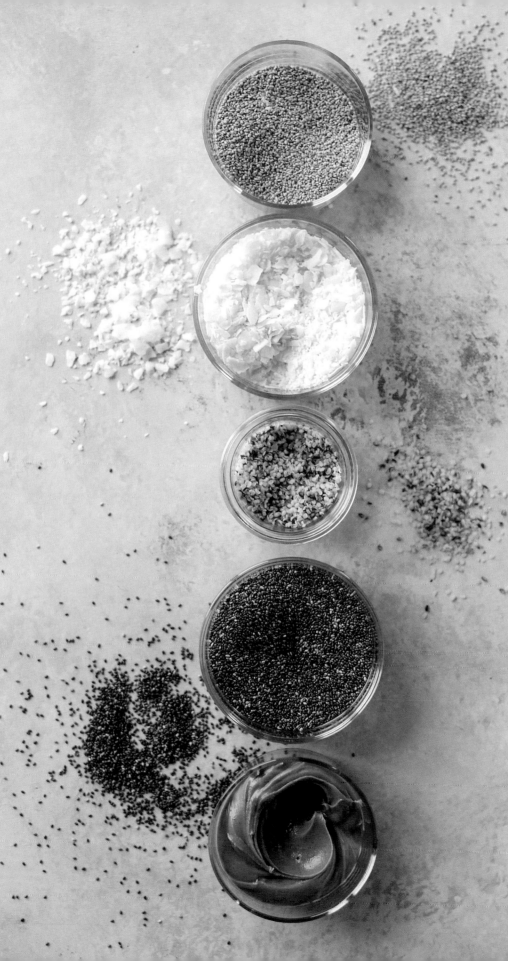

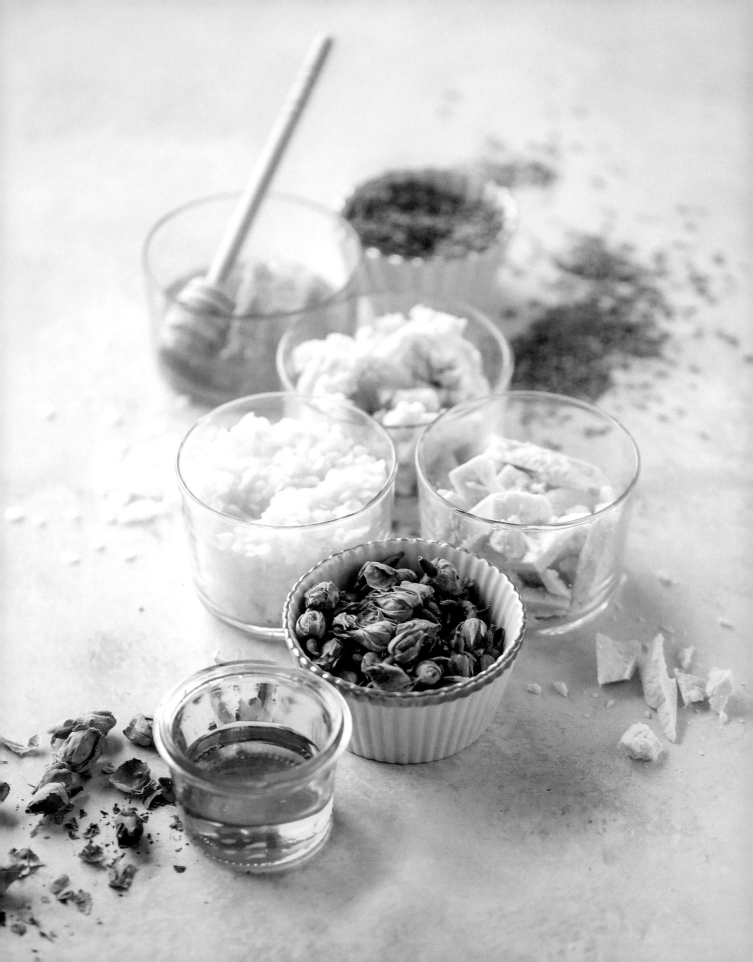

BEAUTY PANTRY STAPLES

If you're looking for ingredients to have on hand so you can always whip up a sugar scrub or homemade lip balm, these are it! Some can stay in the pantry, and some can be stuck in the fridge.

Walnut oil	*Beeswax (I purchase a large bag of beeswax pellets on Amazon!)*
Coconut oil	
Almond oil	*Cocoa butter*
Avocado oil	*Honey*
White sugar	*Dried, culinary-grade flowers (rose, lavender)*
Brown sugar	
Essential oils (peppermint, lavender, eucalyptus, vanilla blend, etc.)	*Plain Yogurt*
	Bananas
Shea butter	*Avocado*

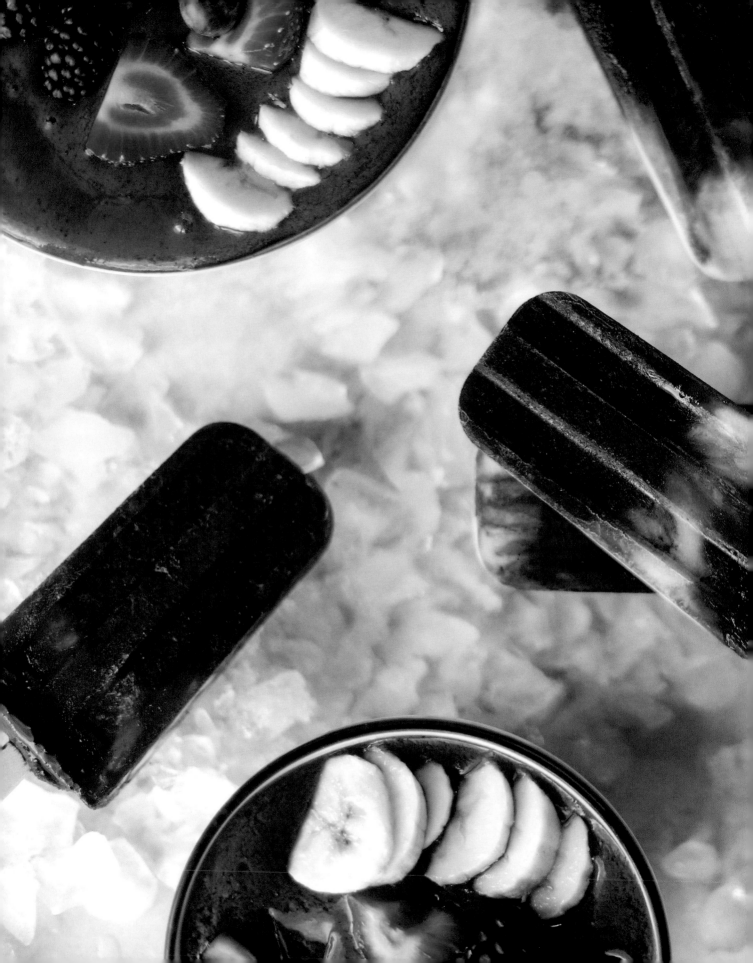

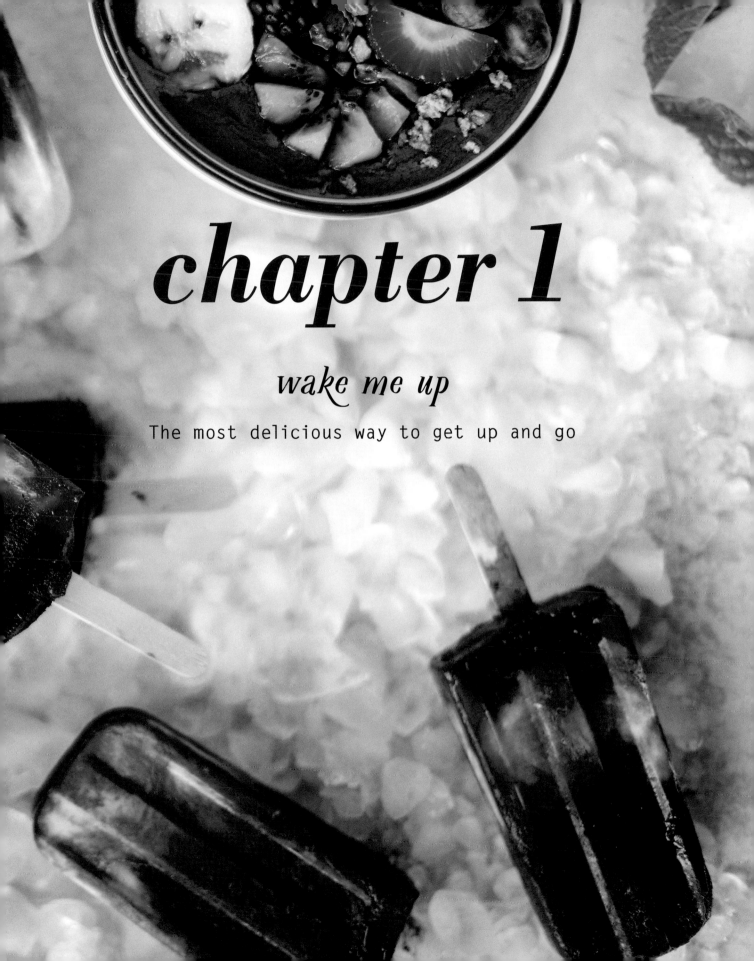

chapter 1

wake me up

The most delicious way to get up and go

IT'S LAUGHABLE TO THINK THAT I COULD actually choose a favorite meal of the day. I love all the meals! And while I wouldn't necessarily consider breakfast to be my favorite meal (it's probably dinner . . . or brunch, because *cocktails*), the food that we traditionally eat at breakfast tends to be my favorite food.

Okay, maybe if I absolutely had to choose, it would be breakfast for dinner? Breakfast foods are just so fantastic. Perhaps it's the comfort food vibe or just my serious obsession with eggs and avocado, but if you forced me to eat breakfast three times a day? I wouldn't complain.

And here's the thing: I come from a long line of breakfast skippers. My mom? Doesn't care about breakfast unless it involves tons of coffee and a slice of cake. Her mom was the same way. Thankfully, that gene didn't make its way to me, because not eating breakfast has never been an option.

In our house, Eddie has his first breakfast super early before leaving the house: a huge green smoothie packed with tons of produce. Max often chooses a smoothie or yogurt for breakfast, with a banana and maybe some granola. I'm on the yogurt train during the week, but I also love overnight oats since I can prep them ahead of time and they keep me full for hours. Occasionally I'll make a smoothie bowl (I don't care how trendy they are!) or eggs (fried or poached are my go-tos) if I have a little extra time.

The weekends are where we tend to splurge a little bit on breakfast, in the form of time and calories. We will often make something on Saturday and/or Sunday that takes a bit longer and is more indulgent, such as pancakes or soft-cooked eggs with bacon. There are lots of options for both of those in this chapter, so get ready to start the day off right!

maple raspberry overnight oats

I find that people fall into two categories in life: the lovers of overnight oats and . . . the haters. It's true that overnight oats have a certain sort of texture and chew to them. It's actually the reason that I love them, but for some it's a deal breaker.

Over the years I have perfected my overnight oats recipe so it's the consistency that I adore. I am a serious texture person and need to have that chew. I also find that adding something crunchy on top helps the breakfast along, as well as some nut butter swirled throughout.

One of the main reasons I love overnight oats, though? And it may make me super weird? It's because I just don't love warm bowls of oats. I like cold overnight oats eaten straight from the fridge. Since we are here in our circle of trust, I'll tell you that I embarrassingly but unapologetically love the flavored packets of instant oatmeal. I still enjoy them to this day. But since they are sugar laden, I try to save them for those times when I really need a hit of comfort food.

I also really adore any sort of recipe that can be constantly customized. As a member of the Internet generation, I'm often bored with the same repetitive choices (while Eddie can eat the same breakfast for six months straight without getting sick of it!), and just one simple change of fruit or topping to my overnight oats is a game changer.

Plus, these jars are wildly satisfying. Overnight oats keep me satisfied for hours—well into lunch-time—and yes, there is always the opportunity to add a little chocolate to them, too. MAKES 2 SERVINGS, IS EASILY MULTIPLIED

1 cup old-fashioned rolled oats

1 cup milk (cow's, almond, coconut, etc.)

1½ tablespoons maple syrup, plus extra for drizzling

1 tablespoon chia seeds

½ teaspoon vanilla extract

1¾ cups fresh raspberries, divided

¼ cup toasted sliced almonds

The night before, in a bowl or jar, stir together the oats, milk, 1 tablespoon of the maple syrup, the chia seeds, and vanilla until combined. Stick it in the fridge and let it sit overnight.

The next morning, mash ¾ cup of the raspberries with the remaining ½ tablespoon maple syrup. Spoon the mashed raspberries evenly into 2 glasses. Scoop the overnight oats into both glasses on top of the mashed raspberries. If you'd like an even creamier consistency, you can add a splash of milk here. Add the whole raspberries, some almonds on top, and another drizzle of maple syrup, if desired. Serve immediately.

TIP: Head to page 258 to find a full method for creating an overnight oats bar for your friends!

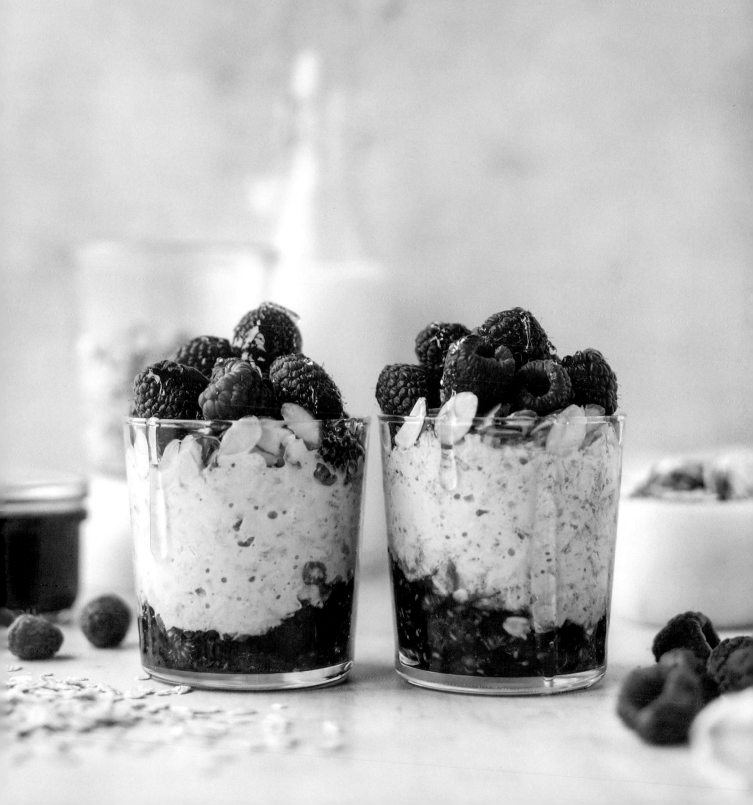

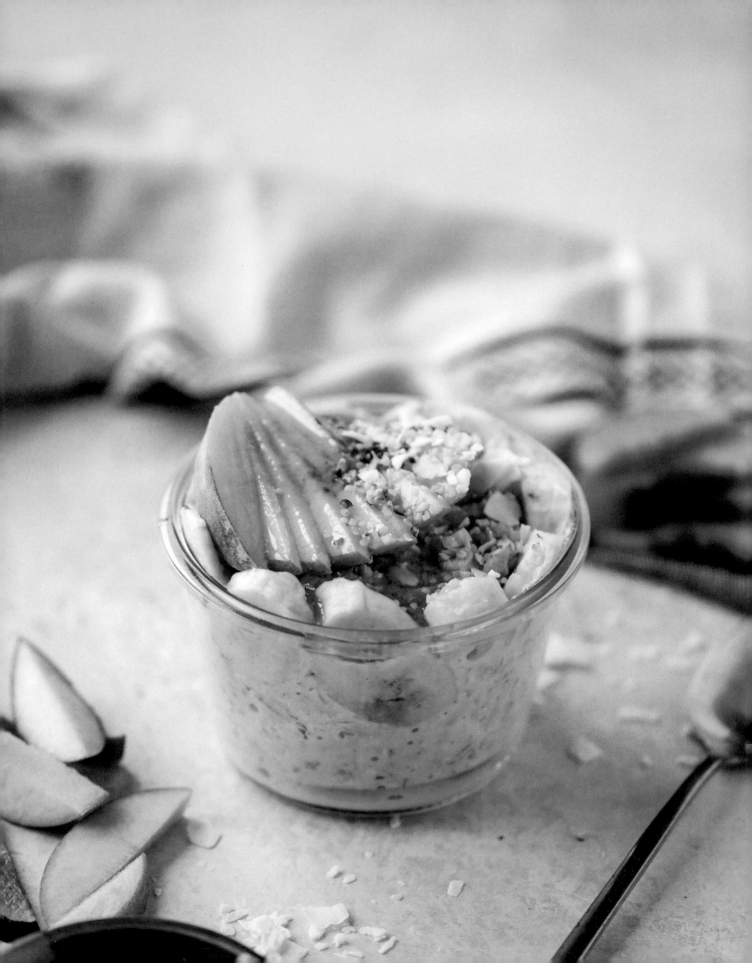

tropical peach overnight oats

One of my favorite combinations that I couldn't resist sharing? Peaches, bananas, and coconut milk. This is one of those standout recipes for me that screams "summer!" and tastes like I'm on a tropical island. Transport me, please. MAKES 2 SERVINGS, IS EASILY MULTIPLIED

1   cup old-fashioned rolled oats

1   cup milk (cow's, almond, coconut, etc.)

2   tablespoons honey, divided

1   tablespoon chia seeds

3   tablespoons flaked unsweetened coconut, divided

½   teaspoon coconut extract

2   bananas, thinly sliced

1   peach, thinly sliced

The night before, in a bowl or jar, stir together the oats, milk, 1 tablespoon of the honey, the chia seeds, 1 tablespoon of the coconut, and the coconut extract until combined. Stick it in the fridge and let it sit overnight.

The next morning, fill 2 glasses with some of the bananas. Add the oats on top of the bananas. Top the oats with the remainder of the bananas and the peach. Drizzle with the remaining 1 tablespoon honey and sprinkle on the remaining 2 tablespoons coconut. Serve immediately.

blood orange ricotta toast

Smear anything on toast and I'm almost bound to eat it. The texture, the crunch—it's the perfect vehicle for all things sweet and savory. In this case, both!

I want to tell you that whipped ricotta is the star of the show here. It's smooth and creamy. It's lighter than cream cheese but slightly more substantial than yogurt. It can take on so many different flavors. But how could I pick the ricotta over stunning blood oranges? These babies have been some of my favorites for years. And not only because they are hot pink. (Although that helps.) They are slightly sweeter than navel oranges. And while they are available for only a few weeks (or months, at best) each year from December to February, I sure as heck make the most of those weeks.

Of course, feel free to use oranges of your choice for this toast if blood oranges are out of season or not available in your area. If you don't have oranges on hand, strawberries are the next best choice, and pineapple works well, too! MAKES 2 SERVINGS

½ cup whole milk ricotta cheese

½ teaspoon vanilla extract (optional)

2 slices bread, toasted

1 blood orange, peeled and segmented

2 tablespoons honey

Pinch of sea salt

In a food processor, combine the ricotta cheese and vanilla, if desired. Process until pureed.

Spread the ricotta evenly over the toast. Add the blood orange segments. Drizzle on the honey and hit the whole thing with the sea salt. Delicious! Tastes best with copious amounts of coffee.

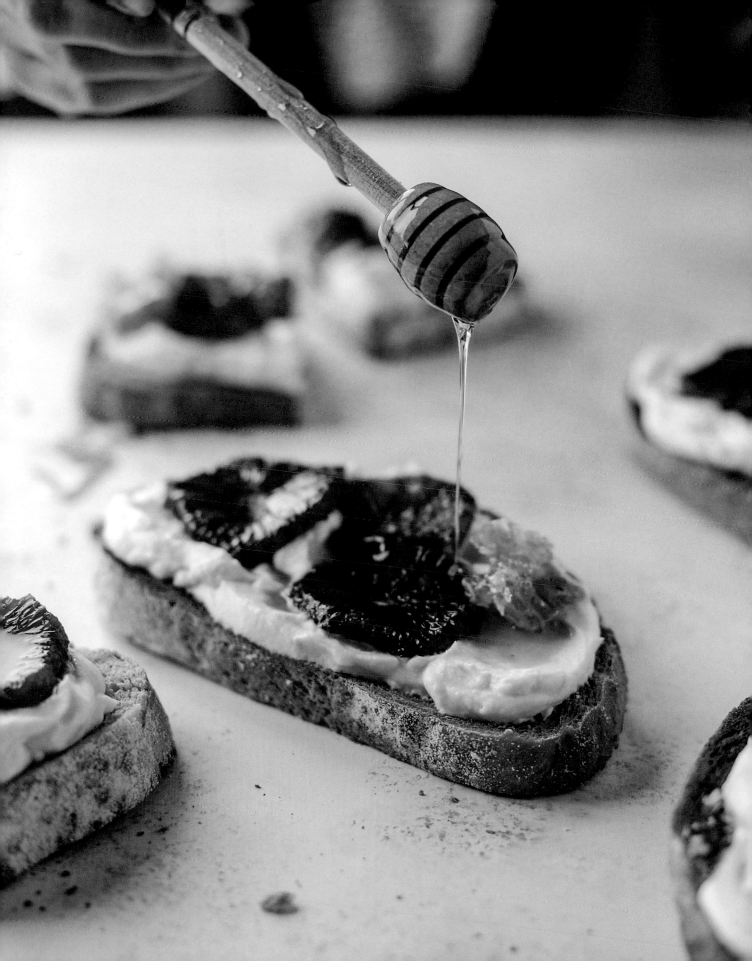

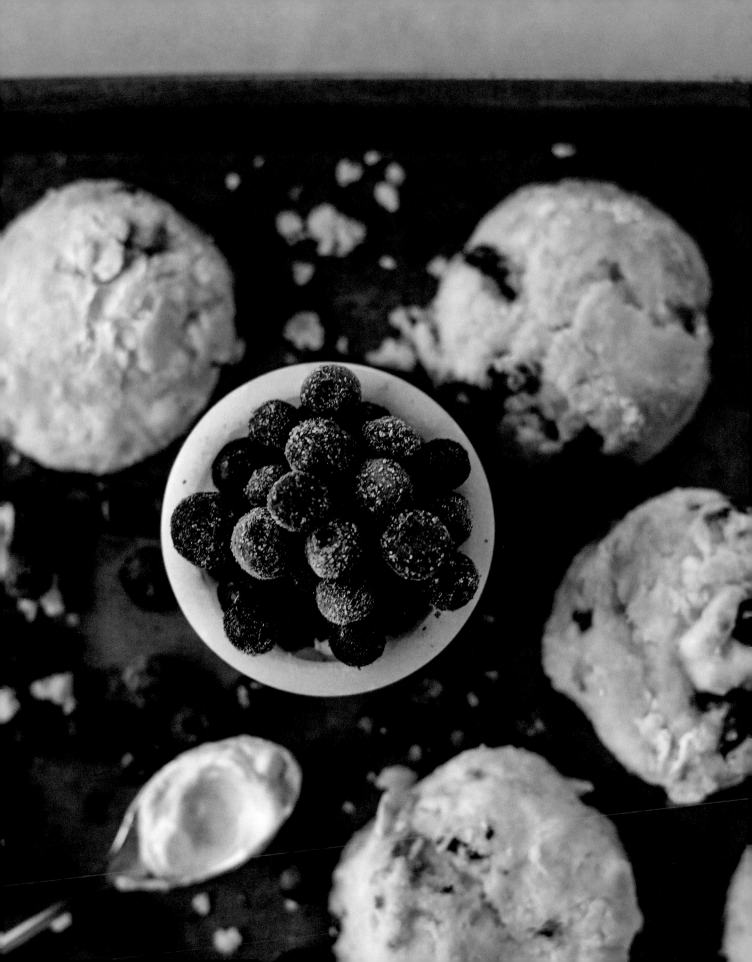

blueberry cream cheese biscuits

WITH SALTED VANILLA BUTTER

Eddie is a serious biscuit lover. We're talking serious.

Biscuits are one of the few foods that he considers to be comfort food. While he loves food, too, he is more of the "eat to live" type than the "live to eat." But biscuits? They are one of the things that he can't resist. And he can never stop at just one.

While he is a biscuit purist and tends to enjoy them plain, I often "ruin" everything by adding flavors and fruits and herbs that he is wary of. In a moment of desperation, he will buy a box of Bisquick and use the age-old recipe, but I always try to squash that from happening with a home-made batch.

These biscuits are a match made in heaven for both of us. I compromised a bit and added only blueberries for flavor. The cream cheese lends a flakiness and a touch of richness that is just so, so good. And the salted vanilla butter? Hello. I'd like to spread that all over my life. Keep a batch in your fridge and use it for everything—toasts, muffins, pancakes, you name it. **MAKES 12 TO 16**

BISCUITS

2¾ cups all-purpose flour

1   tablespoon baking powder

1   teaspoon baking soda

1   teaspoon sugar

½   teaspoon salt

4   ounces cold cream cheese

½   cup cold unsalted butter, cut into tiny pieces

1¼ cups cold buttermilk

⅔   cup fresh or frozen blueberries

VANILLA BUTTER

6   tablespoons unsalted butter, softened

1   teaspoon vanilla bean paste

¼   teaspoon fine sea salt

Preheat the oven to 425°f.

TO MAKE THE BISCUITS

In a large bowl, combine the flour, baking powder, baking soda, sugar, and salt. Add the cream cheese and butter and use a fork, pastry blender, or your hands to mix until coarse little crumbs form. I use my hands and mix for almost 5 minutes. Make a well in the center and pour in the buttermilk. Stir with a large spoon until just combined. Fold in the blueberries. Use your hands if needed to bring the dough together—I do.

Pat the dough into a circle that is about 1½" thick. This will make *tall* biscuits! Using a biscuit or cookie cutter, cut the dough into rounds and place on a nonstick baking sheet. You may need to bring the dough together and flatten it more to get the last few biscuits. Alternately, you could just drop large spoonfuls of batter on the baking sheet and form them that way.

Bake for 10 to 12 minutes, or until the biscuits are golden and high. Let cool slightly before serving.

TO MAKE THE VANILLA BUTTER

In a bowl, mix the butter, vanilla bean paste, and salt until combined. Serve spread on the warm biscuits. You can keep this at room temperature or store it in the fridge for a few days.

banana coconut milk scones
WITH NUTELLA GLAZE

Believe it or not, Nutella is a fairly new ingredient in our pantry. I was never a fan of it until I was pregnant with Max. Even in college, when my roommate would eat it out of the jar with a spoon (she adored it!), I wasn't tempted. I found a chocolate chip covered peanut butter spoon to be the ultimate college splurge (after the coconut rum, of course) and had zero interest in hazelnuts, period.

But then! It's not like I was consuming a pint of ice cream every day or asking for peanut butter and pickle sandwiches (a favorite on my dad's side of the family, eeeek!), but there was just something about Nutella that hooked me. I was adding it to my coffee. I would spread it on hot pancakes so it would melt. I'd add it to yogurt and melt it on top of ice cream. I was a Nutella train wreck, to say the least.

At that time, I remember wondering if the Nutella love would stick. My entire life I had heard about pregnant women who would consume a cheeseburger daily throughout their pregnancy and then, once the baby came, be turned off of cheeseburgers for life.

But I wasn't so lucky with Nutella. The passion stuck, for lack of a better word. In a serious way.

The Nutella kick isn't something that Eddie has caught on to yet. In true wife fashion, I am sure he would love it if he just tried it. Maybe one day? Perhaps these scones? It's my mission to make it happen before the year 2020. **MAKES 12 TO 16**

SCONES
3¼ cups all-purpose flour

⅓ cup loosely packed brown sugar

2½ teaspoons baking powder

1½ teaspoons ground cinnamon

½ teaspoon baking soda

½ teaspoon salt

¾ cup cold unsalted butter,
    cut into pieces

⅔ cup full-fat canned coconut milk

2 teaspoons vanilla extract

2 ripe bananas, mashed

3 tablespoons cream, for brushing

NUTELLA GLAZE
½ cup Nutella

3 tablespoons heavy cream

Drop of vanilla extract

Preheat the oven to 425°F.

TO MAKE THE SCONES
In a large bowl, whisk together the flour, brown sugar, baking powder, cinnamon, baking soda, and salt until combined. Add the butter and use your hands, a fork, or a pastry blender to combine until the butter forms coarse little crumbs. I use my hands, and it usually takes a full 2 to 3 minutes.

Make a well in the center and add the coconut milk, vanilla, and bananas. Mix with a large spoon until a dough forms and comes together—it might be sticky! Flour your hands and work surface. Divide the dough in half and pat each half into a 6" circle on the floured surface. Cut each circle into 6 or 8 wedges. Brush with the cream. Place the scones on a baking sheet and bake for 11 to 13 minutes, or until slightly golden on top.

Let the scones cool slightly on the baking sheet before glazing them.

TO MAKE THE NUTELLA GLAZE
IN A BOWL, WHISK together the Nutella, cream, and vanilla until the Nutella is smooth and drippy. If it is still thick, add more cream 1 teaspoon at a time, whisking well.

Drizzle the Nutella glaze over the scones. Serve immediately!

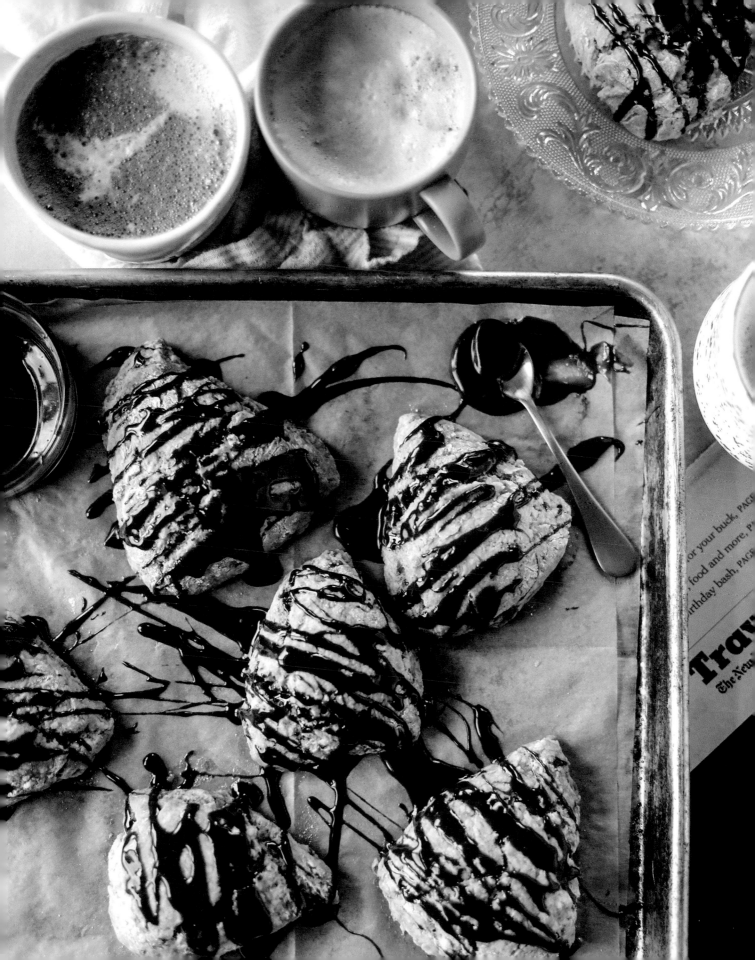

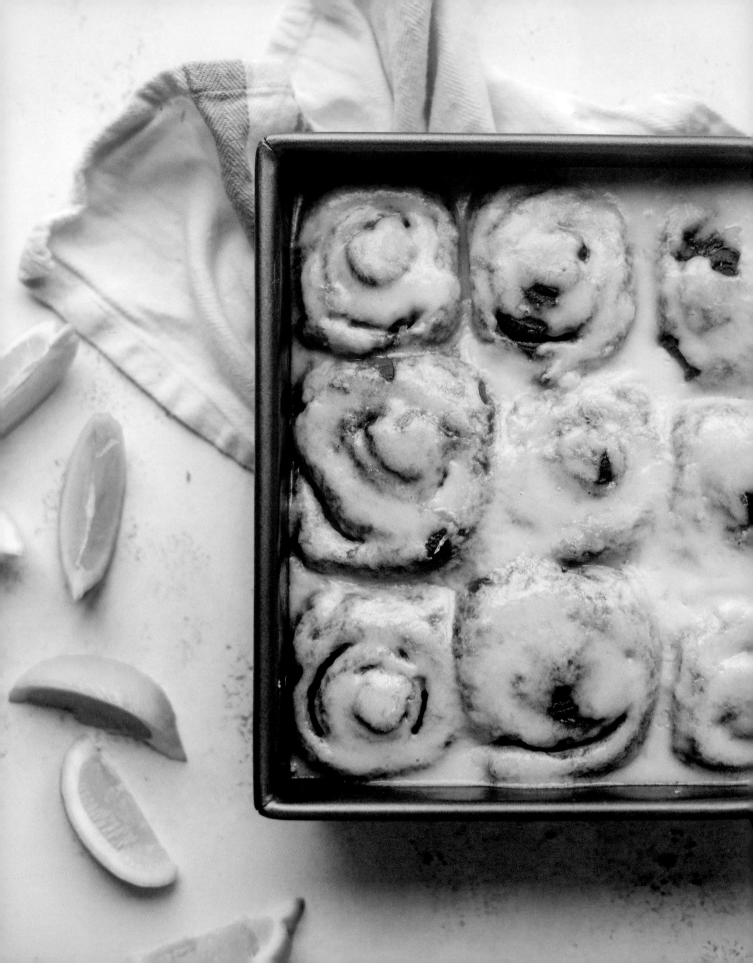

lemon mascarpone sticky buns

I definitely have a dual-sided personality when it comes to sweet things. I'm either in a decadent chocolate mood, or I'm in a lighter lemon mood. But as a kid, I was convinced that lemon desserts and baked goods were only for old people. I never knew another kid who liked lemon anything. I passed up all the lemon things: Jolly Ranchers, Sour Patch Kids, heck, I think I even discarded the yellow Skittles and M&M's. The only person I knew who liked lemon was my grandma. And my mom. And my dad, maybe!

Therefore, in my child brain, lemon desserts meant that you were old.

No offense of course, since I found myself on the lemon-loving train in my early twenties, much to my own dismay. And now I've become a full-blown lemon-loving freak. In fact, I might even go so far as to say that lemon is my favorite flavor.

And with that lighter lemon mood comes my interest in all things mascarpone. If I could eat that stuff with a spoon, I would. This milder version of cream cheese has become a staple in my sweet and savory recipes. MAKES 16

BUNS

- ¾ cup whole milk
- ⅓ cup granulated sugar, divided
- 1 tablespoon active dry yeast
- 2 large eggs
- 1 teaspoon vanilla extract
- 1 teaspoon freshly grated lemon zest
- 3 cups all-purpose flour, plus extra for dusting
- ½ teaspoon salt
- ½ cup unsalted butter, softened and cut into pieces

FILLING

- ½ cup butter, melted, plus extra for brushing
- ½ cup granulated sugar
- 2 tablespoons freshly grated lemon zest
- Pinch of cardamom
- Pinch of salt
- 8 ounces mascarpone cheese, at room temperature

TO MAKE THE BUNS

In a saucepan, heat the milk over medium-low heat until just warm, 105 to 110°F. Stir in 1 tablespoon of the granulated sugar. Sprinkle the yeast over the top and let sit for 5 minutes, or until foamy. Whisk in the eggs until smooth. Whisk in the vanilla and lemon zest.

In the bowl of an electric stand mixer fitted with the paddle attachment, combine the flour, remaining granulated sugar, and salt. Slowly add the milk mixture, mixing on low speed until combined. Add the butter 1 piece at a time, beating until combined. Mix on medium-high speed for 5 minutes, or until the dough is silky and smooth. Transfer the dough to an oiled bowl, then cover with plastic wrap. Let sit for 1 to 2 hours in a warm spot, or until doubled in size.

On a floured work surface, roll the dough out into a large rectangle, about 18" x 12".

TO MAKE THE FILLING

Brush ½ cup of the melted butter all over the dough. In a small bowl, stir together the granulated sugar, lemon zest, cardamom, and salt. Sprinkle the sugar mixture evenly over the dough, leaving a 1" border around the edges. Drop dollops of the mascarpone all over the dough. Tightly roll the dough up from 1 of the long ends into a

(continued)

ICING

8   ounces mascarpone cheese, at room temperature

2   cups powdered sugar

2   teaspoons vanilla extract

1   teaspoon freshly grated lemon zest

4–5 tablespoons milk

long log. Slice into approximately 1" rounds. Place the rounds in a buttered 13" x 9" baking dish. Brush with additional melted butter and cover with plastic wrap. Let rise in a warm place for 30 to 45 minutes.

Preheat the oven to 350°F. Bake the buns, uncovered, for 45 to 50 minutes, covering them with foil if they start to brown too much. You want the bottom to be bubbling and the buns to be set.

TO MAKE THE ICING

In a large bowl, whisk the mascarpone until creamy. Whisk in the powdered sugar, vanilla, and lemon zest. Gradually stream in the milk and stir until a glaze forms. You will have to stir for a minute or 2 to remove any lumps and bring the glaze together. If the mixture still seems too thick, add more milk 1 tablespoon at a time, whisking well until smooth. Pour over the hot sticky buns. Serve immediately!

pretzel puff pastry cheater's croissants

The elusive pretzel croissant. Ahhhh. The flavor has haunted all of my dreams since I had my first bite in 2012 at City Bakery in New York City. The overly salty (in the best way), flaky layers are easily one of the best things I've eaten in all my years, as simple as they may be.

Yes, I'm declaring those croissants to be one of my favorite meals, even if a croissant doesn't necessarily constitute a meal. But meal memories are a thing for me. And I remember that moment so vividly.

The pretzel croissant I ate that day was paired with a smooth latte, which sounds like a very weird combination (salt plus creamy coffee? I don't know) but just worked. I have aimed to re-create that moment so many times in so many coffee shops in the last few years, but the moment is just unbeatable.

Croissants themselves hold a special meaning for me. That's something only a true foodie would say, right? But my first croissant was eaten in Boyne City, Michigan, when I was a kid, and every summer following that, my grandma and I would enjoy fresh croissants while on vacation each morning.

I've made real, legit croissants a handful of times in my life. But after I had a child, the option to do so has been pretty slim. Croissants are so time and labor intensive that they require a full day devoted only to croissant making, and with another babe on the way, I have no idea when the next time will be.

So I did the next best thing. If you're a reader of my blog, it's no secret to you that I'm a major fan of frozen puff pastry. It's just so . . . easy. I use it to top pot pies, to make homemade pop tarts, and to make personal pizzas. It's practically foolproof and full of delicious, buttery layers. And you don't have to do the work!

This cheater's pretzel croissant is something that took me a few tries to get right. It's never going to be as delicious as the City Bakery staple, but it comes close and gives you the general giddy feeling if you live states away and find yourself mid-craving. The secret is a sesame seed salt mix for the top. It adds the perfect burst of flavor that makes you think "pretzel!" MAKES 8 TO 10

(continued)

2 sheets frozen puff pastry, completely thawed

¼ cup cold European butter (it has that fat content you need!), cut into pieces

1 large egg + 1 teaspoon water, lightly beaten

2 tablespoons toasted sesame seeds

½ teaspoon coarse sea salt

Preheat the oven to 425°F. Line a baking sheet with parchment paper.

Place 1 sheet of puff pastry on a very lightly floured work surface. Cover the sheet with the pieces of butter, then top it with the second sheet. Use a lightly floured rolling pin to roll the pastry into a much larger, thinner rectangle—at least double the size if you can. Be patient and gentle with the pastry since it can tear easily. You need it to be as thin as possible, or the inside will not cook and the outside will burn. If this intimidates you, you can simply roll out 1 plain sheet of pastry, slice it into triangles, and roll it up. It won't be quite as buttery, but it will still be delish!

Once you have your large rectangle, use a pizza cutter or knife to cut triangles in the dough in a zigzag pattern from top to bottom. Starting at the bottom, roll each triangle up into a croissant-like shape. Place on the baking sheet.

Brush the tops of the croissants with the beaten egg wash. In a bowl, stir together the sesame seeds and salt. Sprinkle each croissant liberally with the sesame salt mixture.

Bake the croissants for 20 minutes. After 20 minutes, check on the doneness of the croissants. The outsides will start to look golden, but the insides might remain raw. Return the croissants to the oven and bake for 5 to 10 minutes, or until the tops start to get really golden. Gently cover the croissants with a piece of foil so they don't burn, and bake for 10 minutes more. You want to make sure the insides are done! You can even cut 1 open to see if you'd like. If it's still doughy, continue baking in 5-minute increments (still covered with foil) until done.

Let the croissants cool slightly before serving.

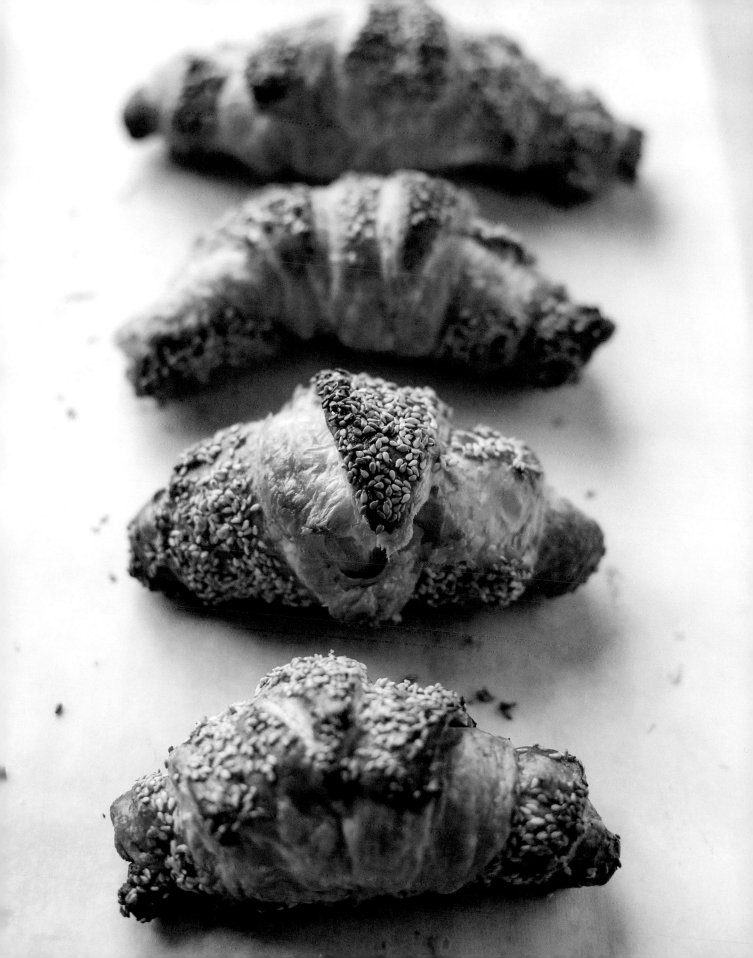

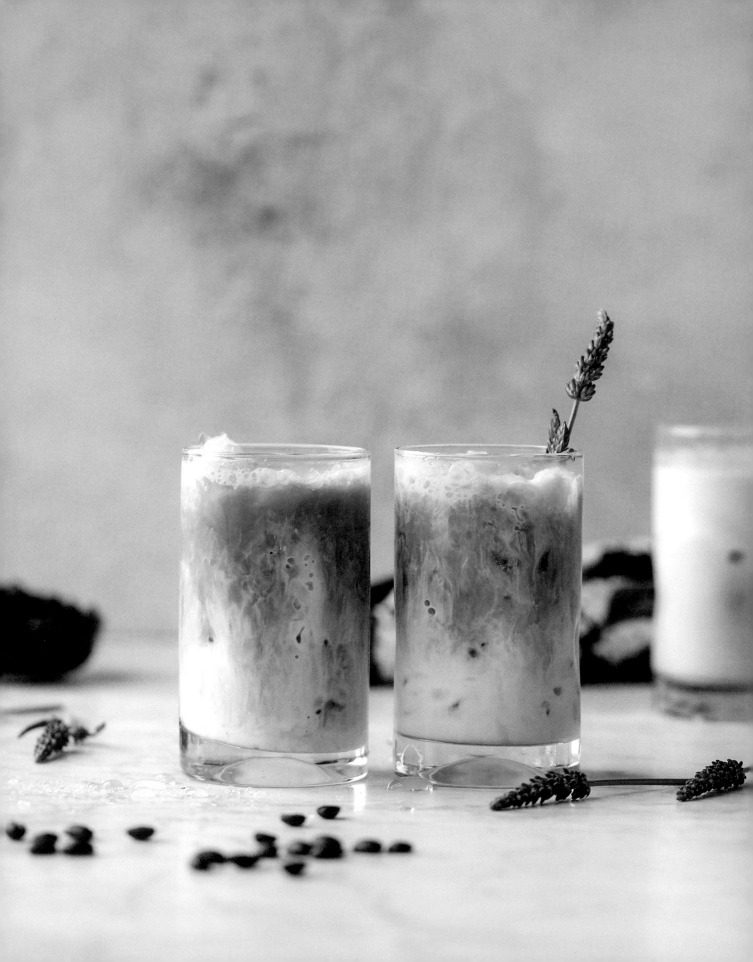

iced lavender vanilla latte

Coffee and I have a history (to put it mildly). It goes so deep that once I wrote a post on my blog titled "If you don't like coffee, but love coffee ice cream, then I love you."

This is my plight.

The scent of coffee is wildly nostalgic for me. If you haven't grasped it by now, I am such a nostalgic, sentimental person. The slightest hint of flavor or scent yanks me into memories that are 20 years old. And coffee is one of those.

The scent alone reminds me of daily life when I was growing up. The coffee would be brewing early for my parents, and the scent is comforting. But it wasn't until around five years ago that I fell in love with it myself.

I will forever be an iced coffee person. It's my favorite way to consume it. It's the way I learned to love it. I order iced coffee when it's 7 degrees outside without batting an eye. It's just so good!

One of my favorite local places in Pittsburgh has a seasonal lavender vanilla latte, and it is just divine. I have always thought that the combination of lavender and vanilla smells like an ice cream shop . . . as long as it's a little heavy on the vanilla. Which this of course is.

P.S. You can absolutely keep extra syrup on hand for delicious things like cocktails . . .

Just a thought. MAKES 1 SERVING, IS EASILY MULTIPLIED

LAVENDER VANILLA SYRUP

½   cup sugar

½   cup water

2   teaspoons dried culinary lavender

2   sprigs fresh lavender

1   vanilla bean, split in half

½   teaspoon vanilla extract

LATTE

2   shots espresso

2   tablespoons lavender vanilla syrup

6   ounces milk (cow's, almond, coconut, etc.)

Fresh lavender sprig, for garnish

TO MAKE THE LAVENDER VANILLA SYRUP

In a saucepan over medium-low heat, combine the sugar, water, dried and fresh lavender, and vanilla bean. Whisk until the sugar dissolves. Bring the mixture to a simmer, and cook for 1 minute. Turn off the heat and set the saucepan aside until the mixture has cooled completely. Strain the mixture through a fine-mesh sieve to remove the lavender and vanilla bean. Stir in the vanilla. Store in a sealed container in the fridge. The recipe will make ½ cup of syrup.

TO MAKE THE LATTE

Fill a large glass with ice. Add the espresso and syrup and stir together well. Pour in the milk and stir. Garnish with the lavender sprig. Serve immediately!

pistachio latte

Yes, I know that I just ranted about my love for iced coffee, but I make a few exceptions. Much like my thoughts on lemon-flavored desserts and coffee beverages, pistachio was a flavor I came to love later in life.

And by "later in life," I mean when I was about 30 years old. You can slap me if you wish.

Pistachio desserts are always the business. I can't get over their nutty richness. I don't care if there are actual pistachios in the dessert, but the flavor alone? Oooooh baby. I love it.

Hence this delicious (and simple!) pistachio syrup. Take it a step further and use pistachio milk if you'd like. It doesn't exactly froth up as well as cow's milk, but the flavor pretty much makes up for it. Now if only I could get this naturally green . . . MAKES 1 SERVING, IS EASILY MULTIPLIED

PISTACHIO SYRUP

½ cup sugar

½ cup water

⅓ cup chopped pistachios

¼ teaspoon almond extract

LATTE

2 shots espresso

2–3 tablespoons pistachio syrup

6 ounces steamed milk (cow's or pistachio)

Chopped pistachios (optional)

TO MAKE THE PISTACHIO SYRUP

In a saucepan over medium-low heat, combine the sugar, water, and pistachios. Whisk until the sugar dissolves. Bring the mixture to a simmer, and cook for 2 minutes. Turn off the heat and set the saucepan aside until the mixture has cooled completely. Strain the mixture through a fine-mesh sieve to remove the pistachios. Stir in the almond extract. You can keep the syrup in a sealed container in the fridge for about a week. The recipe will make ½ cup of syrup.

TO MAKE THE LATTE

In a mug, combine the espresso and syrup and stir together. Pour in the steamed milk. Sprinkle with chopped pistachios, if desired. Serve immediately!

PISTACHIO MILK

1 cup shelled, roasted pistachios (or raw if you can find them!)

4½ cups filtered water

½ teaspoon almond extract

2 tablespoons honey (optional)

Place the pistachios in a bowl and cover them with water. Soak overnight or for at least 6 hours. Drain.

In a blender, combine the soaked pistachios, filtered water, and almond extract. Blend until smooth and creamy. Taste the milk and, if desired, add the honey and blend again. Store in the fridge for up to 1 week.

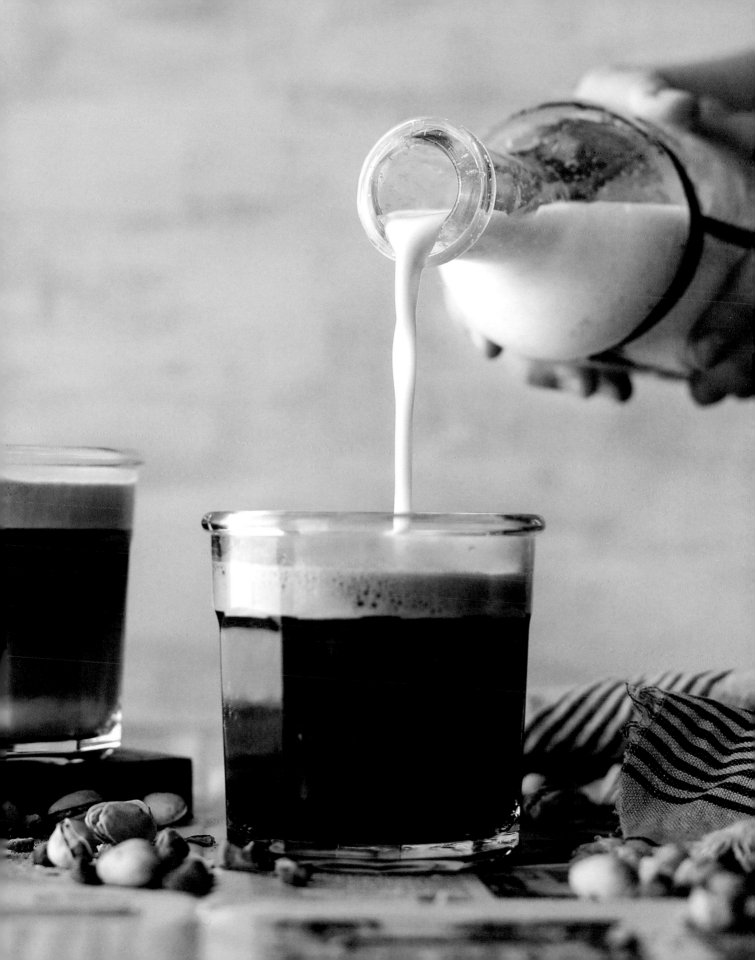

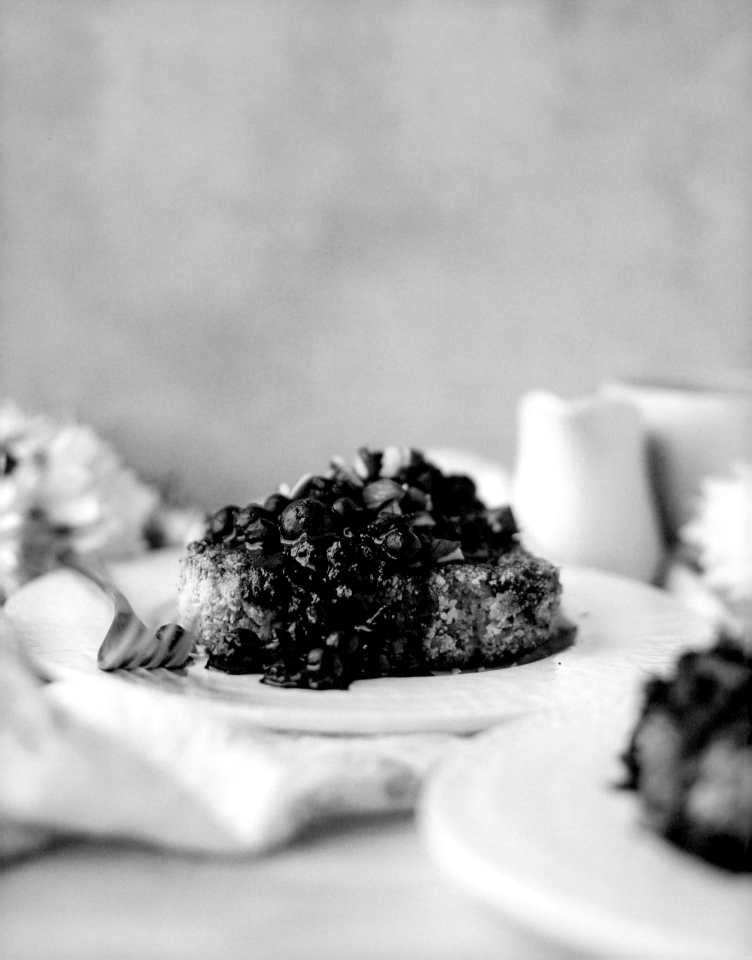

almond-crusted french toast
WITH BLUEBERRY SYRUP

French toast with an extra crunch is something that I crave. Being the huge texture person that I am, coating some brioche bread in creamy custard and crunchy almonds before frying it in butter is music to my . . . tastebuds?

I love making this "extra" French toast on mornings when we have a bit more time and can enjoy a leisurely brunch at home. French toast is so perfect for serving a crowd because it doesn't necessarily need to be piping hot, and you can serve it as you make it.

Paired with a blueberry syrup, this is one heck of an indulgent way to start the day. And with all those almonds, it's satisfying, too. MAKES 2 TO 4 SERVINGS

FRENCH TOAST

3   whole eggs
¼   cup milk
2   tablespoons sugar
2   tablespoons butter, melted
1   teaspoon vanilla extract
½   tablespoon ground cinnamon
Pinch of salt
1   cup crushed almonds
4   thick slices brioche bread
Unsalted butter, for frying

BLUEBERRY SYRUP

1½ cups fresh or frozen blueberries
⅓   cup maple syrup

TO MAKE THE FRENCH TOAST

In a shallow bowl, whisk together the eggs, milk, sugar, melted butter, vanilla, cinnamon, and salt. Place the almonds on a plate.

Heat a large skillet or griddle over medium heat. Place a slice of bread in the egg mixture. Turn to coat the other side, making sure every inch is covered. Dip it in the crushed almonds, pressing gently so they adhere to the bread. Turn to coat the other side. Repeat with the remaining bread.

Melt a tablespoon of butter in the skillet before frying each slice. Cook the bread, 1 slice at a time, for 6 minutes, turning once, or until golden brown on both sides. Repeat with the remaining slices.

TO MAKE THE BLUEBERRY SYRUP

In a saucepan, combine the blueberries and maple syrup. Heat over low heat until bubbling. Cook for 5 to 6 minutes, or until the blueberries break down and the mixture is syrupy. You can mash the blueberries with a fork if needed!

NOTE: I find the easiest way to crush the almonds is in my food processor. I blend them until just before they turn into crumbs.

ricotta scrambled eggs

I told you that I am a serious egg lover! And I don't discriminate. I'll eat them any way you serve them, as long as they aren't runny when scrambled. That's one thing I just cannot handle.

I'm always looking for the best way to fluff up my scrambled eggs, though. Something to make them special, even if they really are just scrambled eggs. I believe that I've found the biggest secret, and it all lies in lovely ricotta cheese.

Tossing some of this stuff into your eggs while you scramble them yields such a fluffy, creamy texture, all while fully cooking the eggs. That's a win in my book. The ricotta also adds a richness that I can't quite pinpoint. It's not the same as butter, but it gives the eggs something extra. And when these eggs are piled high on toast, they are sure to be a hit.

Give them a little chive shower, too, for some of that garden flavor. Seriously, couldn't you eat this every single day?! **MAKES 2 SERVINGS**

1   tablespoon unsalted butter
4   large eggs
¼   teaspoon salt
¼   teaspoon ground black pepper
⅓   cup ricotta cheese
2   tablespoons snipped fresh chives
Toasted, buttered baguette slices, for serving

In a large skillet, melt the butter over medium heat. In a bowl, whisk together the eggs, salt, and pepper.

Add the eggs to the skillet and let them set a bit, then gently push them around with a spatula to scramble them. Once they are almost fully cooked, add in the ricotta cheese and continue to stir with the spatula for another minute or so until the eggs are done and no longer runny.

Serve the eggs with a sprinkle of chives on top and some buttered toast.

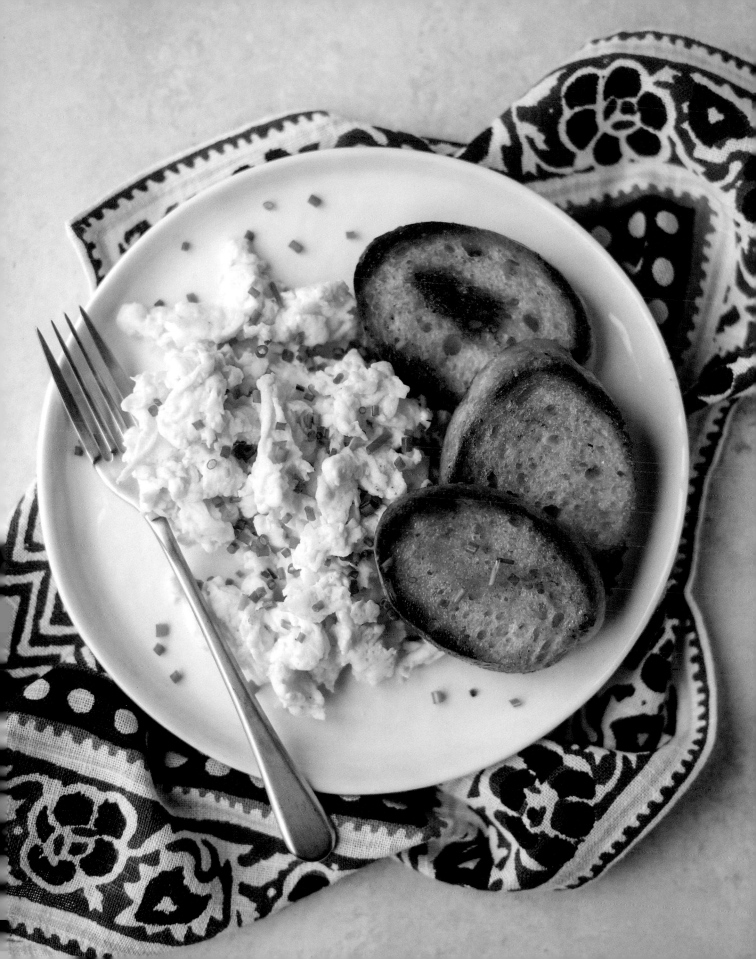

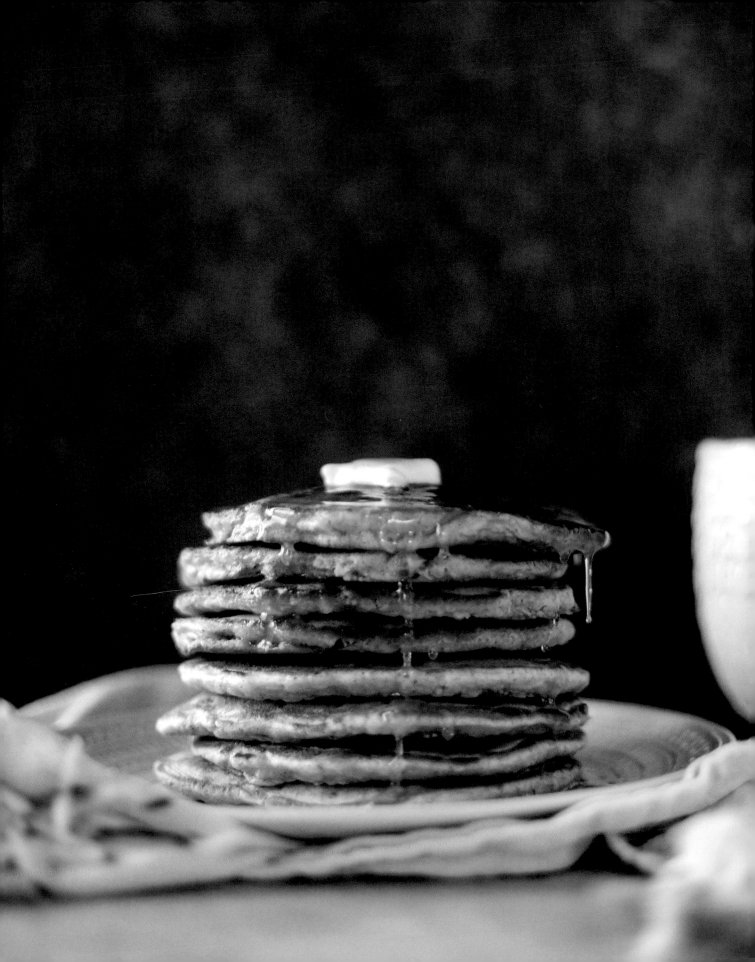

zucchini bread pancakes

Zucchini bread is one of those special baked goods because you'll ask yourself: Is it cake? Or is it bread? Is it dessert? Or is it a snack? Can I eat it for breakfast and still be an adult? Can I smother it with Nutella or cinnamon butter and still consider it a balanced snack? If I just take a few bites from one single piece, but don't consume the entire piece, do the calories still count?

There are so many questions surrounding this tender, cinnamony quick bread that I figured I'd make it into breakfast so we could stop asking questions. Sounds fair, right?

Also, I have excellent news. There is a vegetable in your pancakes! You know what this means, right?

Extra butter and syrup all around.   **MAKES 4 SERVINGS**

1½   cups all-purpose flour

2   tablespoons brown sugar

2   teaspoons baking powder

1   teaspoon baking soda

1   teaspoon ground cinnamon

¼   teaspoon freshly grated nutmeg

¼   teaspoon salt

2   large eggs, lightly beaten

1¼   cups milk

1   teaspoon vanilla extract

2   tablespoons unsalted butter, melted

1   cup freshly grated zucchini

Unsalted butter, for cooking the pancakes (optional)

Maple syrup, for serving

In a large bowl, combine the flour, sugar, baking powder, baking soda, cinnamon, nutmeg, and salt. Whisk together until well combined. In a small bowl, whisk together the eggs, milk, vanilla, and melted butter. Add the wet ingredients to the dry, mixing until smooth and combined. Fold in the zucchini.

Heat a large skillet or electric griddle over medium heat. Add a bit of butter, then pour ¼ cup of batter on the hot skillet and repeat, leaving 1" between pancakes. Cook for 2 minutes, or until the pancakes bubble on the top and edges. Turn and cook for 1 to 2 minutes, or until golden and set. Repeat with the remaining batter.

Serve immediately with maple syrup.

chocolate oatmeal bowls

I haven't always loved hot oatmeal. I still don't always love hot oatmeal.
But.
If there just happens to be a lot of chocolate in my hot oatmeal?
I really like hot oatmeal.   **MAKES 2 SERVINGS**

1   cup old-fashioned oats

2   cups milk (cow's, almond, or coconut), divided

½   teaspoon salt

Pinch of ground cinnamon

3   tablespoons unsweetened cocoa powder

2   tablespoons maple syrup

2   ounces bittersweet chocolate, chopped, plus extra for garnish

1   teaspoon vanilla extract

In a saucepan, combine the oats and 1½ cups of the milk and place over medium-low heat. Add the salt and cinnamon and stir to combine. Cook, stirring often, for 15 minutes, or until the oats are super creamy. Remove from the heat. Stir in the cocoa, maple syrup, chocolate, and remaining ½ cup milk. Stir in the vanilla.

Serve with extra chopped chocolate on top.

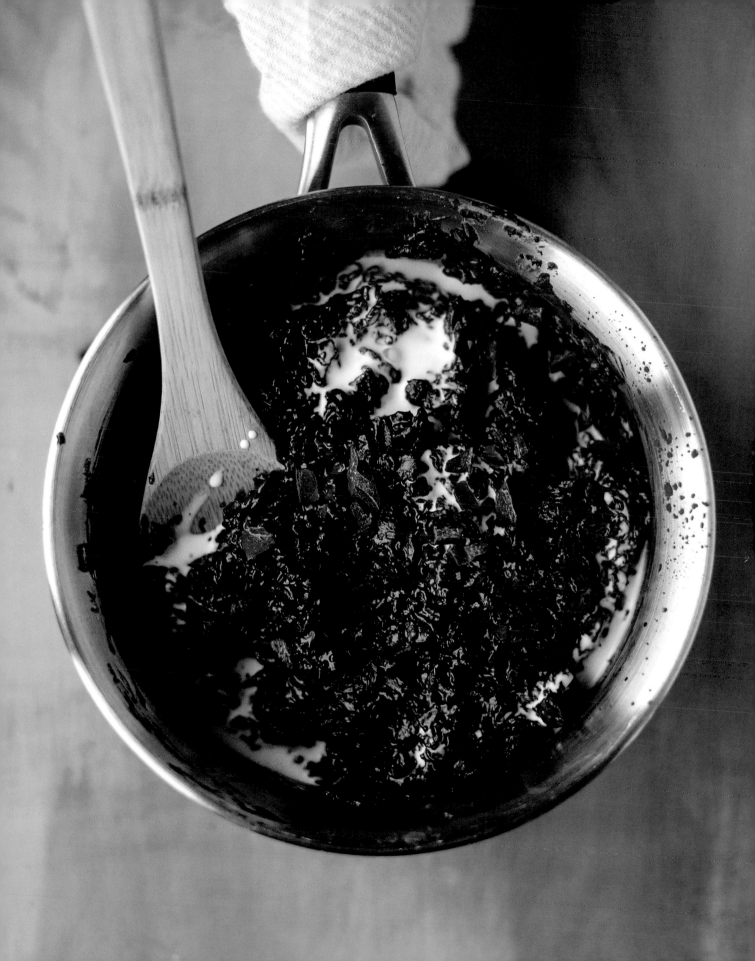

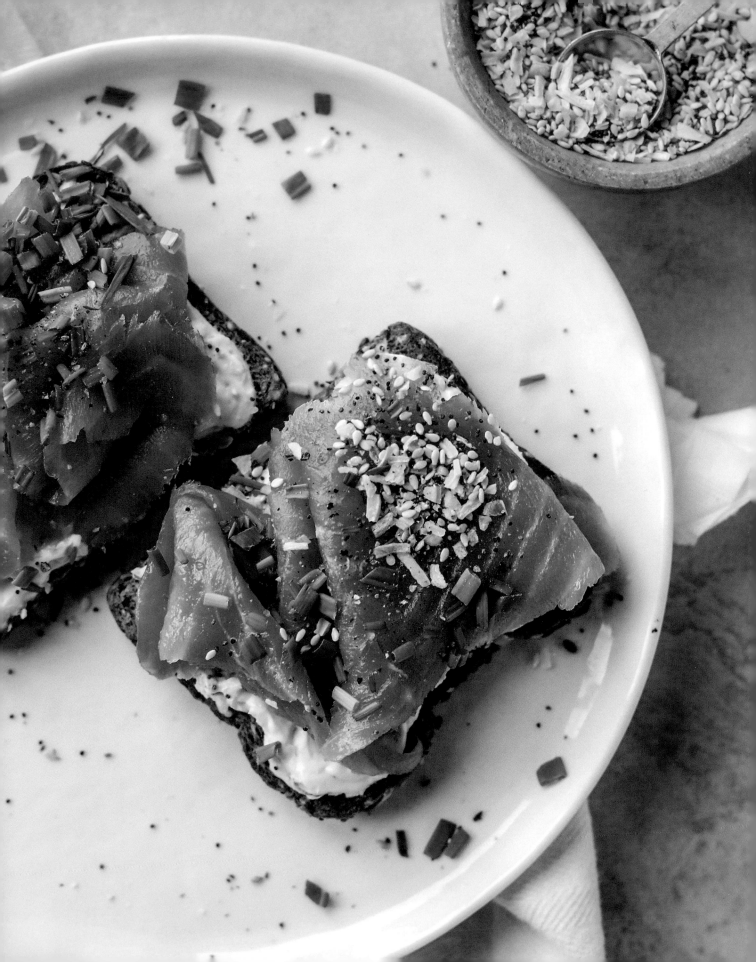

salmon lox toast

Another recipe, another toast obsession. This recipe should come as no surprise, but it might be a little change of pace since it's not on a bagel!

There are few things I love more than an at-home girls' brunch with everything bagels, smoked salmon, and cream cheese. I took that same combo but threw it on some toast with our own "everything" seasoning I've been using since I first shared the recipe. This seasoning is so flavorful and instantly amps up any meal. MAKES 2 TO 4 SERVINGS

4   slices seedy, whole grain bread, toasted

⅓   cup whipped cream cheese

2   tablespoons Everything Seasoning (below)

4   ounces smoked salmon

3   tablespoons snipped fresh chives

Spread each slice of toast with 1 to 2 tablespoons of the cream cheese. Sprinkle each slice with ½ tablespoon of the Everything Seasoning. Add 1 ounce of salmon on top of each and sprinkle with the chives. Serve immediately.

EVERYTHING SEASONING

2   tablespoons dried minced onion

2   tablespoons toasted sesame seeds

1   tablespoon poppy seeds

1   tablespoon dried minced garlic

1   teaspoon flaked sea salt

¼   teaspoon ground black pepper

In a small bowl, stir together the onion, sesame seeds, poppy seeds, garlic, salt, and pepper until combined. You can keep this mixture stored in a sealed container in your spice cabinet for a few weeks.

birthday cake waffles

Happy birthday to you! Cake batter waffles are only made better when studded with neon sprinkles. Am I right?

Okay, wait, with a scoop of ice cream on top, of course. Celebrate! **MAKES 4 SERVINGS**

2 eggs

1½ cups all-purpose flour

¼ cup sugar

1 tablespoon baking soda

Pinch of salt

1½ cups milk

½ cup unsalted butter, melted

1 tablespoon vanilla extract

½ cup assorted sprinkles,
   plus extra for topping

Whipped cream or ice cream,
   for serving

Separate the egg yolks from the whites. Set the yolks aside. Place the whites in the bowl of an electric stand mixer and beat until fluffy and stiff peaks form.

In a large bowl, whisk together the flour, sugar, baking soda, and salt. In a small bowl, whisk together the milk, butter, vanilla, and reserved egg yolks. Whisk the wet ingredients into the dry. Using a spatula, fold the egg whites into the batter. Gently fold the sprinkles into the batter.

Heat a waffle iron to your desired setting. Following the manufacturer's directions, pour batter into the center and cook until the waffle is set. Repeat with the remaining batter. Top with whipped cream or ice cream and sprinkles!

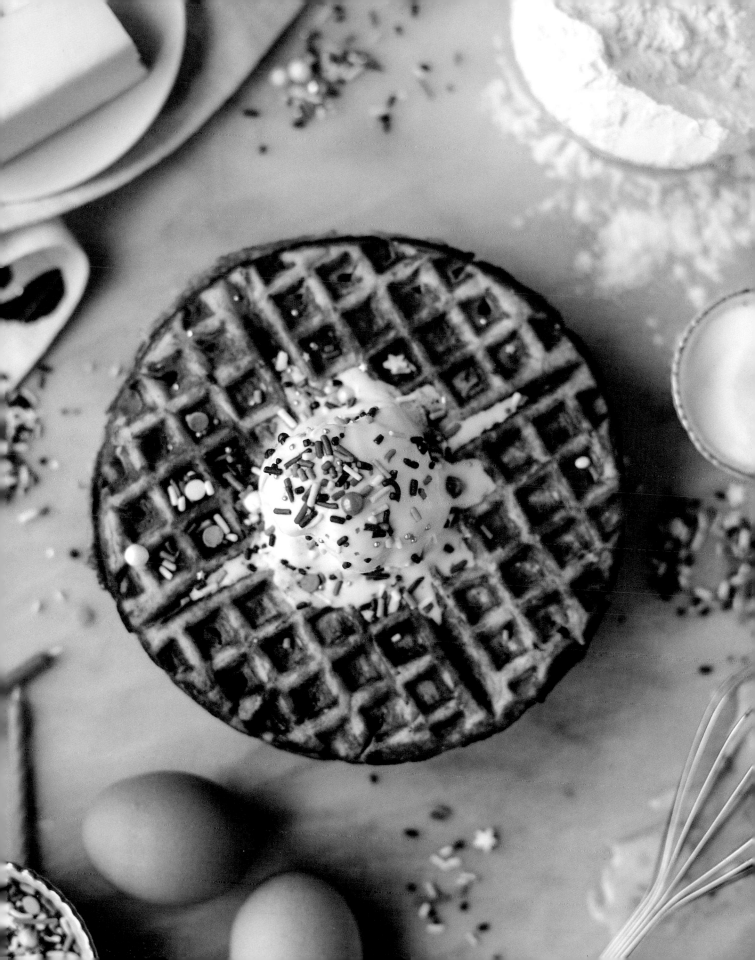

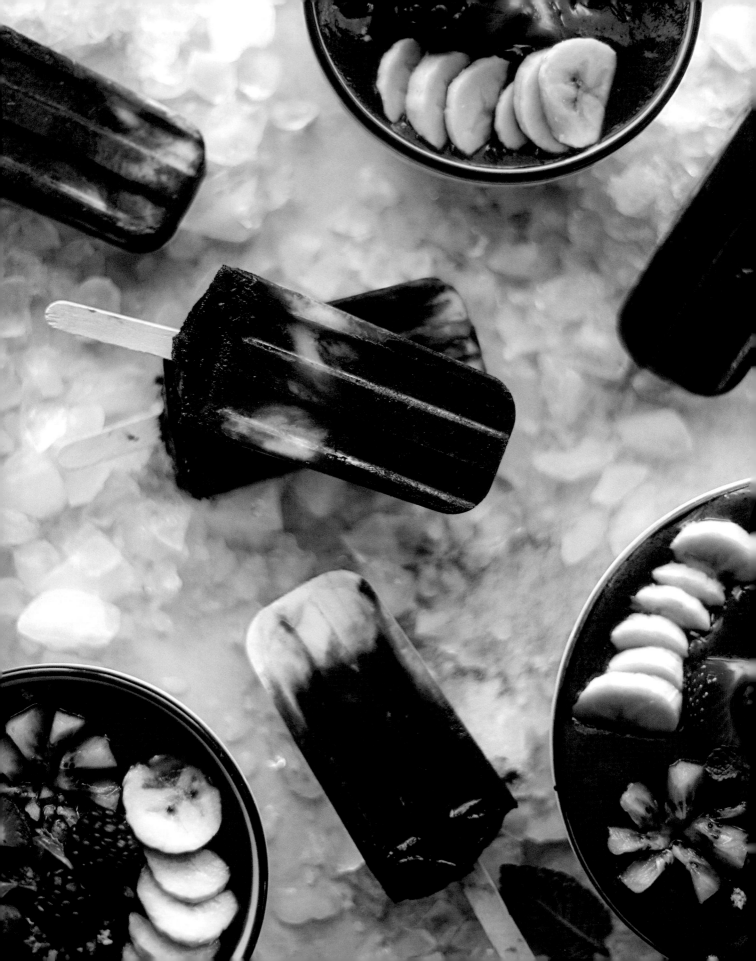

superfood pitaya popsicles

(AND MY FAVORITE PITAYA BOWL RECIPE!)

I have fallen for the smoothie bowl trend, and I have fallen hard. Of course, in true Jessica fashion, there are a few stipulations. The smoothie must be the consistency of ice cream so it's spoonable and similar to frozen yogurt. I have no interest in consuming liquid on a spoon. It also must have a few healthy ingredients. And it has to have a little crunch on top.

Pink dragon fruit, otherwise known as pitaya, is my favorite ingredient to use for smoothie bowls because of its wild (natural!) neon pink color. It makes eating the bowl so much more fun.

I'm sharing below my favorite method for bringing a pitaya bowl together as a little bonus, but what I really want to tell you about here are breakfast popsicles. These are super fun to consume in the summertime, on hot sunny mornings, and even better if you're at the pool or on the beach.

The creamy coconut milk blends perfectly with the slightly tart yet sweet pitaya. Who doesn't want a popsicle for breakfast? **MAKES APPROXIMATELY 8, DEPENDING ON YOUR MOLD**

1 package (3.5 ounces) frozen pitaya
½ cup frozen blueberries
¼ cup milk
1 can (14 ounces) full-fat coconut milk, shaken and whisked (so there is no separation)

In a blender, combine the pitaya, blueberries, and milk. Blend until creamy and smooth.

Spoon the pitaya mixture into popsicle molds, alternating with the coconut milk. You can make them half and half, layer them, or just fill the tops and bottoms with coconut!

Freeze for at least 6 to 8 hours before serving.

PITAYA BOWL

1 package (3.5 ounces) frozen pitaya
½ cup frozen peaches
½ frozen banana
½ cup milk (cow's, almond, coconut, etc.)
1 tablespoon chia seeds
1 tablespoon hemp seeds

TOPPING
Sliced banana
Berries
Granola

In a high-powered blender, combine the pitaya, peaches, banana, milk, chia seeds, and hemp seeds. Blend until thick and creamy. Scoop the smoothie into a bowl and top with sliced banana, berries, and granola. Eat immediately! **MAKES 1 GENEROUS SERVING**

coconut oil brûléed cinnamon toast

Though this is the simplest recipe in this cookbook, and therefore possibly the most embarrassing, it is still one that I must share with you due to the extreme nostalgia it brings me.

When I was a kid and we stayed overnight at my grandparents' house, my grandma would always make me cinnamon toast. The cinnamon toast of that day was toasted bread that was smeared with butter and covered in cinnamon sugar. The key, however, was the cinnamon sugar shaker.

She had one of the old-school Domino cinnamon shakers that had a bear on the front, and it always made our cinnamon toast sprinkle special. I've almost gone as far as buying the shaker off of ebay for the full nostalgic experience.

In an attempt to modernize the cinnamon sugar toast treat, I spread my whole wheat bread with coconut oil and add a mix of ground cinnamon and raw turbinado sugar on top. The technique has changed from using the toaster to using the broiler, which provides not only toasted, crispy bread, but a crunchy, crème brûlée–like topping of sugar. It is absolutely divine. And such a simple treat!

MAKES 2 TO 4 SERVINGS

3 tablespoons raw turbinado sugar
1 teaspoon ground cinnamon
4 slices of your favorite bread
4 tablespoons coconut oil

Preheat the oven to 375°F. In a bowl, stir together the sugar and cinnamon.

Spread 1 side of each slice of bread with 1 tablespoon of the coconut oil. Sprinkle on the cinnamon sugar. Place the bread slices on a baking sheet and bake for 10 minutes. Turn the broiler on high and broil for 1 to 2 minutes, watching closely so the toast doesn't burn. You want the sugar to get crunchy and delicious!

Let cool slightly before serving.

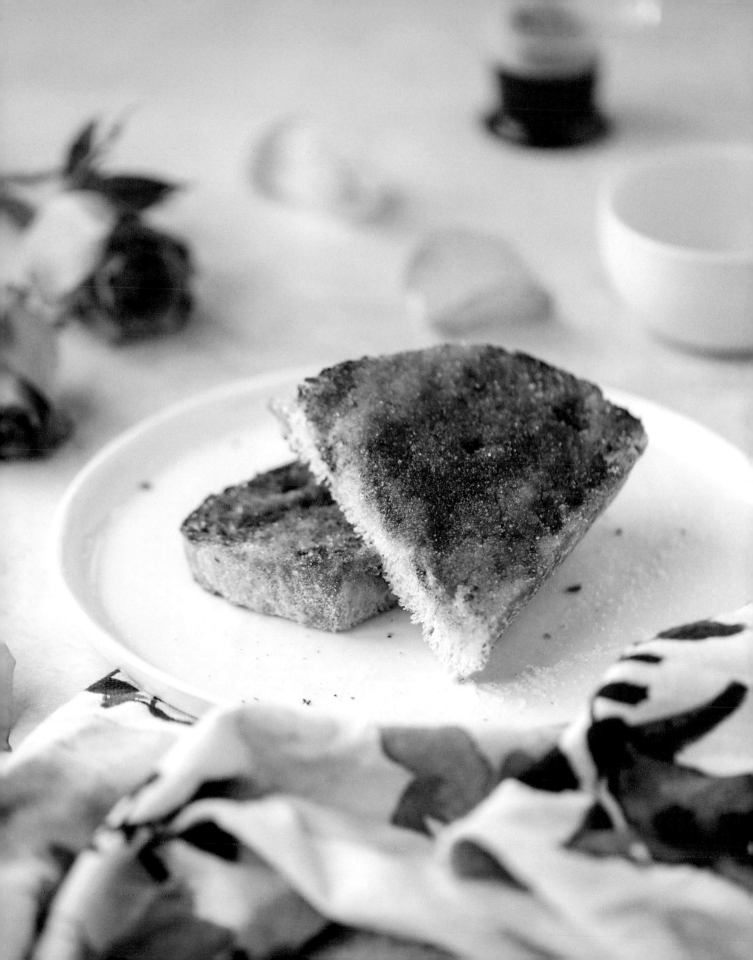

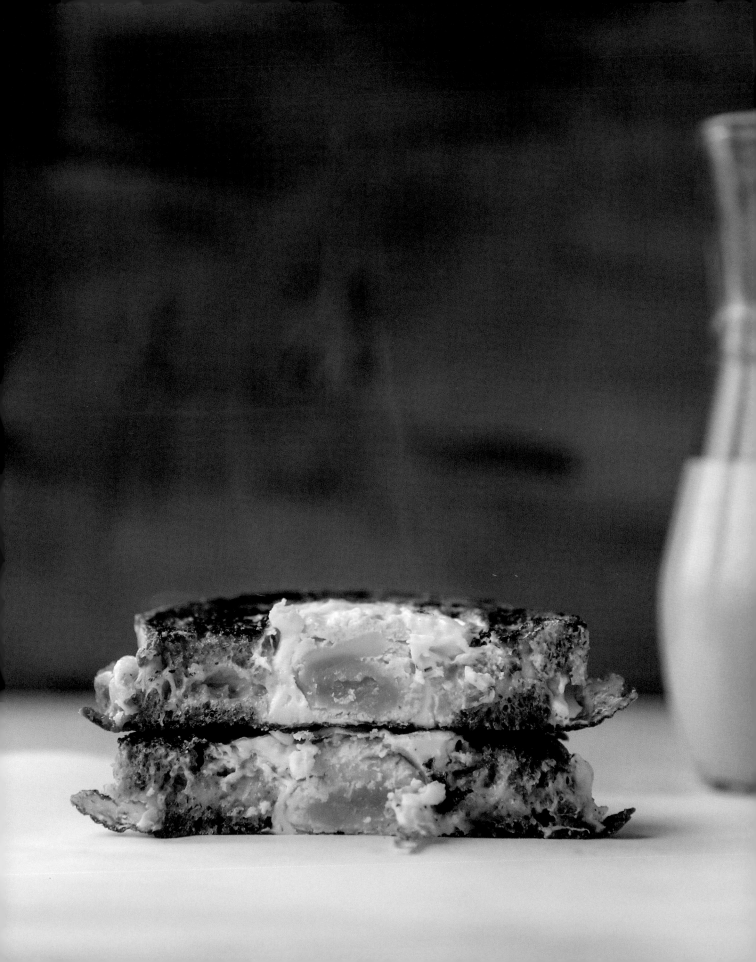

egg in a hole grilled havarti cheese

Let's talk about what a brat I am.

I feel completely deprived since I was never given Egg in a Hole toast as a kid. Sure, it comes with lots of different names: Toad in the Hole (ummm, no thanks), Egg in a Basket (not terrible), Frog in the Hole (still no), Egg in the Nest (eh?), One-Eyed Jack (what!), and more, but I prefer the whole Egg in a Hole thing.

I never had this until I was in my early twenties. Clearly, I still can't get over not having this as a child, and don't worry, I ask my mom about it constantly. Especially because she always made us toast and eggs! How did she miss this method?

There are not many meals that I find more comforting than eggs on toast. It is satisfying and tastes like home. And I will never know the reasoning, but I enjoy the egg in the toast so much more. Perhaps it's because I use a little extra butter than I do with regular toast, so the bread is more golden, is a bit more flavorful, and just has a little extra somethin' somethin'. I also love that the egg in the center tends to remain "dippy" and that you can use your bread cutout for dipping. I believe that dippy eggs are a Pennsylvania term, but they are something that I would request for breakfast constantly as a child. Basically, they're over-easy eggs with lots of toast for dipping in the yolk. And I never wanted to eat the egg whites.

One thing I love almost as much as eggs and toast? Grilled cheese. The simple version has made its reappearance in my life lately due to my toddler. And while I've trashed up my fair share of grilled cheese sandwiches over the years, cutting out the center and adding an egg is by far my new favorite.

MAKES 2 SERVINGS

4   slices bread
2   tablespoons softened butter, for spreading
6   ounces Havarti cheese, freshly grated
2   large eggs
1   teaspoon butter

Heat a large skillet over medium heat. Spread 1 side of each slice of bread with the softened butter, all the way to the edges. Turn the bread and divide the cheese among 2 of the slices. Cover with the remaining slices, buttered sides up. Place the sandwiches in the skillet, buttered sides facing down and up. Cook until golden on both sides and the cheese is melty.

Transfer the sandwiches to a work surface. Use a biscuit cutter or a paring knife to slice a hole in the center. Place the sandwiches back in the skillet. Add a drop of butter in the center of each and crack an egg into each center. Cook for 5 minutes, or until the eggs are almost set. You can cover the skillet to help cook the top.

Turn the sandwiches and cook until the eggs reach your desired degree of doneness. The longer they cook, the more done the yolks will be, of course. With the melty cheese, I like my egg yolk around medium to firm.

Remove the sandwiches and slice in half. Serve immediately with the cheese cutouts.

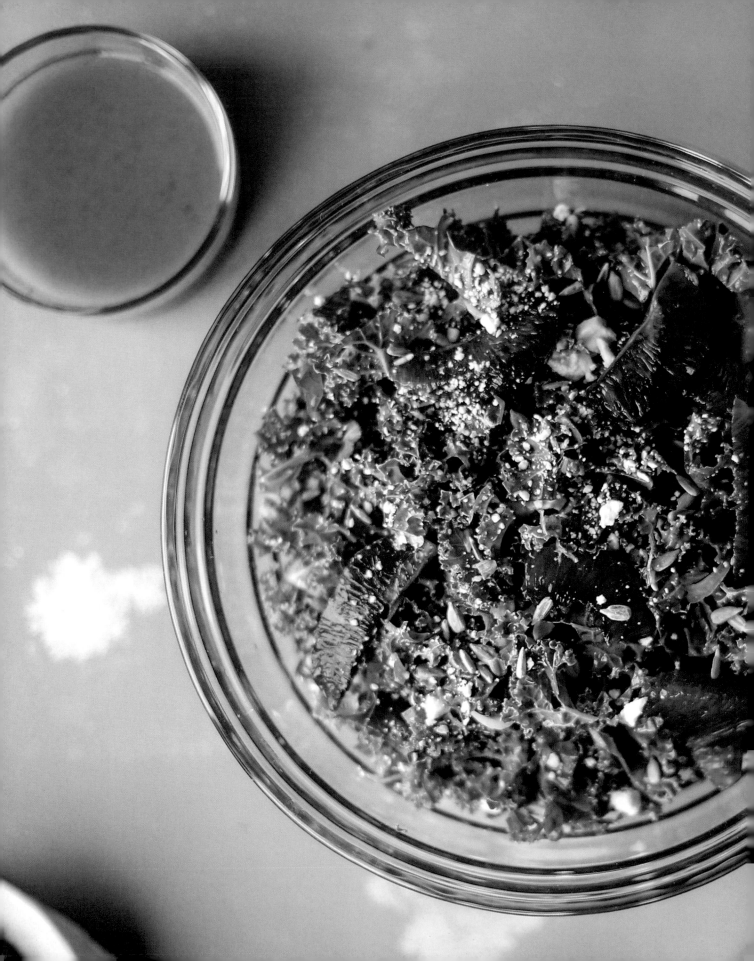

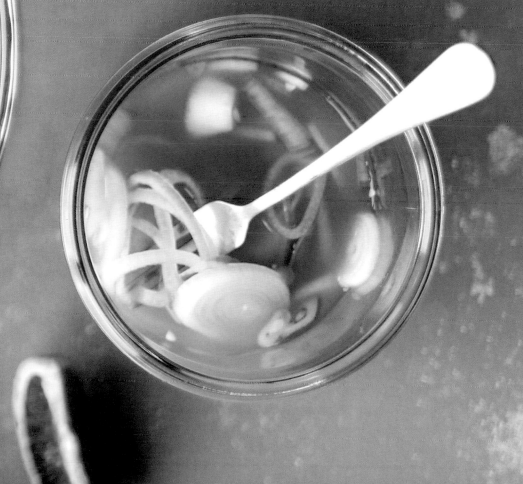

chapter 2

book club and beyond

All the snacks and apps you need
for gatherings and everyday life

I AM, PERHAPS, THE BIGGEST PROPONENT of a cheese plate that you may ever meet. Cheese boards make the world go 'round. They are *theeeee* ideal starter for any sort of party or gathering, and the best part is that the phrase "cheese board" is all encompassing.

Want to load it up with veggies? Go for it.

Tons of dried fruit and nuts? Knock yourself out.

Crackers, chips, pretzels—whatever you can find in that pantry is a go.

As long as your cheese board has, well, cheese on it, you're free to use the term!

Now, of course, this chapter isn't *all* about cheese boards (however, now I'm having second thoughts and wishing that I did center one entire chapter on that luxurious snack). It's filled with a few of my favorite snacks, salads, and party appetizers, most of which can be prepared ahead of time for easy transporting.

Some are ideal for parties or late summer dinners with your family outside on the patio, when it's too hot to do anything but snack and nibble. Others are go-tos that I make for my family to munch on throughout the week, like granola bars and nut butter quesadillas. Either way, they are all the sort of snackage that we love. Snacks can totally make a meal!

feta cheeseball

Basically, it's not a party in our family if there isn't a cheeseball of some sort. My grandmother was the queen of the cheeseball, perfecting that old-school one filled with pimientos and olives and then rolled in chopped walnuts. She made it for every occasion, and as simple as it was, guests always went crazy for it. I always went crazy for it.

My mom has taken on the role of making that cheeseball for special occasions these days. Heck, sometimes she even makes it for herself to snack on throughout the week! Even the biggest olive-haters (I'm looking at you, Eddie) and walnut-haters (both of my brothers, always) eat this cheeseball with gusto. It's one of those things that taste like childhood. It's comforting party food, if I do say so myself. It's simple to make, and it's simple to eat.

I shared that traditional recipe on my blog many moons ago. And since then, I've made it my mission to make all sorts of different cheeseball flavors, much to my mom's dismay. It's not that she doesn't like my cheeseball experiments. She just loves the "regular" one so much and at the same time, like me, hates change. I've added different vegetables to the cheeseballs, even used dried fruits, rolled them in all sorts of nuts (pistachios are tops), and sometimes made mini versions just so I could call them cheese truffles.

Really. Who wouldn't want to eat a cheese truffle?

This version is semi-Greek inspired. It's loaded with feta, which may be my favorite cheese because it's incredibly versatile. It's filled with roasted red peppers, kalamata olives, and artichokes, then rolled in crushed almonds. It tastes fantastic with crackers or pita chips, and it even makes me want to eat some raw veggies, too. Cucumbers and carrots are winners! **MAKES 8 SERVINGS**

6 ounces feta cheese, crumbled

1 package (8 ounces) cream cheese

1 clove garlic, minced

¼ cup chopped kalamata olives

2 tablespoons chopped roasted red peppers

2 tablespoons chopped artichoke hearts

Pinch of salt

Pinch of ground black pepper

½ cup finely chopped marcona almonds

Crackers and pita chips, for serving

Veggies, for serving

Place the feta in a food processor and pulse into small crumbs. Transfer to a large bowl. Add the cream cheese, garlic, olives, red peppers, artichokes, salt, and black pepper and stir until combined.

Mold the mixture into a big ball as best you can. Roll it in plastic wrap and refrigerate for 30 minutes.

After 30 minutes, mold the cheese into a smoother ball. Spread the almonds on a plate or baking sheet and roll the ball through them, using your hands to press them into all the cracks and crevices.

Serve immediately or keep it in the fridge until ready to use. The cheeseball can be made 1 to 2 days beforehand, wrapped in plastic wrap, and stored in the fridge. Serve with crackers, chips, and veggies.

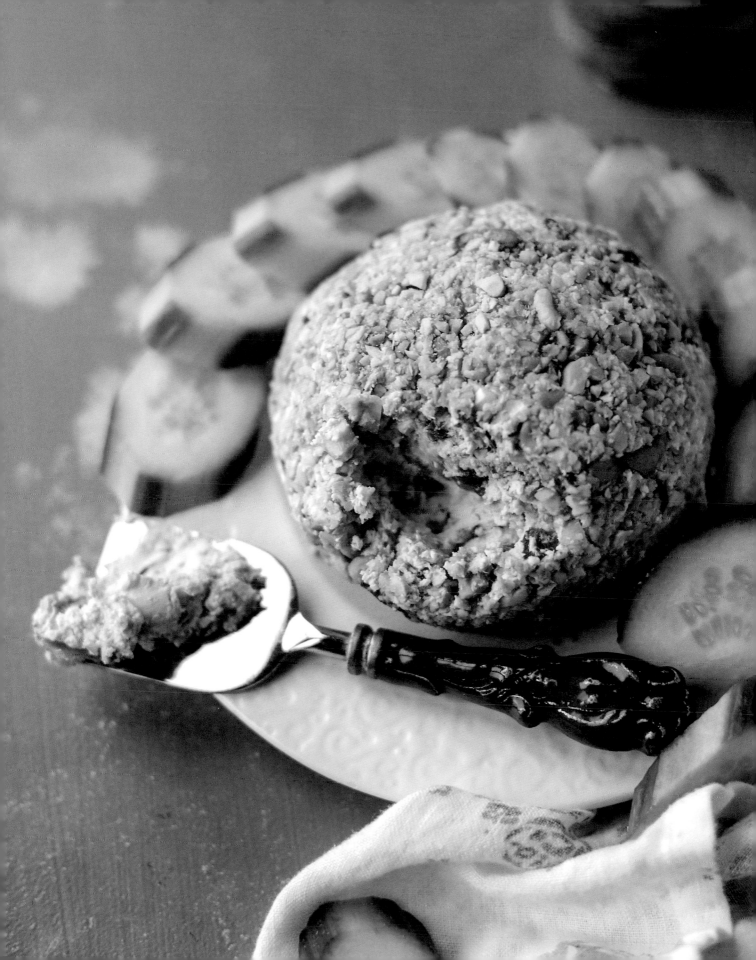

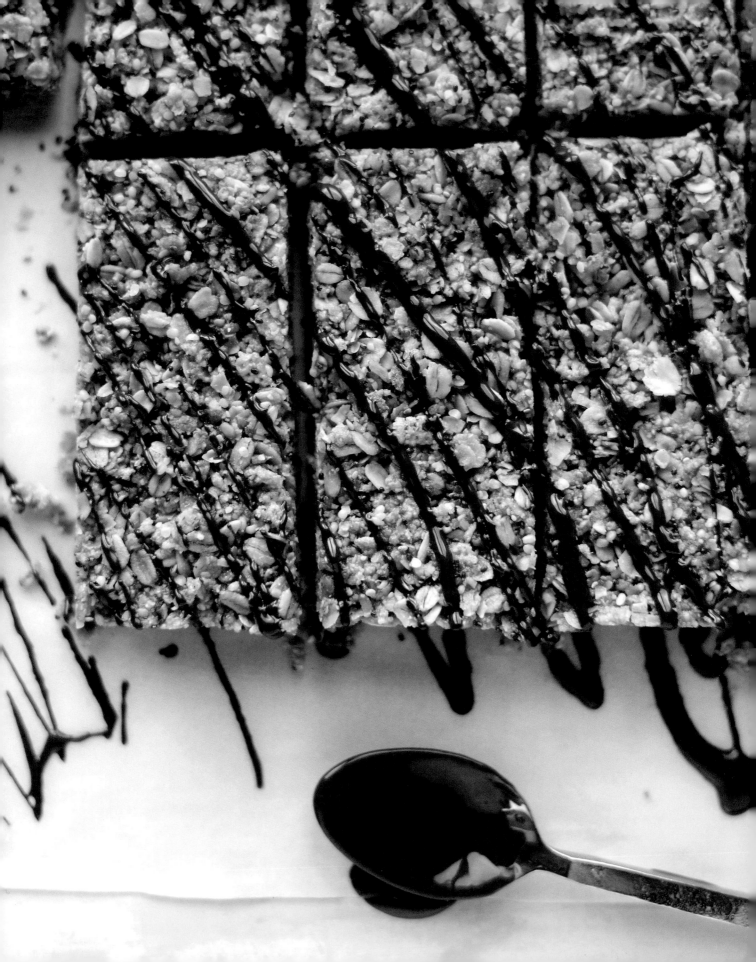

chocolate-drizzled tahini granola bars

Oh tahini! How I love you.

My first experience with tahini was in hummus, naturally. It was never an ingredient we were exposed to growing up, so as soon as I hit my twenties and entered a full-blown hummus obsession, I fell in love.

As a general fan of all things sesame, it wasn't long before I started experimenting with tahini in other savory and sweet ways.

I use almond, cashew, and walnut butter all the time to make granola bars (and regular granola), so I was determined to use tahini in this same way, too. I love the bit of savory flavor that the tahini lends these bars. Paired with the chocolate drizzle, it feels like you're eating a treat. My favorite time to make these is on Sunday afternoon to prepare for the week ahead, and once they are sliced, I wrap them in plastic wrap or parchment and stick them in the fridge. MAKES ABOUT 12

6   tablespoons unsalted butter

6   tablespoons tahini

½   cup honey

¼   cup firmly packed light brown sugar

2   teaspoons vanilla extract

1   cup old-fashioned rolled oats

1   cup quick-cooking oats

1½ cups brown rice cereal

3   tablespoons ground flaxseed

2   tablespoons chia seeds

2   tablespoons hemp hearts

½   teaspoon salt

1   cup chocolate chips, melted, for drizzling

3   tablespoons sesame seeds, for topping

Line a 13" x 9" dish with parchment paper. Spray the paper with cooking spray.

In a saucepan, heat the butter, tahini, honey, and sugar over low heat. Whisk until the butter melts, the sugar dissolves, and the mixture is warm. Remove the pan from the heat and stir in the vanilla.

In a large bowl, stir together the oats, cereal, flaxseed, chia seeds, hemp hearts, and salt. Pour the butter mixture over the dry ingredients and use a spatula to gently combine until everything is moistened. Press the mixture into the pan. Drizzle with the melted chocolate. Sprinkle the sesame seeds over the top. Refrigerate the bars for 4 hours, or until set.

Remove from the fridge and lift the parchment out of the dish. Slice the bars into squares or triangles.

fried burrata

This savory treat needs no explanation. Creamy, cheesy goodness with a crispy crust. It is truly one of the best things I have ever eaten. **MAKES 4 SERVINGS**

⅔ cup seasoned bread crumbs

½ teaspoon garlic powder

¼ teaspoon crushed red-pepper flakes

1 large egg, lightly beaten

2 tablespoons grapeseed oil

1 ball (8 ounces) cold burrata cheese

1 cup chopped cherry tomatoes

Pinch of salt and ground black pepper

Red-pepper flakes, for sprinkling

Sliced baguette or crackers, for serving

In a shallow dish, stir together the bread crumbs, garlic powder, and red-pepper flakes. In another shallow dish, lightly beat the egg.

In a skillet, heat the oil over medium heat. Dip the burrata in the beaten egg and then into the bread crumb mixture, pressing gently to adhere. Place the cheese in the hot oil and cook for 2 minutes, turning once, or until golden on both sides but not melted. Carefully remove and set on a plate.

Arrange the tomatoes around the cheese and season with the salt and pepper. Sprinkle on the red-pepper flakes. Serve with a sliced baguette or your favorite crackers.

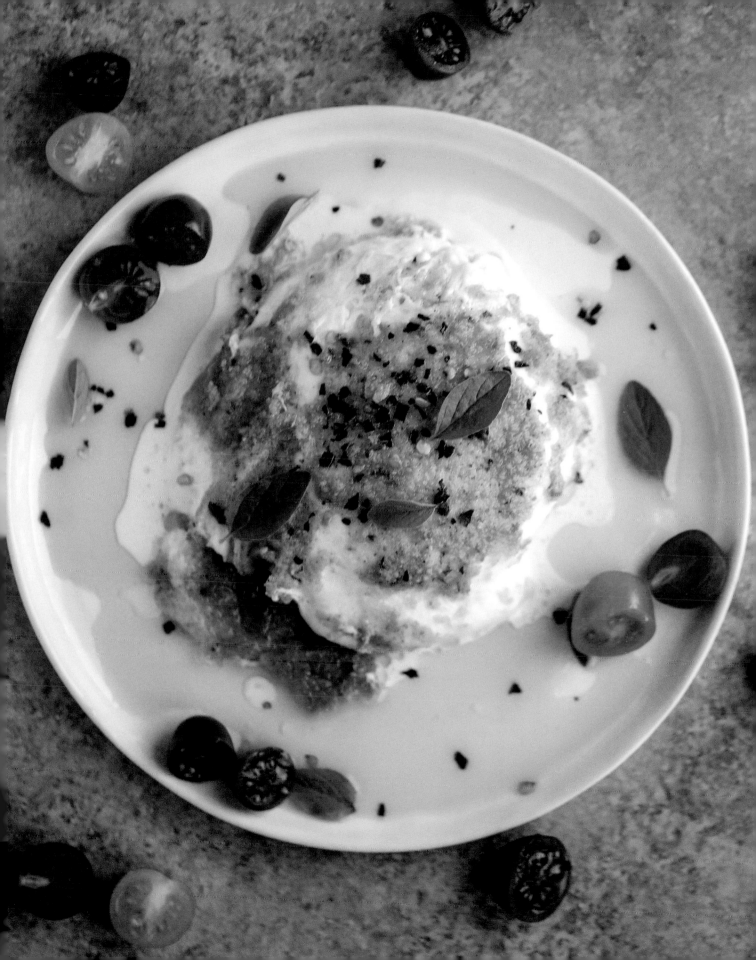

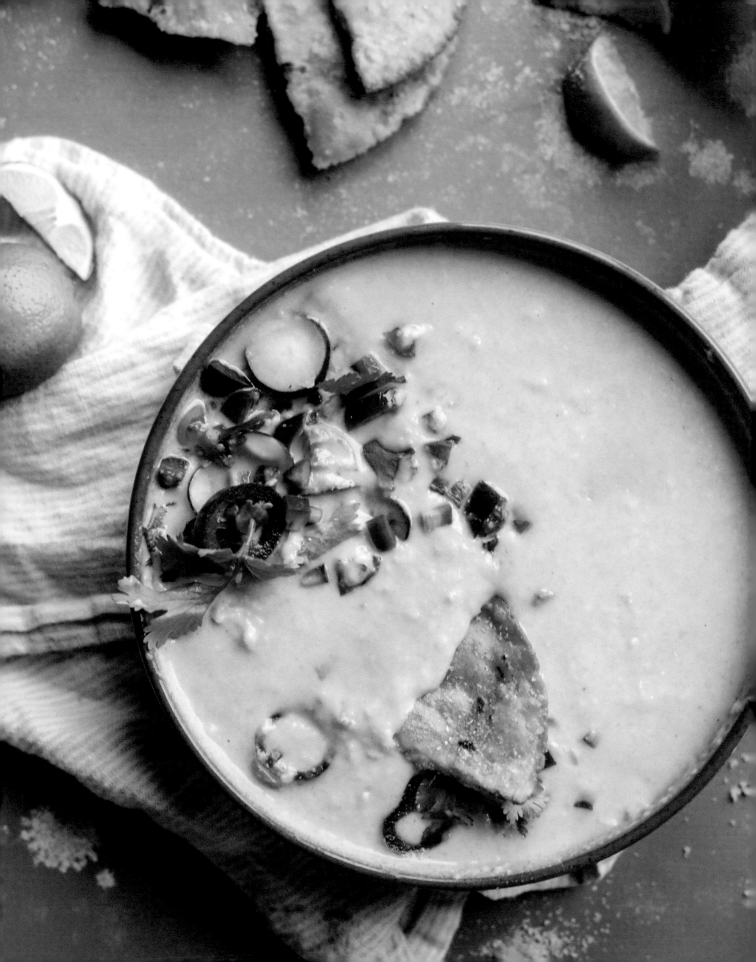

butternut squash queso
WITH RUSTIC TORTILLA CHIPS

I cannot even tell you the number of times my husband and I have to decide between guacamole or queso as a starter at our local Mexican restaurant. Of course, most times we want both. Just like any other normal human.

Around here, any sort of guacamole side or queso dip is always extra. Saying that "it's worth it" is probably the understatement of the year because I don't think I know one person who doesn't want to dip all of their tortilla chips in cheese sauce. Do you?

This version of queso takes my butternut squash love into account. At the same time, it slightly lightens up the dip, because vegetables. But that's not the plan here. The end goal is to still have a wonderfully cheesy, melty dip with just a hint of squash flavor that is perfect for sharing with friends. And when paired with your own homemade little corn tortilla chips?

I want nothing else, ever. **MAKES 4 TO 6 SERVINGS**

BUTTERNUT SQUASH QUESO

2½ cups cubed butternut squash

4 tablespoons olive oil, divided

½ teaspoon salt

½ teaspoon ground black pepper

½ teaspoon garlic powder

1 tablespoon unsalted butter

2 jalapeño chile peppers, chopped

½ sweet onion, diced

2 cloves garlic, minced

⅛ teaspoon salt

⅛ teaspoon ground black pepper

1½ cups half-and-half, divided

1 tablespoon cornstarch

16 ounces sharp white Cheddar cheese, freshly grated

8 ounces Monterey Jack cheese, freshly grated

Cilantro, for topping

Radish slices, for topping

Chopped tomatoes, for topping

RUSTIC TORTILLA CHIPS

Canola oil

12 corn tortillas (4" diameter), torn into pieces

Salt, for sprinkling

TO MAKE THE BUTTERNUT SQUASH QUESO

Preheat the oven to 425°F. Line a baking sheet with parchment paper. In a bowl, toss the squash with 3 tablespoons of the olive oil, salt, black pepper, and garlic powder. Spread the squash on the baking sheet and bake for 30 minutes, tossing the squash halfway through, or until tender when pierced with a fork.

Transfer the squash (and any drippings) to a food processor. Blend until pureed and smooth. Set aside.

In a saucepan, melt the remaining 1 tablespoon olive oil and the butter over medium heat. Stir in the jalapeño peppers, onion, and garlic. Season with the salt and black pepper. Cook for 5 to 6 minutes, or until the onion softens. Slowly stream in 1 cup of the half-and-half, whisking the entire time. In a bowl, whisk together the remaining ½ cup half-and-half and the cornstarch until no lumps remain to create a slurry. Stir the slurry into the saucepan and cook for 1 minute, or until the mixture thickens. Reduce the heat to low.

Stir in the cheeses, 1 small handful at a time, until melted. Stir in the squash until combined. Transfer the mixture to a crock, large bowl, or a small slow cooker set on low.

Serve with the cilantro, radishes, and tomatoes on top.

TO MAKE THE RUSTIC TORTILLA CHIPS

Heat a cast-iron skillet over medium-high heat and add the canola oil. Add the tortilla pieces in batches (however many your skillet can hold in a single layer) and fry for 2 to 3 minutes, or until golden brown. Transfer to a paper towel to drain excess grease. Sprinkle the chips with salt and repeat with the remaining tortilla pieces.

pimiento cheese–stuffed olives

It's time to confess something: I almost threw these olives in the deep fryer. Yes, deep-fried, pimiento cheese–stuffed olives. My heart beats for that!

For a few years, my cousin Chris has been telling me about these delicious fried pimiento cheese olives he gets at a local bar. As a lover of both pimiento cheese and olives, the idea has haunted me, and I am so desperate to try them.

I took matters into my own hands. I whipped up our favorite pimiento cheese, which Eddie refused to eat until last year, since he was convinced that there were actually olives in the cheese. Spoiler alert: There are not! Ever since he learned the truth, pimiento cheese has been an indulgent treat that we make once or twice a year.

These olives go like hotcakes on a cheese board. They go like hotcakes even if they are just sitting in a bowl! People go crazy over them because they are so packed with flavor. And even though Gorgonzola may be a little classier than pimiento cheese, I like to think that these are the modernized take on blue cheese–stuffed olives.

Plus, they make a killer dirty martini garnish. Turn to page 221 for the recipe! **SERVES A CROWD**

6   ounces sharp white Cheddar cheese, freshly grated

2   ounces (½ of 4-ounce jar) pimientos, drained

2   ounces cream cheese, softened

¼   cup mayonnaise

½   teaspoon garlic powder

½   teaspoon onion powder

¼   teaspoon salt

¼   teaspoon ground black pepper

1   jar (12 ounces) jumbo pitted green olives

In a large bowl, combine the Cheddar, pimientos, cream cheese, mayonnaise, garlic powder, onion powder, salt, and pepper. Mix well.

Stuff the olives with the pimiento cheese using a teaspoon or a small condiment spoon. Serve!

NOTE: These can be made successfully a few hours ahead of time.

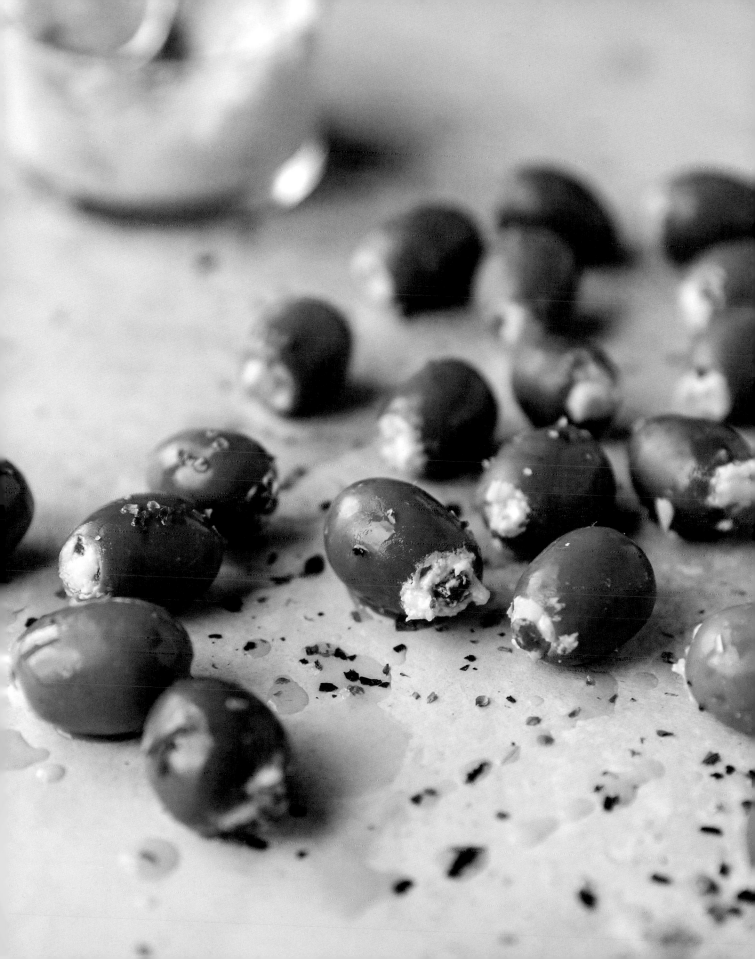

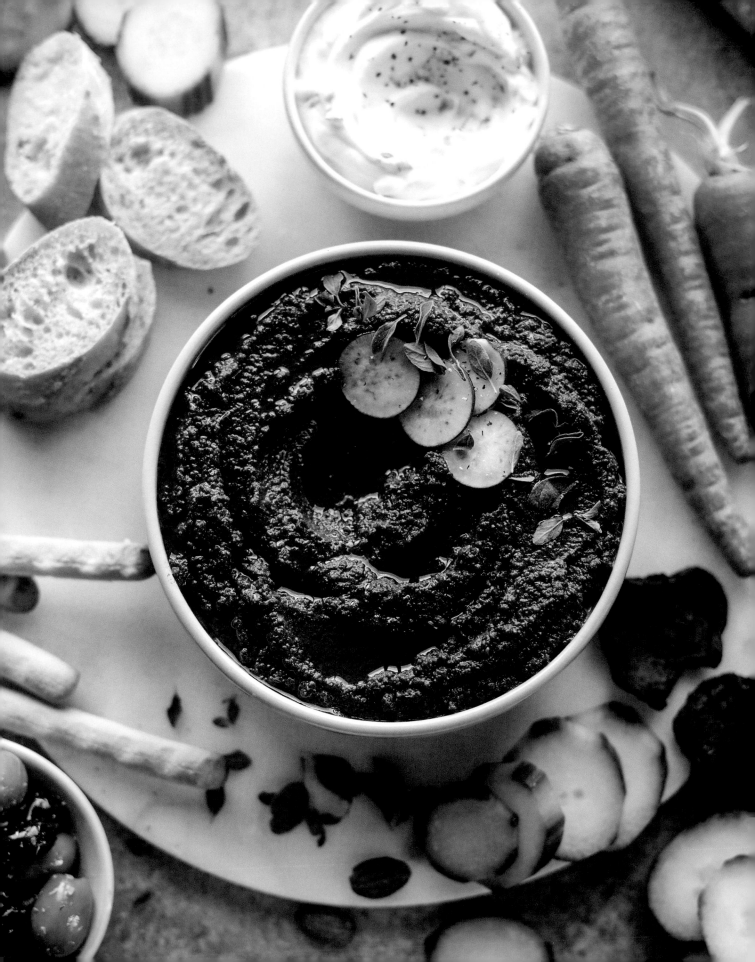

hot pink hummus platter

If the color of this hummus alone doesn't sell you, I don't know what will.

Here's the thing. I know that beets can be very polarizing. You either love 'em or hate 'em, and I get it. I really do.

Eddie taught me to enjoy beets a few years ago, and I shared our favorite beet recipe, a salad with roasted beets, creamy goat cheese, and honey, in my first cookbook. Since then, we've gone out of the box a little and tried to enjoy beets in different ways.

Specifically, this hot pink hummus! If you know someone who isn't a beet lover, start them out on this. Make a beautiful, colorful platter that is chock-full of dippers and whip some beets and chickpeas together in your food processor. The flavor is an absolute delight!

Beet dreams do come true, you guys.   MAKES 4 TO 6 SERVINGS

2   medium red beets, scrubbed

1   tablespoon + ½ cup olive oil

1   cup chickpeas, rinsed and drained

½   cup tahini

2   cloves garlic, minced

½   teaspoon salt

½   teaspoon ground black pepper

3–4   tablespoons ice water

Pita triangles and crackers,
    for serving

Cucumber rounds, carrots, and
    radishes, for serving

Olives, for serving

Preheat the oven to 375°F. Rub the beets with 1 tablespoon of the oil and wrap them tightly in foil. Roast for 60 to 90 minutes, or until they are fork-tender and the skin can be rubbed right off. Chop the beets into pieces.

In a food processor, combine the beets, chickpeas, tahini, and garlic. Blend until smooth and pureed. With the processor running, stream in the remaining ½ cup oil and continue to blend until the hummus is smooth. Add the salt and pepper and blend a bit more. Taste and season with additional salt and pepper if needed. With the processor running, stream in the ice water and blend until smooth.

Scoop the hummus into a bowl and serve with a variety of dippers.

spicy corn and peach salsa

My love for fruit salsa knows no bounds. It's similar to my love for tacos. I will put anything in a taco and call it a taco and eat that taco. Just like I will put any fruit in my salsa and call it salsa and eat that salsa.

The best thing about fruit salsa is that it's incredibly versatile. Sure, it goes great on said tacos, but I also use it as a simple dip, a salad topping, a burger topping, a fish topping, or Eddie's favorite: eating it off a spoon as if it's a side dish. I don't blame him. The options are endless!

This salsa is packed with sweet, juicy peaches, sweet corn, poblano peppers, diced red onion, and jalapeño peppers for some extra heat. It's essentially spicy summer in a bowl. Pair it with a few home-made tortilla chips and an icy margarita. I can't think of anything better. **MAKES ABOUT 1½ CUPS**

3   ears corn, grilled or roasted
2   peaches, diced
1   poblano chile pepper, diced
1   jalapeño chile pepper, diced
1   clove garlic, minced
½   red onion, diced
Juice of 2 limes
3   tablespoons chopped cilantro
½   teaspoon salt
¼   teaspoon ground black pepper

In a bowl, combine the corn, peaches, chile peppers, garlic, onion, lime juice, cilantro, salt, and black pepper. Stir well. Let sit for a few minutes at room temperature so the flavors can come together. Use with grilled fish or chicken or serve with tortilla chips!

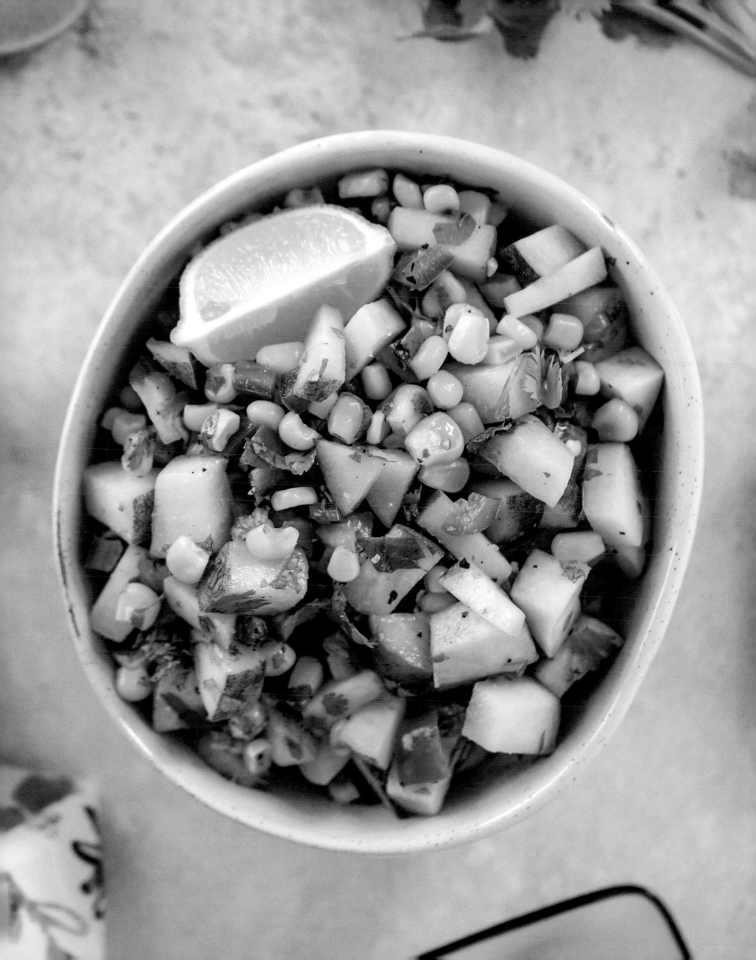

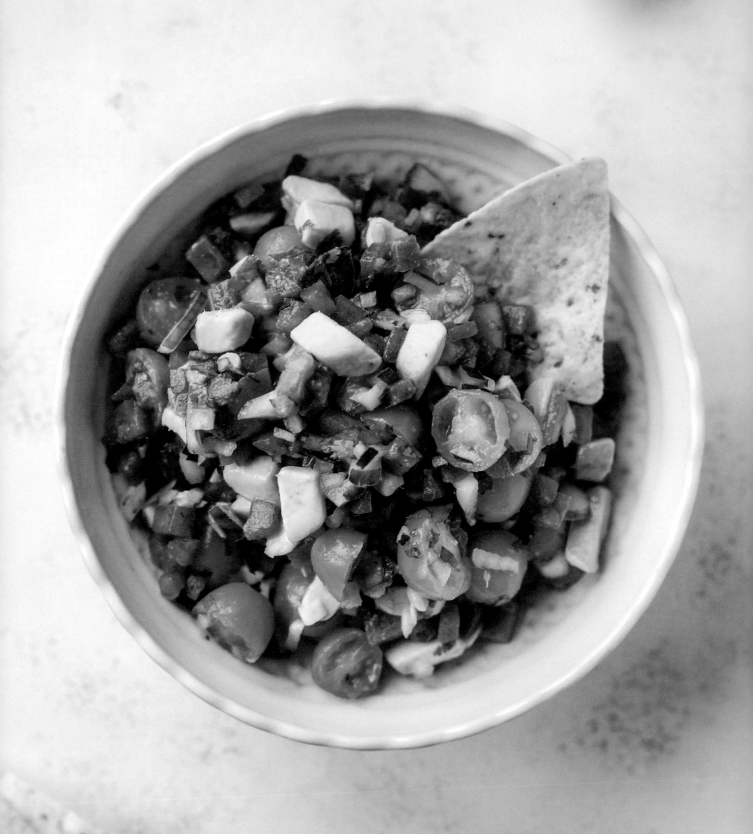

watermelon avocado salsa

Here is another take on a fruit salsa that we love so much. Sweet watermelon, sweet onion, diced jalapeño, and everyone's favorite ingredient: avocado.

A tip on using avocado in the salsa: If you want it to stay pretty and not turn brown, add the avocado right before serving. As the salsa sits, the avocado adds creaminess to the salsa. While it's still delish, it can turn the salsa into an unappealing shade. Toss in those avo chunks right before serving, and you're good to go! MAKES ABOUT 2 CUPS

1½ cups diced watermelon

1 cup cherry tomatoes, quartered

½ red onion, thinly sliced

½ jalapeño chile pepper, thinly sliced

3 tablespoons chopped cilantro

Juice of 2 limes

½ teaspoon salt

¼ teaspoon ground black pepper

1 avocado, diced

In a medium bowl, combine the watermelon, tomatoes, onion, jalapeño pepper, cilantro, lime juice, salt, and black pepper. Stir well. Right before serving, stir in the avocado. Serve this with fish or chicken—or serve with tortilla chips for dipping!

sweet and spicy pretzels

WITH MAPLE BEER MUSTARD

There are no bones about it: I am a mustard freak. I have loved the briny, vinegary condiment since I was a kid. Maybe even a toddler. My tastebuds love vinegar-based dressings and sauces, so all forms of mustard are immediately in my favorites category.

In my middle school days, my after-school snack would be pretzel sticks dipped in mustard. Sometimes with olives on the side. Not much has changed since then, except my pretzels have received a little homemade spice boost and my mustard has booze in it. Sounds fair to me!

These pretzels are baked with a buttery spice rub on them, imparting a delicious addictive flavor. These sweet and spicy pretzels are a spin on the classic whiskey pretzels that I always make around the holiday season—a recipe you may have tried over the years due to its popularity.

The mustard needs to be made ahead of time, but we're only really talking the night before. It has to set so it's not super liquidy, and I promise you . . . it's totally worth it.   **MAKES 8 SERVINGS**

PRETZELS

1   bag (9 ounces) large sourdough pretzels

½   cup unsalted butter, melted

3   tablespoons firmly packed brown sugar

2   teaspoons smoked paprika

2   teaspoons garlic powder

½   teaspoon cayenne pepper

MAPLE BEER MUSTARD

¼   cup brown mustard seeds

3   tablespoons yellow mustard seeds

⅓   cup ground mustard powder

1   teaspoon salt

1½ tablespoons maple syrup

½   cup beer (use your favorite; I like a wheat or amber ale)

3   tablespoons apple cider vinegar

TO MAKE THE PRETZELS

Preheat the oven to 300°F. Line 2 baking sheets with parchment paper. Spread the pretzels evenly over both sheets. You don't want to layer them.

In a bowl, whisk together the butter, sugar, paprika, garlic, and cayenne pepper. Pour the mixture over the pretzels and use your hands to toss everything together really well. Bake for 25 minutes, tossing the pretzels after the first 15 minutes. Let cool completely on the sheets.

TO MAKE THE MAPLE BEER MUSTARD

Place the mustard seeds in a mortar and grind them up a bit with a pestle.

In a bowl, stir together the mustard seeds, mustard powder, salt, maple syrup, and beer. Let the mixture sit for 20 minutes, then stir in the vinegar. The mustard will be runny, but let it sit overnight in the fridge and it will thicken. Serve with the pretzels!

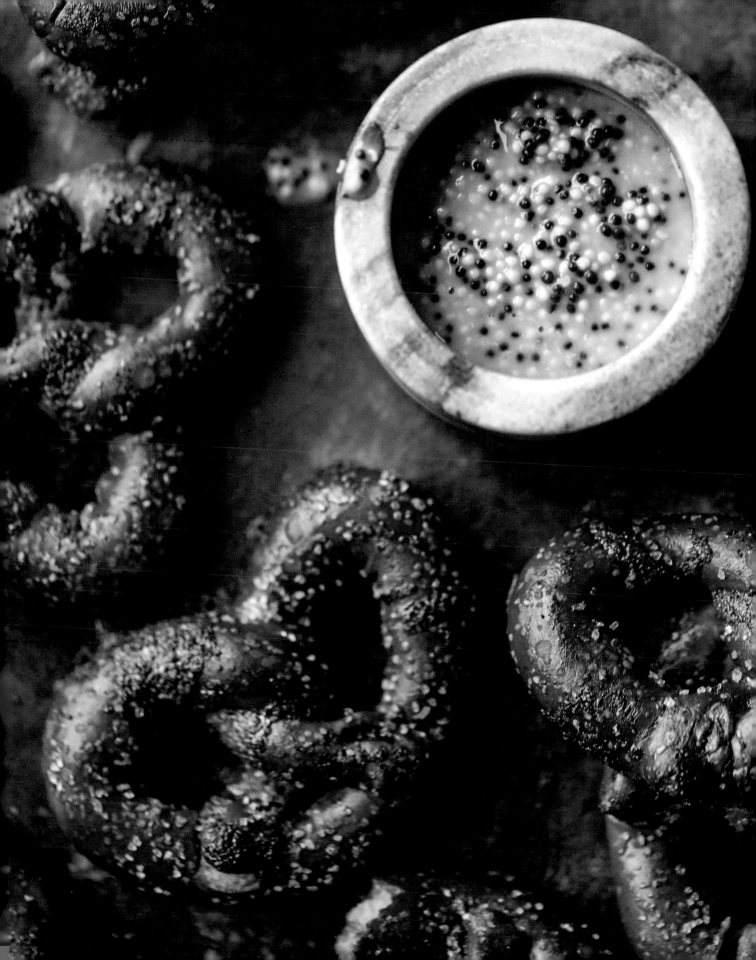

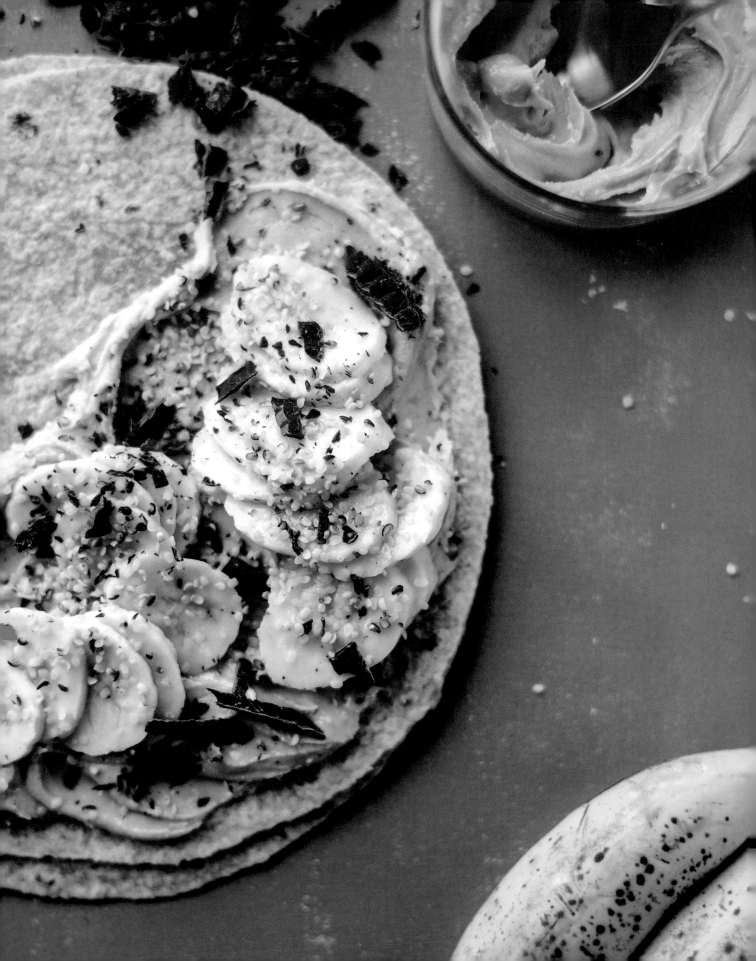

cashew banana quesadilla

WITH CRUNCHY HEMP

There has never been a time in my life when nut butter and bananas weren't staple foods. From the time I was a young kid, this combination was solidified in my brain as one of the best snacks of all time.

It's not just the flavor, or the multiple combinations that we can make these days with all the varieties of nut butter that are available. It's the way it's so satisfying and energy giving. I love the combination as a pre- and post-workout snack, as a simple breakfast, and as a lighter before-dinner treat.

In my tween years, I would make "banana boats" with my brother. We'd slather a piece of bread with peanut butter, wrap it around a banana, and secure it together with pretzel sticks. This is sort of my high-end version of that.

A soft tortilla is spread with cashew butter (which I'm always convinced is one flavor step away from vanilla cake). Banana slices go in next. And if you want to toast this quickly in a skillet? I suggest opting for the teeniest amount of freshly chopped dark chocolate for decadence. Finally, I love to sprinkle crunchy hemp hearts over top. They not only give it a bit of texture, but protein for that satiety factor. This is my sort of health food! **MAKES 1 SERVING**

1   whole wheat flour tortilla
    (8" diameter)

2–3 tablespoons cashew butter

1   banana, thinly sliced

½   ounce dark chocolate, chopped
    (optional)

1   tablespoon hemp hearts

Spread 1 side of the tortilla with the cashew butter and layer on the banana slices. If desired, sprinkle on the chopped chocolate and then the hemp hearts. Fold the tortilla over and serve!

roasted garlic hummus & bean salad

I've come to a terrible point in my life where hummus just isn't hummus anymore without the addition of some crazy topping. We can probably thank the Internet (and Instagram!) for that, but there is just something so wonderful about creamy, smooth hummus being topped with extra beans, herbs, glugs of olive oil, and even cheese.

For this recipe, I decided to keep it on the lighter side and go with a marinated bean salad. To say that I adore beans would be an understatement. I'd even go so far as to say that they are one of my favorite foods! They are creamy and light, yet when placed on the hummus, they add that tiny bit of chew that is so wonderful with warm, soft pita.

A bonus: You can make the hummus and beans ahead of time and store them separately. Get to your destination (i.e., a party . . . maybe in your own kitchen! With yourself!) and transfer the beans to the top of the creamy dip. So much yes. **MAKES 4 TO 6 SERVINGS**

ROASTED GARLIC HUMMUS

- 2 bulbs garlic
- 2 teaspoons + 3 tablespoons olive oil
- 1 can (14 ounces) chickpeas, rinsed and drained
- 1 cup tahini paste
- Juice of ½ lemon
- ½ teaspoon salt
- ½ teaspoon ground black pepper
- 4– 5 tablespoons ice water

BEAN SALAD

- ½ cup chickpeas
- ½ cup cannellini beans
- ½ cup pinto beans
- 2 tablespoons olive oil
- 1 teaspoon apple cider vinegar
- 2 tablespoons chopped fresh herbs (such as oregano and parsley)
- 1 clove garlic, minced
- Pinch of salt and ground black pepper

TO MAKE THE ROASTED GARLIC HUMMUS

Preheat the oven to 350°F. Slice off the top portion of the garlic bulbs to reveal the cloves. Lightly run your fingers back and forth on each garlic bulb to remove any excess paper. Pour 2 teaspoons of the olive oil over the bulbs. Wrap the bulbs tightly in foil and roast for 45 to 60 minutes, or until the cloves are caramelly and golden in color. (You can do this step ahead of time. I will keep roasted cloves in my fridge for 2 to 3 days.) When ready to use, squeeze the roasted garlic cloves out of the bulbs.

In a food processor, combine the roasted garlic cloves, chickpeas, tahini, lemon juice, salt, and pepper. Puree until the chickpeas break down and the mixture starts to come together (it won't be smooth yet). Make sure to scrape the sides with a spatula. Drizzle in the remaining 3 tablespoons olive oil with the food processer running. Drizzle in the ice water while the processor is going. The hummus should become really smooth. If you need a little more water, add it 1 tablespoon at a time.

Scoop the hummus into a large bowl for serving.

TO MAKE THE BEAN SALAD

In a medium bowl, combine the chickpeas, cannellini beans, and pinto beans. In a small bowl, whisk together the oil, vinegar, herbs, garlic, salt, and pepper. Drizzle the dressing over the beans and toss.

Top the hummus with the bean salad before serving.

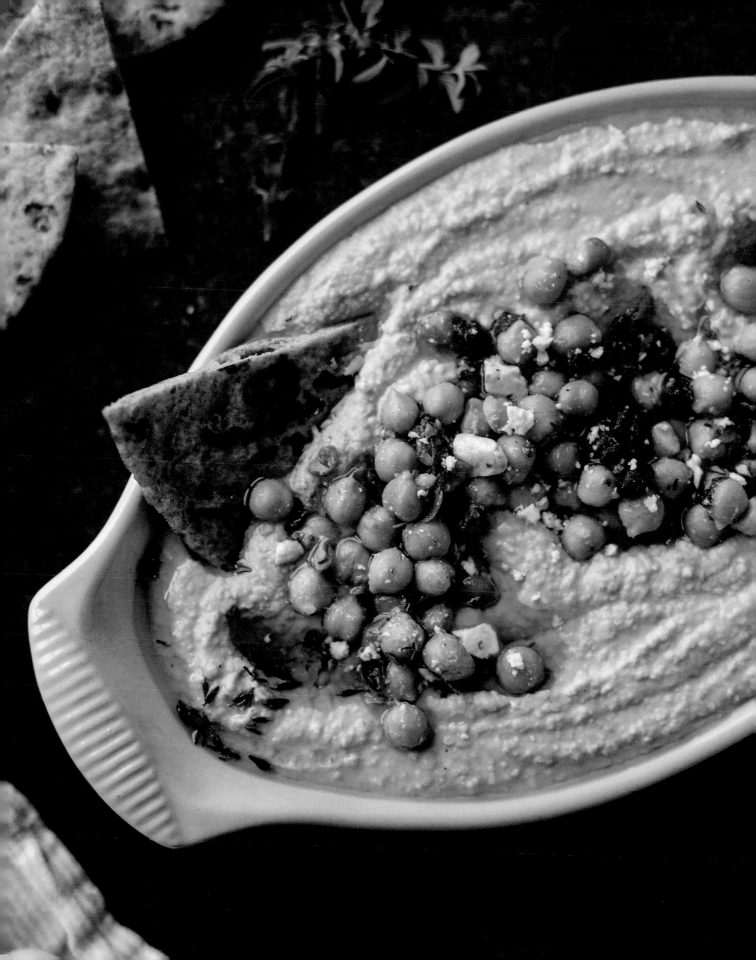

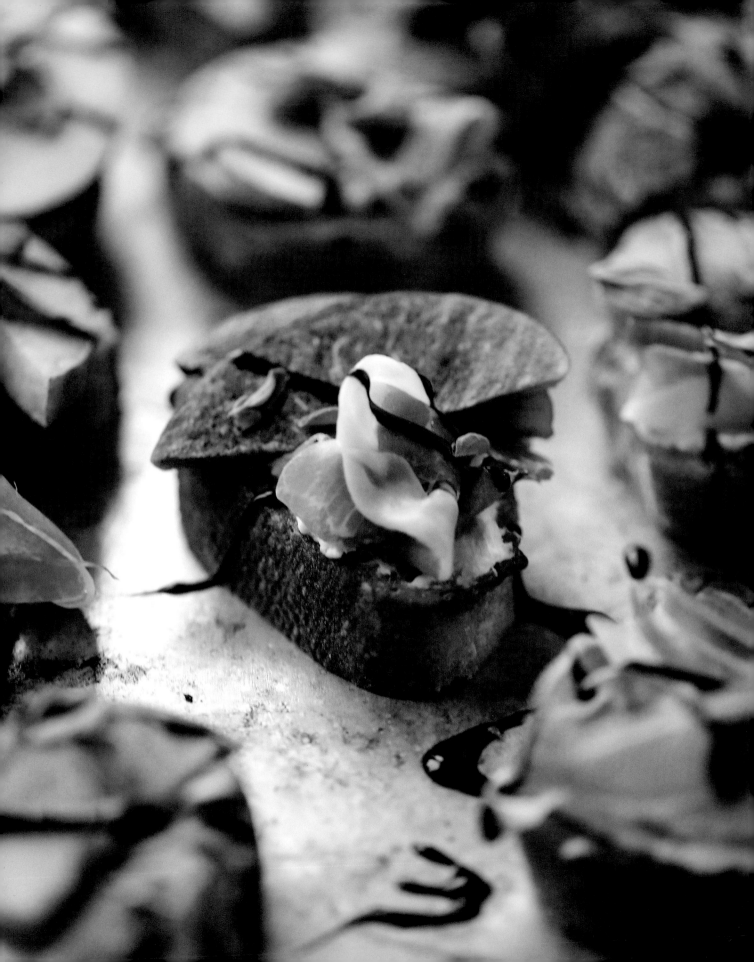

prosciutto, goat cheese, and nectarine crostini

I love giving you options. One of the reasons that I enjoy cooking so much is because I love inspiring others. I enjoy seeing what people can come up with based on a simple recipe I may share. I love to see others' takes on my own creations, and since I'm technically a millennial, and therefore usually bored with all the options in front of me after one use, I take inspiration from what others have tried with my own recipes.

Let's use this as an example. There are a few ways that we can serve these crostini, and what you choose will all depend on your tastebuds and the time you have to prepare it.

We can use an untoasted sourdough baguette, which will be wonderfully chewy. We could toast that baguette in the oven until it's crunchy, or we could even grill it for some smoky flavor.

If the bread is toasted and warm, the cheese will be melty and delightful. If it's sliced, fresh bread? The cheese will be smeared on top in a delicious layer.

We can use the prosciutto as is, or we could crisp it up in a skillet, similar to bacon. It's totally your call.

And finally! The nectarines. The fruit lover inside of me is fine with slicing these fresh. I eat so many slices as I prep the crostini that I usually buy extra. But you could take it a step further and grill your nectarines, so they are warm and caramelly and again . . . a little smoky.

See? It's all in what we love and what we have time to do. This combination of sweet and savory is a winner no matter what. **MAKES 6 TO 8 SERVINGS**

1   sourdough baguette, sliced into rounds

6   ounces goat cheese

8   ounces prosciutto, thinly sliced and torn into pieces

2   nectarines, thinly sliced

Balsamic glaze, for drizzling

Fresh herbs (such as basil, oregano, or parsley), for topping

Spread each bread slice with a smear of the goat cheese. Top each with a piece of prosciutto and 1 or 2 nectarine slices. Drizzle the slices with balsamic glaze and cover with fresh herbs. Serve immediately.

watermelon fruit pizza

Welcome to what I can easily declare as my favorite summer snack of all time. After ice cream, of course.

Guys. This is incredibly refreshing. It is super fun to make. Kids go crazy for it, but even kids who masquerade as adults (such as myself) love it, too.

You can make this big watermelon wedge into whatever the heck you want. Slice a big round circle and cover it in your yogurt of choice. Plain, unflavored, whatever you love will work. Pile on your fruits, which may differ based on the summer months. I love peaches, strawberries, kiwifruit, and blueberries. I like to add a touch of granola and a drizzle of honey or melted almond butter, too. Crushed almonds, pistachios, or cashews add the best crunch. Lime zest is lovely, and if you want to go the savory route? Feta cheese is perfect.

And finally, fresh mint leaves for some fresh flavor. You cannot beat this. I just hope you forgive me for calling it pizza. **MAKES 2 TO 4 SERVINGS**

I large round slice watermelon (about 1" thick)

½ cup vanilla Greek yogurt

1 peach, thinly sliced

¼ cup blueberries

2 tablespoons almond butter, melted

1 tablespoon honey

2 tablespoons sliced almonds, toasted

½ ounce dark chocolate, chopped

1 handful fresh mint, for topping

Place the watermelon round on a large plate or platter. Spread the yogurt all over the round, leaving space at the edges to grab the slices. Add the fruit on top, then drizzle with the almond butter and honey. Sprinkle with the almonds, chocolate, and mint. Serve!

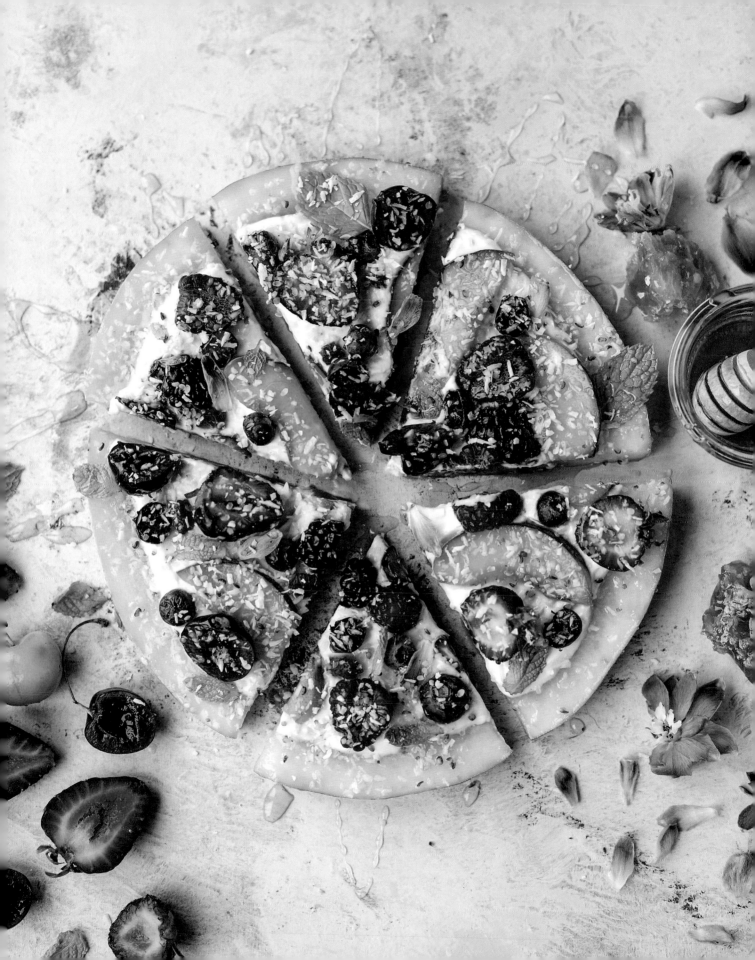

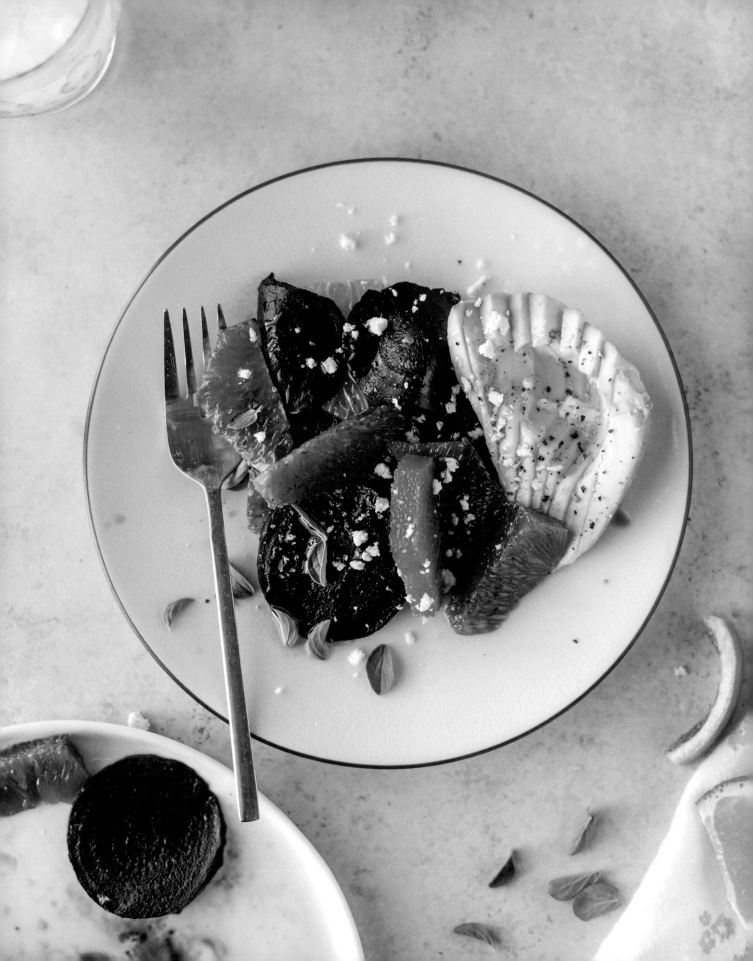

blood orange, avocado, and beet salad

How could you say no to such beautiful, natural colors on your plate? It's impossible. This salad just begs you to make it.

I will admit that I tend to prefer a "heartier" salad on the regular. It's rare that I serve a lettuce-less salad when hosting because most of our family expects and hopes for some sort of "normal" salad, and I aim to freak them out with only one dish per event.

In this case, I make an exception. There is no need for lettuce in this beauty. The flavors mesh together perfectly. The beets are a bit earthy. The blood oranges are tangy and sweet. The avocado is creamy and mild. This satisfies all those tastebud dreams! Plus, it's practically neon.

Prepared beets are so easily found in grocery stores these days that this salad can come together in a matter of minutes. I've included the instructions for roasting the beets below, but if you plan on serving this at a dinner party or on a holiday, I suggest roasting them the day before and sticking 'em in the fridge.

Nature is so beautiful!　**MAKES 2 SERVINGS**

2　red beets, scrubbed

3　tablespoons extra-virgin olive oil, divided

2　blood oranges, segmented

1　avocado, thinly sliced

¼　teaspoon salt

¼　teaspoon ground black pepper

2　ounces goat cheese, crumbled

Juice of 1 lime

1　tablespoon chopped fresh oregano

Preheat the oven to 375°F. Rub the beets with 1 tablespoon of the olive oil and wrap them tightly in foil. Roast them for 60 to 90 minutes, or until they are fork-tender and the skin can be rubbed right off. Slice the beets into pieces.

To assemble the salad, place the beets on a plate or serving platter. Add the orange segments and avocado slices. Season with the salt and pepper. Crumble the goat cheese over top.

Drizzle with the remaining 2 tablespoons olive oil and then spritz with the lime juice. Sprinkle on the oregano. Serve immediately.

chopped kale salad
WITH BLOOD ORANGE VINAIGRETTE

I still surprise myself with my love for kale. In a world where some of the last veggies people get into are kale and Brussels sprouts, both remain favorites for me. I can pass on carrots and celery, but give me all the greens!

Kale in all forms finds its way into my family's diet. We don't mind it in smoothies, as long as it's pureed without little extra green bits. We love kale roasted into kale "chips," and the three of us can easily finish off a baking sheet's worth of them. But the way that we eat kale weekly is in salad form. Once some olive oil or dressing is massaged into chopped kale, the texture is chewy but fabulous. The bitterness is gone, and all the other flavors shine.

If you haven't realized it by now, I'm a bit of a blood orange fanatic. I know that this can pose a problem when we are all craving blood oranges in the late summer and they are nowhere to be found, so just remember that any sort of orange is an easy swap. If it isn't blood orange season, then Cara Caras are next on my list.

Feta cheese is an easy salad favorite, but if that isn't your thing, feel free to switch it up. And don't forget the crunch. I love sunflower seeds here, but any nut or seed that you adore works. **MAKES 2 SERVINGS**

QUICK PICKLED SHALLOTS

½ cup water

⅓ cup apple cider vinegar

1 tablespoon sugar

1 teaspoon salt

2 shallots, thinly sliced

BLOOD ORANGE VINAIGRETTE

⅓ cup blood orange juice

¼ cup golden balsamic vinegar

1 clove garlic, grated or pressed

¼ teaspoon salt

¼ teaspoon ground black pepper

⅓ cup olive oil

CHOPPED KALE SALAD

4 cups chopped curly green kale

1 tablespoon olive oil

2 blood oranges, segmented and chopped

1 avocado, chopped

2 ounces feta cheese, crumbled

2 tablespoons sunflower seeds

TO MAKE THE QUICK PICKLED SHALLOTS

In a small bowl, whisk together the water, vinegar, sugar, and salt. Place the shallots in a jar or container and pour the vinegar mixture over top. Let sit at room temperature for 20 to 30 minutes before using—or store in the fridge for about a week! These can easily be made ahead of time.

TO MAKE THE BLOOD ORANGE VINAIGRETTE

In a small bowl, whisk together the orange juice, vinegar, garlic, salt, and pepper. Slowly stream in the olive oil while whisking until the dressing is emulsified. This stores great in the fridge for 3 to 4 days.

TO MAKE THE CHOPPED KALE SALAD

In a large bowl, combine the kale with the olive oil and massage it with your hands for a few minutes, making sure to get all the pieces coated. Let the kale sit for 5 minutes.

Add in the oranges, avocado, some of the pickled shallots, and the feta. Drizzle with the vinaigrette and toss. Sprinkle with the sunflower seeds. Serve with more vinaigrette on the side.

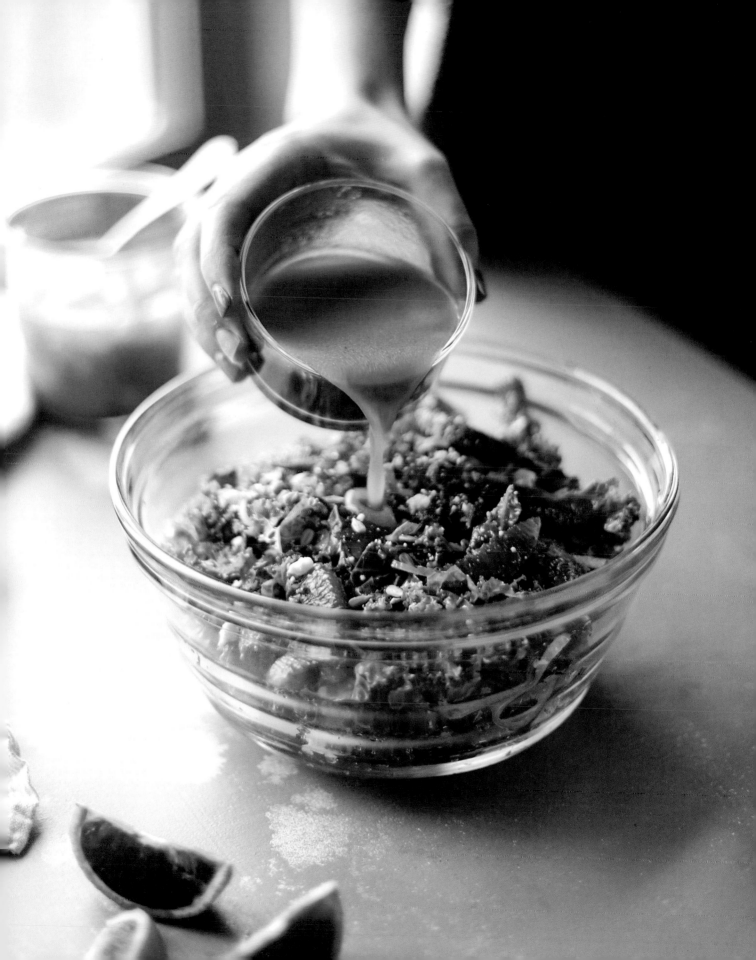

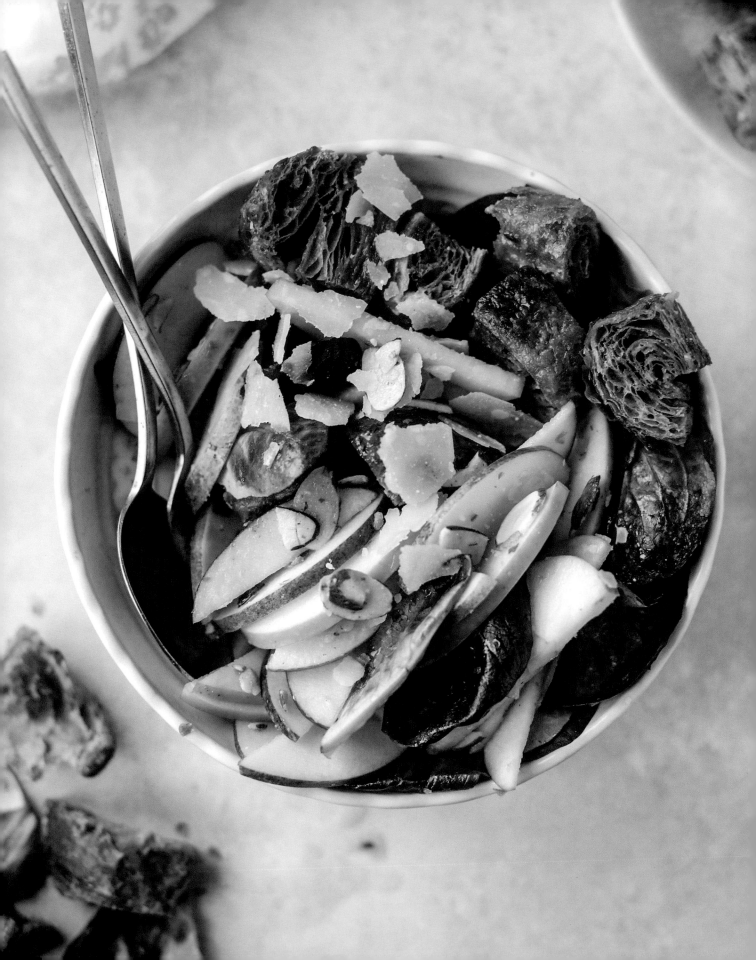

apple croissant panzanella salad

Bread in salad changed the game for me. And no, we aren't talking croutons. When I came across my first panzanella salad recipe, I knew that I could finally become a salad lover. Gone were the days of chopped iceberg, hard carrots, tiny black olive rings, and flavorless tomatoes. Salads with tons of flavor and texture could be a thing. And a thing that I so thoroughly enjoyed.

The difference between panzanella salads and simple croutons is that unlike croutons, where the cubes are a simple topping, toasted bread pieces are a major part of the salad and doused in dressing, where the flavor hides like a bomb. The texture is lovely! The taste is even better.

In what I determined was a brilliant stroke of genius, I decided to use croissants in said bread salad. Croissants. Oh yes. In fact, I even used whole grain croissants that I can find at a local bakery, which just makes me feel better about life in general. All that butter, man . . . it's good.

This fall-inspired salad also comes complete with juicy apples, creamy Brie cheese, and sliced almonds. And an apple cider and cinnamon vinaigrette. My life is complete. MAKES 2 TO 4 SERVINGS

4   croissants, cut into cubes

6   cups butter lettuce

Pinch of salt and ground black pepper

1   green apple, thinly sliced

2   Gala or Fuji apples, thinly sliced

3   ounces Brie cheese, cut into pieces

2   ounces Parmesan cheese, shaved

3   tablespoons sliced almonds

APPLE CIDER CINNAMON
VINAIGRETTE

¼   cup apple cider vinegar

2   tablespoons apple cider

1   tablespoon honey

2   cloves garlic, finely minced or pressed

¼   teaspoon salt

¼   teaspoon ground black pepper

⅛   teaspoon ground cinnamon

½   cup extra virgin olive oil

Preheat the oven to 350°F. Place the croissant cubes on a baking sheet. Bake for 10 to 15 minutes, tossing once or twice, or until lightly toasted and golden. Let cool completely.

Chop the lettuce into pieces and place in a large bowl. Toss it with a pinch of salt and pepper. Add the croissant cubes, apples, Brie, Parmesan, and almonds. Toss together.

TO MAKE THE APPLE CIDER CINNAMON VINAIGRETTE
In a small bowl, whisk together the vinegar, apple cider, honey, garlic, salt, pepper, and cinnamon. Stream in the olive oil while whisking until the dressing emulsifies. (This dressing stays great in the fridge for about a week!)

Drizzle the dressing over the salad, toss, and serve.

bacon, blue cheese, and shrimp chopped salad

Why are chopped salads so satisfying to eat? It must be because we truly get a taste of each ingredient in almost every bite, right? There is no slicing and serving or frustration while attempting to cut your lettuce before eating. Everything is cut up into bite-size pieces right in your little bowl.

It wouldn't be a stretch to say that this is one of my favorite recipes in the entire book. Yes, I might be the queen of favorites (how could I ever choose just 1?), but with one bite, you'll understand. This salad is quintessential summer.

The flavor is unreal. The bacon is fried, and the shrimp and garlic are subsequently cooked in the bacon grease. The butter lettuce, corn, and tomatoes lend a fresh feel to the otherwise hearty salad, and there isn't one thing that's missing here in flavor town. Except maybe your Watermelon Michelada (page 241) on the side. **MAKES 2 TO 4 SERVINGS**

8 slices bacon, chopped

1 pound raw shrimp, peeled and deveined

4 cloves garlic, minced

12 ounces butter lettuce, chopped

½ cup grilled or roasted corn (page 131)

4 ounces blue cheese, crumbled

½ pint cherry tomatoes, halved

1 avocado, chopped

Heat a large skillet over medium heat and add the bacon. Cook until crispy and the fat is rendered. With a slotted spoon, transfer the bacon to a paper towel–lined plate to drain any excess grease. Remove all but 2 tablespoons of the bacon grease from the skillet.

Add the shrimp and garlic to the skillet. Cook for 2 to 3 minutes, or until the shrimp are opaque. Remove the shrimp from the skillet and chop into pieces.

To assemble the salad, in a large bowl, toss the lettuce, bacon, shrimp, corn, blue cheese, tomatoes, and avocado together. Serve immediately.

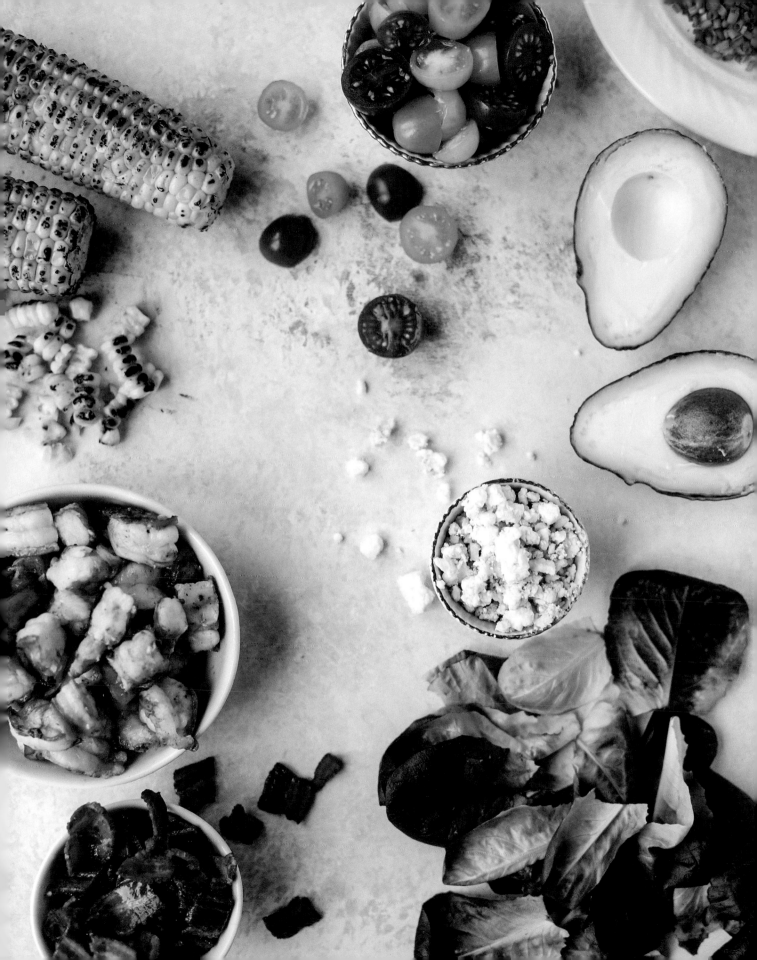

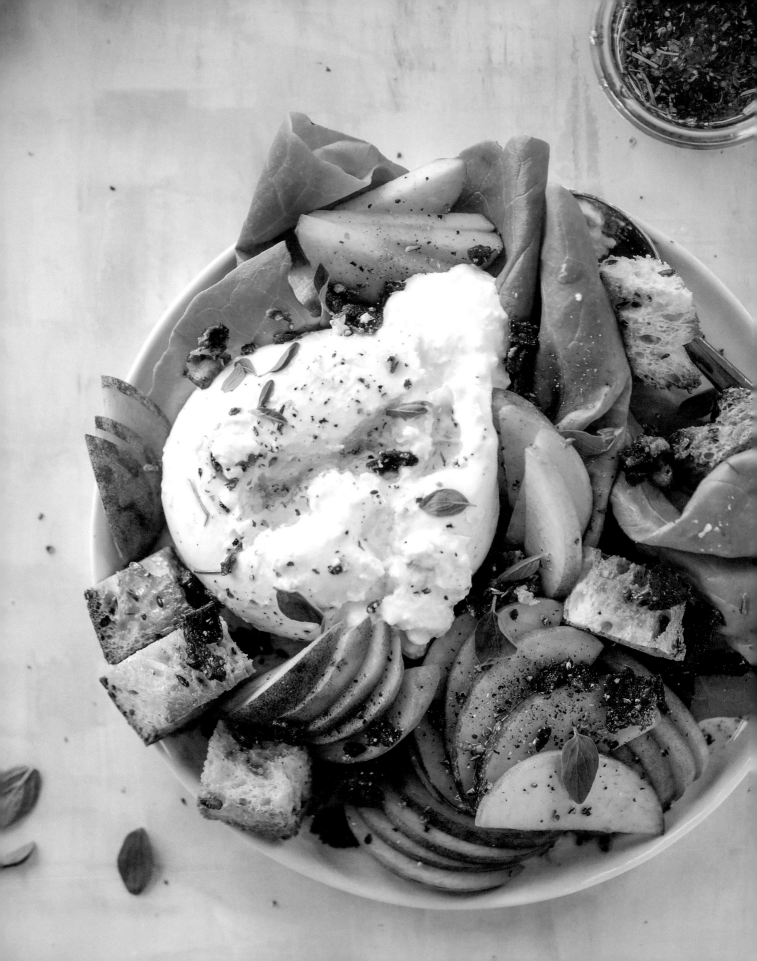

peach panzanella salad with bacon and burrata

WITH HOUSE VINAIGRETTE

One of the things that I'm known for in our family is my constant combination of the sweet and the savory. When I was a young girl, my parents probably would have told you that I had a major sweet tooth, and well . . . it wasn't a lie.

As I've grown up, I've learned to appreciate and even crave savory flavors more than I once did. In fact, I couldn't even tell you right now if I'm more of a sweet or savory person. It all totally depends on my mood, the situation that we're in, what else I've consumed that day, and how I'm feeling.

Therefore, I almost always like to have the option of both. Options are what makes life go 'round! And in this case, I love to pair fresh peaches with bacon. Or fresh peaches with cheese. Or fresh peaches with bacon and cheese!

Are you sensing a trend here? I can barely serve a salad unless it contains bacon. My apologies.

Traditional sourdough works best in this recipe because it doesn't take away from the flavorful peach and powerful smokiness of the bacon. As a dressing, a classic vinaigrette is my favorite—in fact, this is a take on my own personal "house dressing" that we whisk up constantly. I like to think that it can go with any and all salads, but that will of course depend on your personal preference.

MAKES 2 TO 4 SERVINGS

3   cups sourdough bread cubes

2   peaches, thinly sliced

1   handful fresh butter lettuce leaves

1   ball (8 ounces) burrata cheese

3   slices bacon, cooked and crumbled

HOUSE VINAIGRETTE

¼   cup golden balsamic vinegar

1   tablespoon honey

1   teaspoon Dijon mustard

2   cloves garlic, finely minced or pressed

¼   teaspoon salt

¼   teaspoon ground black pepper

½   teaspoon crushed red-pepper flakes

½   cup extra-virgin olive oil

To assemble the salad, place the bread, peach slices, and lettuce on a plate. Top with the burrata, pull it apart, and sprinkle on the bacon.

TO MAKE THE HOUSE VINAIGRETTE

In a bowl, whisk together the vinegar, honey, mustard, garlic, salt, black pepper, and red-pepper flakes. Stream in the olive oil while whisking until the dressing emulsifies. (This dressing stays great in the fridge for about a week!)

Drizzle the dressing over the salad, toss, and serve.

meatball salad

Ohhh yes. I went there. I threw a meatball in a salad. In this case . . . a couple of meatballs!

One of my local restaurants has a meatball salad on their menu. It may sound totally weird, but paired with some creamy ricotta on the side and fresh bread, it makes for a great lunch or even a light dinner.

The key is using hearty greens, like baby spinach, plus some cherry tomatoes for sweetness and, of course, a bit of Parmesan.

I have never been a meatball lover, but they are one of Eddie's favorite meals, so they are often in the rotation at home. Even he goes crazy over this salad. It's a great weeknight meal when you don't feel like adding in a large bowl of pasta or a heavy white roll to make meatball subs. MAKES 2 TO 4 SERVINGS

MEATBALLS

½ pound lean ground beef

1 egg

2 tablespoons grated Romano cheese

1 clove garlic, minced

½ teaspoon dried basil

½ teaspoon dried parsley

¼ teaspoon salt

¼ teaspoon ground black pepper

3 tablespoons panko bread crumbs

1 tablespoon olive oil

⅔ cup marinara sauce

SALAD

6 cups baby spinach

2 cups spring greens

1 cup chopped cherry tomatoes

3 ounces Parmesan cheese, shaved

Ricotta, for serving (optional)

1 tablespoon finely grated Parmesan cheese

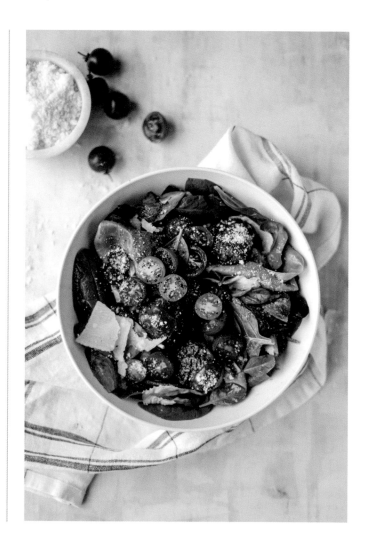

PARMESAN BASIL VINAIGRETTE

¼ cup red wine vinegar

3 tablespoons finely grated Parmesan cheese

1 teaspoon honey

1 teaspoon Dijon mustard

2 cloves garlic, finely minced or pressed

½ teaspoon dried basil

¼ teaspoon salt

¼ teaspoon ground black pepper

¼ teaspoon crushed red-pepper flakes

½ cup extra-virgin olive oil

TO MAKE THE MEATBALLS

In a large bowl, combine the ground beef, egg, Romano, garlic, basil, parsley, salt, pepper, and bread crumbs. Mix, gently tossing a few times with your hands. Don't overmix, which will result in tough meatballs! Form the mixture into 6 or 8 meatballs, depending on what size you would like in your salad.

In a large skillet, heat the olive oil over medium heat. Cook the meatballs on all sides, turning them over often, for 10 minutes, or until the outsides are browned and the insides are no longer pink. You can cover the skillet to help the process along. Add in the marinara sauce and reduce the heat to low. Cover the skillet and cook for 10 minutes.

TO ASSEMBLE THE SALAD

In a large bowl, combine the spinach and greens. Top with the meatballs and add the tomatoes and shaved Parmesan. Add a scoop of ricotta on the side, if you wish.

TO MAKE THE PARMESAN BASIL VINAIGRETTE

In a small bowl, whisk together the vinegar, Parmesan, honey, mustard, garlic, basil, salt, black pepper, and red-pepper flakes. Stream in the olive oil while whisking until the dressing emulsifies. (This dressing stays great in the fridge for about a week!)

Drizzle the dressing over the salad and sprinkle on the grated Parmesan. Serve immediately.

charred pineapple salad

We may be pushing the limit here calling this a salad, but smoky charred pineapple on a bed of butter lettuce is my new salad favorite.

This is definitely a lighter option that can stand on its own, as there are only a few other dishes that I'd serve after this. One is any sort of whitefish, something citrusy or light. A seafood dish like scallops or maybe some simple grilled chicken would be a few other options, but I love when this salad stands out by itself.

Of course, you can always skip the greens if you really want to. You don't have to convince me. Charred pineapple topped with chopped, roasted cashews does sound pretty fantastic. MAKES 2 SERVINGS

1 pineapple, peeled and cut into slices or wedges

1 tablespoon honey

1 tablespoon grapeseed, canola, or vegetable oil

Pinch of sea salt

4 cups butter lettuce, torn

2 kiwifruit, peeled and sliced

1 avocado, thinly sliced

¼ red onion, thinly sliced

¼ cup chopped roasted, salted cashews

Salt and ground black pepper

PINEAPPLE VINAIGRETTE

¼ cup red wine vinegar

3 tablespoons pineapple juice

1 teaspoon honey

1 clove garlic, finely minced or pressed

¼ teaspoon salt

¼ teaspoon ground black pepper

½ cup extra-virgin olive oil

Preheat the grill to the highest setting. Drizzle the pineapple on both sides with the honey and oil. Grill the pineapple for 4 to 6 minutes, turning once, or until golden and charred on both sides. Transfer the pineapple to a plate. Season with the salt. (Alternately, you can cook the pineapple in a skillet over medium-high heat until it caramelizes.)

To assemble the salad, place the butter lettuce on a plate. Top with the pineapple, kiwifruit, avocado, onion, and cashews. Season with salt and pepper to taste.

TO MAKE THE PINEAPPLE VINAIGRETTE: In a small bowl, whisk together the vinegar, pineapple juice, honey, garlic, salt, and pepper. Stream in the olive oil while whisking until the dressing emulsifies. (This dressing stays great in the fridge for about a week!)

Drizzle the salad with the dressing and serve.

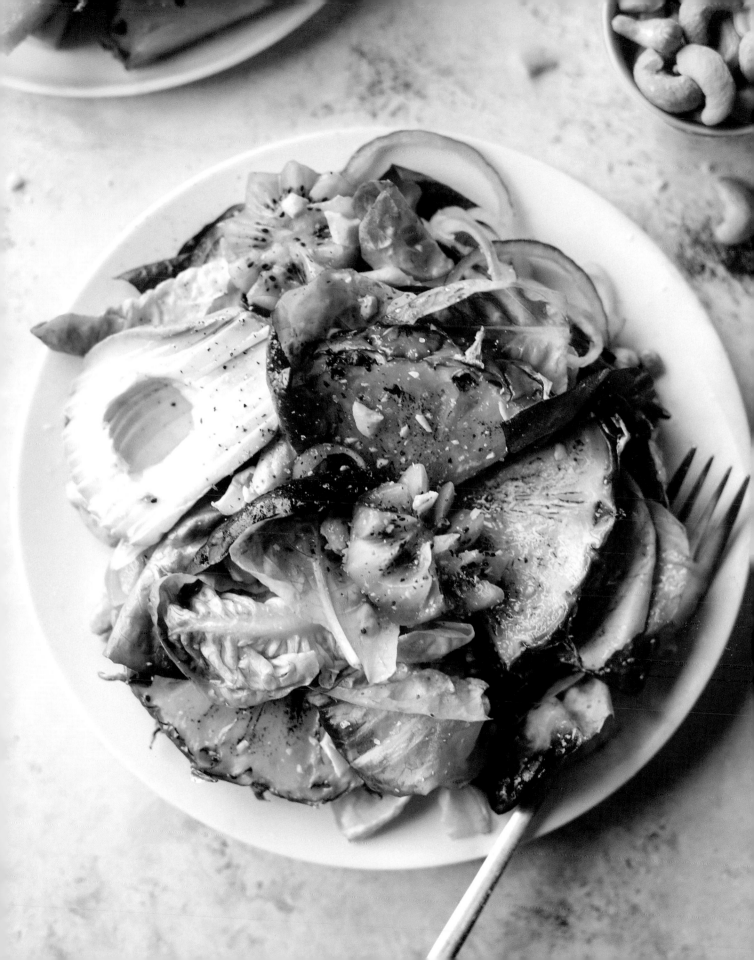

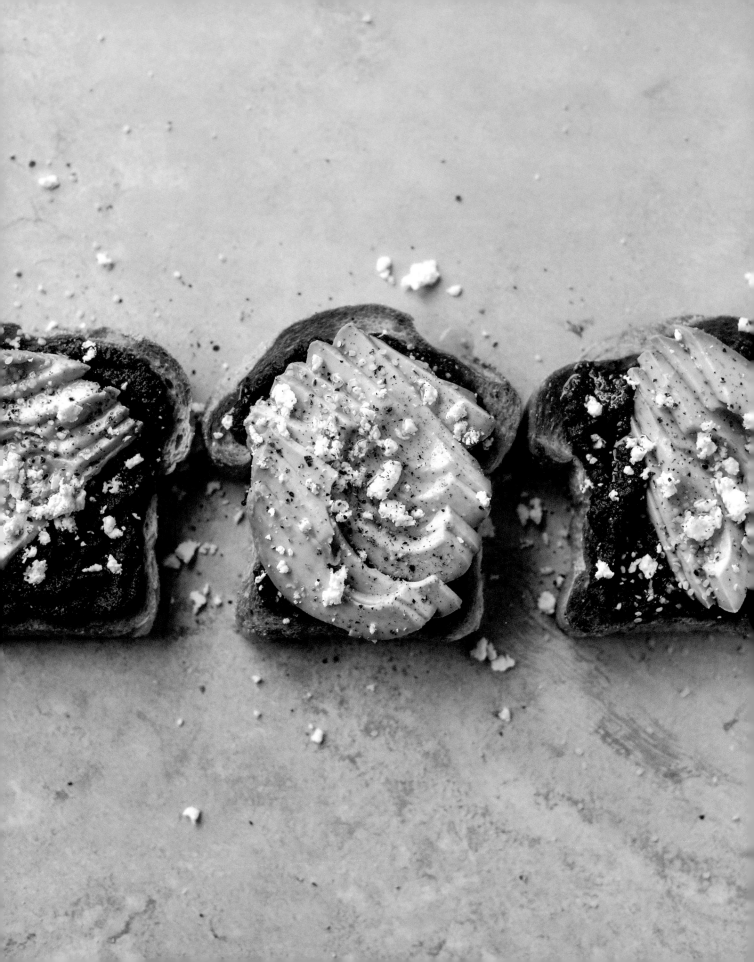

hot pink hummus avocado toast

Say hello to the prettiest toast that you just might ever eat! I can hardly stand the beauty here on a slice of bread. The colors make me so happy. Food already makes me happy, but when it's naturally so stunning? I melt into a puddle of love.

I first had toast like this on a retreat in Park City, Utah. I was initially drawn to the appearance, my inner 13-year-old Lisa Frank–loving heart absolutely losing it over the green and the pink, but once I took a bite, the flavor sold me.

This is such a lovely addition to your regular avocado toast—not to mention, it's more satisfying. It's fun to eat this for lunch every day, but I really love serving these toasts for a girls' brunch or holiday breakfast because of their beautiful color. No one can resist them! **MAKES 4 SERVINGS**

4   slices bread (your favorite
    variety), toasted

½   cup Hot Pink Hummus (page 57)

2   avocados, thinly sliced

¼   teaspoon salt

¼   teaspoon ground black pepper

1   tablespoon extra-virgin olive oil

3   ounces goat cheese, crumbled

Spread each slice of toast liberally with the hummus. Top each slice with one-quarter of the avocado. Season with the salt and pepper, then drizzle on the olive oil. Cover with the goat cheese and serve. Perfect!

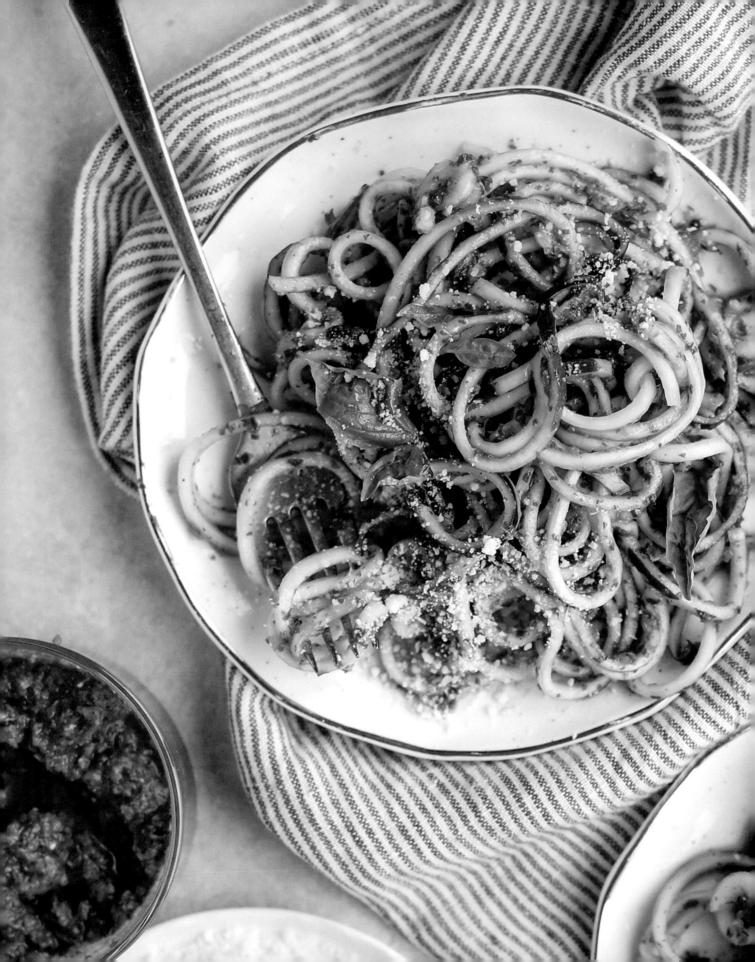

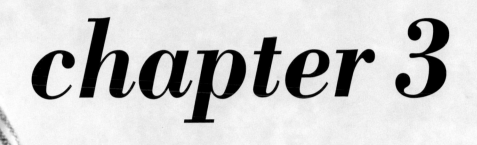

chapter 3

main meals for your main self

All of the dishes for dinner that
we want to eat all the time

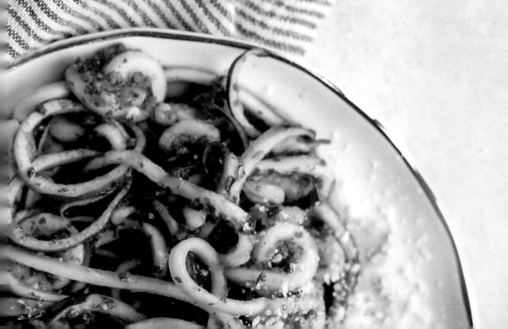

THE RECIPES IN THIS CHAPTER ARE WHAT I like to call my bread and butter. Sure, they might not contain bread. Or butter. But they are the recipes that I find myself pulling together most often for friends and family. They are the recipes that allow us to *finally* sit down together around the table.

Or should I say, stand around the kitchen island and chat? What is it about everyone gathering in the kitchen? It's fabulous and it's the center of our home. But half the time, I have to force everyone to sit down around the table. Fortunately, pretty décor goes a long way!

Even if breakfast and brunch contain the foods that I love the most, it's rare that we entertain at that time of day, unless it's a holiday. Our gatherings are more spontaneous and weekend-based, and they tend to happen in the late afternoons or evenings. And while you will never see me turn down breakfast for dinner (only the best meal to ever exist!), it's not something I cook up for guests on the fly.

I was raised with dinner as the largest, family-based meal in our home. Sure, studies today may show that it's technically healthier to have a large breakfast and a smaller dinner, but with timing and busy schedules, evenings are the most convenient time for my family to be together, or if we have guests, it's the best time for me to see my girlfriends and for

us to cook and eat well into the night. There is just something so special to me about having friends and family around the table, well after the meal is over, laughing and talking until long after the sun goes down.

To share the most personal peek into my cooking, this chapter is broken into two parts. First, there are meals you would make on Monday, Tuesday, and Wednesday. You know—when you're feeling your healthiest self and super motivated in the kitchen to create balanced meals.

The second half of the chapter is perhaps my favorite section in the whole book because it's all about comfort food. It's where my favorite taco recipes live, as well as the soups that I love to share, and some delicious compound butters for every season. These are the recipes that make Thursdays, Fridays, and the weekends taste so much better.

I hope these recipes bring the same sort of joy to your dinner table!

meals for monday, tuesday, and wednesday: things we eat when we want to feel balanced

Behold! This section details all of my favorite healthier and simpler recipes, including entrées and side dishes.

baked whitefish
WITH OLIVES AND TOMATOES

This recipe comes from close family friends of mine. When I was first entertaining new recipe ideas for this book a few summers ago, they shared the delicious dinner they had made the night before. It was simple, healthy, and flavorful. They raved about it and said we had to go home and try it.

We love to eat seafood, but I often get in a rut when it comes to preparation. My memories of flaky whitefish are strong and vivid, from eating it freshly caught in Northern Michigan while vacationing with my family every summer. My dad would catch small fish off the dock in front of our condo, but only one or two of them, and fry them up in a beer batter for us just so we could have a taste. It was fabulous.

This dish could not be simpler to prepare—and it's easy enough to make for a crowd! Prepping the parchment packets takes no time at all, especially if you have your topping ingredients ready to go. Get the freshest fish that you can—even salmon will work, though I love to pick up flounder, halibut, or even cod here in Pennsylvania. **MAKES 2 SERVINGS**

12 ounces whitefish or other mild fish, such as flounder or halibut

¼ teaspoon salt

¼ teaspoon ground black pepper

2 tablespoons olive oil

2 tablespoons chopped kalamata olives

1 cup cherry tomatoes

Juice of 1 lemon

1 tablespoon capers

Preheat the oven to 375°F.

Place the fish in the middle of a piece of parchment paper. Sprinkle with the salt and pepper. Drizzle with the olive oil, then top with the olives, tomatoes, lemon juice, and capers. Fold the parchment up around the fish and secure with a piece of tape if needed. Place the parchment on a baking sheet.

Bake for 15 to 20 minutes, or until the fish flakes easily with a fork. Serve immediately with an extra wedge of lemon. I really love this with rice or Winter Rice Bowls (page 104).

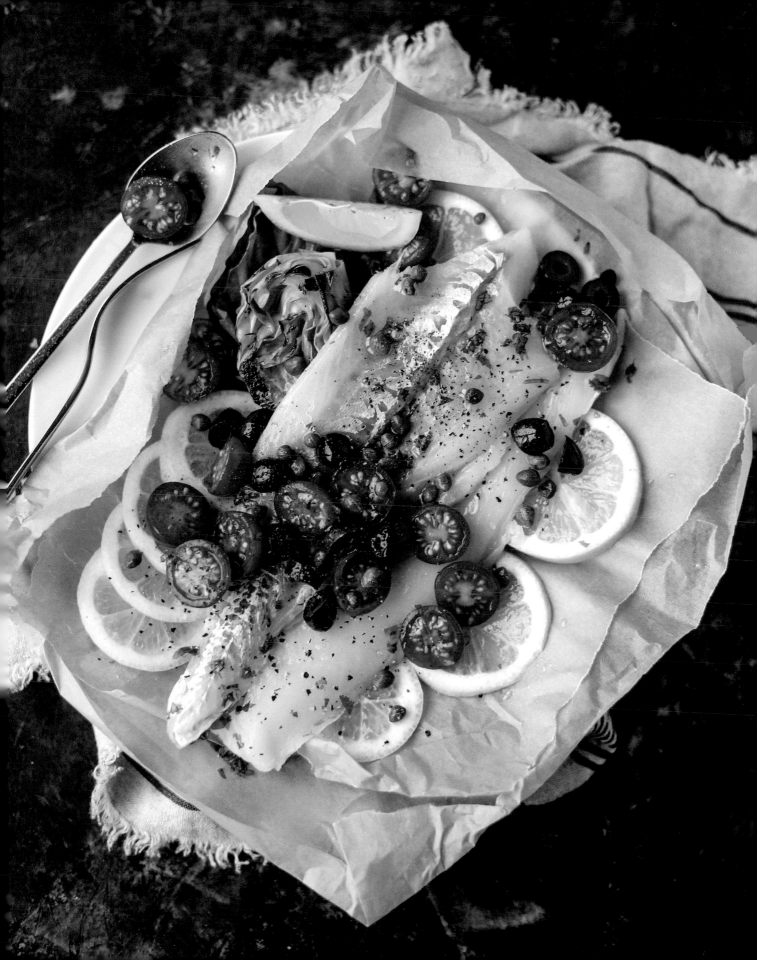

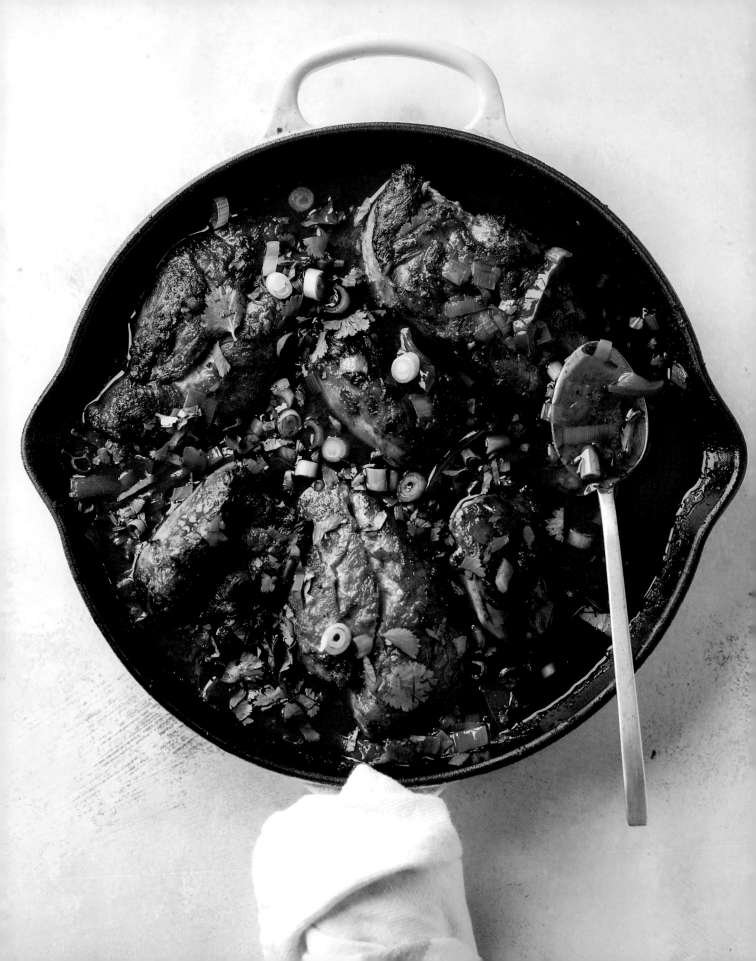

coconut curry braised chicken skillet

One of the newer comfort foods that I was introduced to later in life is coconut curry sauce and rice. It doesn't matter what is in the coconut curry—vegetables, pineapple, shrimp, chicken—I could eat a bowl of it alone. So decadent and flavorful.

This is my take on a simpler weeknight chicken skillet braised in coconut curry. The idea of the skillet chicken works better for us than a soupy pot of curry with chicken chunks, which isn't Eddie's favorite. He likes the flavor, but he'd rather have a whole chicken breast and eat it as he chooses.

Here, we both get what we love. There is certainly enough sauce to drizzle over rice or potatoes. Heck, it even works on salad. But there is also enough chicken that you can slice it and use it for leftovers without the curry overpowering everything. I like to use a mix of chicken breasts and boneless, skinless thighs, but you can use whatever you love here. It's the new comfort food!

P.S. Freshly sliced sourdough bread makes for an excellent sauce dipper. **MAKES 4 SERVINGS**

1½ pounds boneless, skinless chicken thighs or breasts (or both!)

½ teaspoon salt

½ teaspoon ground black pepper

2 tablespoons coconut oil

1 red bell pepper, thinly sliced

1 leek, thinly sliced

2 cloves garlic, minced

½ teaspoon grated fresh ginger

2 tablespoons red curry paste

1 can (14 ounces) full-fat coconut milk

3 tablespoons torn fresh cilantro

Rice, for serving (optional)

Sliced sourdough bread, for serving (optional)

Preheat the oven to 375°F. Season the chicken with the salt and black pepper.

In a large ovenproof skillet, melt the coconut oil over medium-high heat. Add the chicken and sear on both sides until deeply golden brown. Transfer to a plate.

Reduce the heat to medium low. Add the bell pepper, leek, garlic, and ginger. Stir to combine. Cook for 2 minutes, or until slightly softened. Stir in the curry paste. Cook for 5 minutes, stirring often. Slowly pour in the coconut milk while stirring to combine. Return the chicken to the skillet.

Place the skillet in the oven and cook for 25 minutes, or until a thermometer inserted in the thickest portion of the chicken registers 165°F and the juices run clear. Top with the cilantro. Serve with rice and fresh sourdough bread for mopping up the sauce, if desired.

fall-spiced pesto

Pesto is a staple in our freezer. I say in "our freezer" because every September, I hoard the rest of my fresh basil like a freak and make a giant batch of basil pesto to store all winter long. It's a nice taste of summer, even in the coldest months.

My use for pesto doesn't stop with pasta. Sure, I often toss hot pasta with it because it's a surefire way to add perfect flavor, but I also love to add it to soups, salad dressings, sauces, and even butter.

Given my love for all things autumn, a fall-spiced pesto has played out in my mind for years. Instead of basil, this version has arugula, along with pumpkin puree, toasted pepitas (pumpkin seeds), and some spices that just scream October! It's fabulous over bucatini or penne and even better when drizzled over caramelized squash. It's irresistible straight off a spoon, too. **MAKES ABOUT 1½ CUPS**

⅔ cup raw, unsalted pepitas (pumpkin seeds)

3 cups arugula

¼ cup pumpkin puree

½ cup finely grated Parmesan cheese

3 cloves garlic

½ teaspoon salt

½ teaspoon ground black pepper

¼ teaspoon crushed red-pepper flakes

¼ teaspoon freshly grated nutmeg

¼–⅓ cup olive oil

2–3 tablespoons cold water (optional)

Heat a large skillet over medium heat. Add the pepitas and toast until slightly golden and fragrant, stirring often and shaking the pan so they don't burn.

In a food processor, combine the pepitas, arugula, pumpkin, Parmesan, garlic, salt, black pepper, red-pepper flakes, and nutmeg. Pulse until combined and blended. With the processor on, stream in the olive oil, starting with ¼ cup. The mixture will be thick, but you want it to be able to coat hot pasta. You can add more olive oil if you'd like it thinner or if it is too chunky. If desired, blend in cold water to help bring the pesto together.

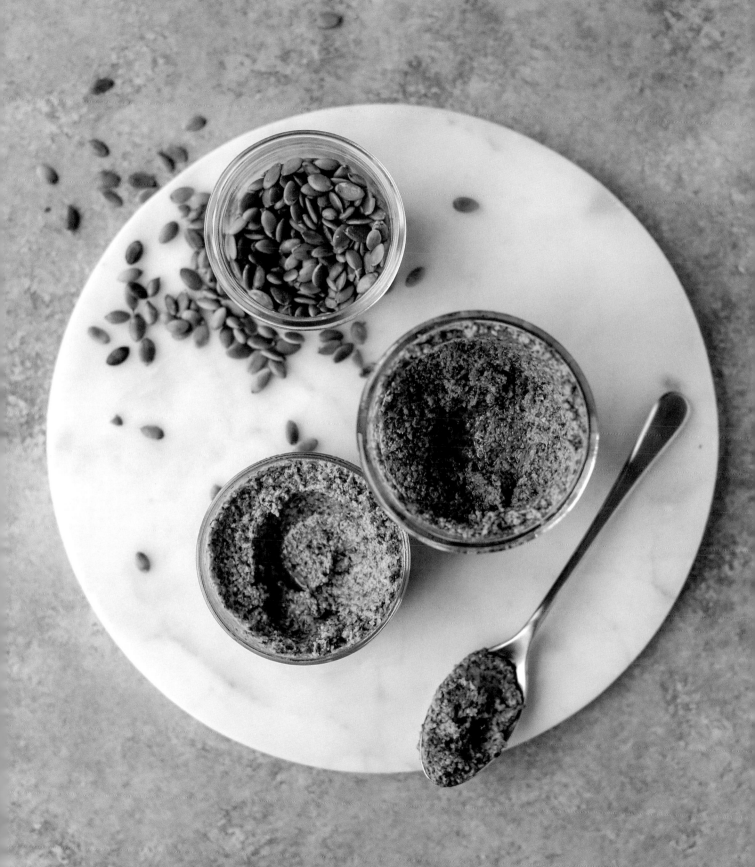

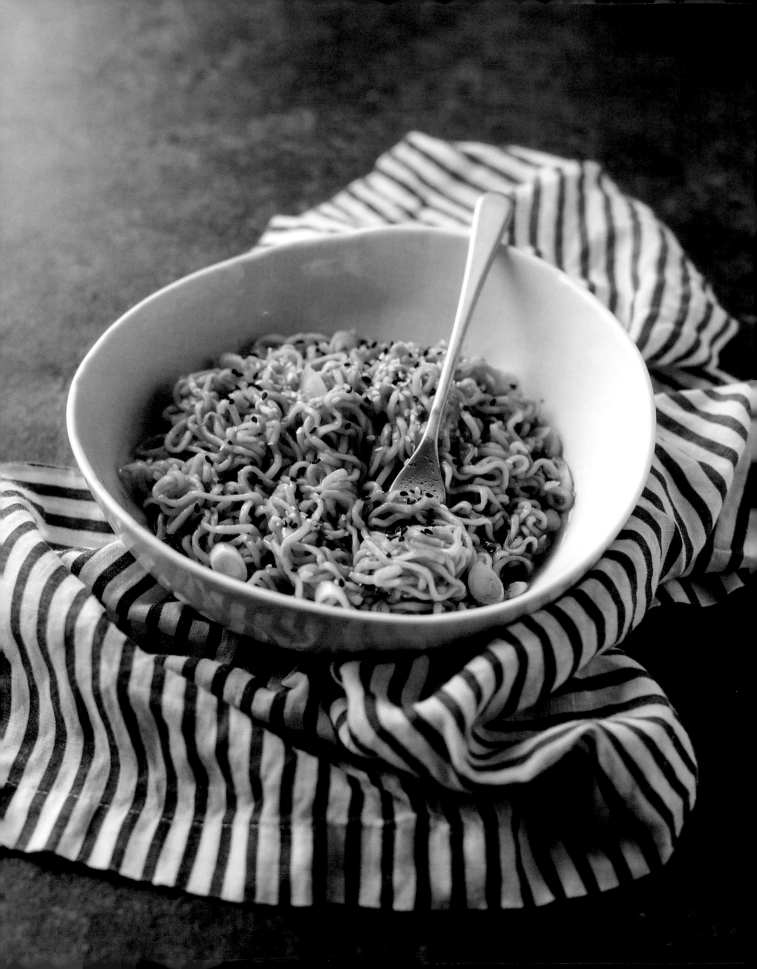

quick sesame ramen noodles

I am definitely a fan of the ramen noodle bowl trend and would gladly eat a bowl weekly if I had the chance. The hot, comforting soup, often packed with veggies, meat, and a soft-cooked egg, is perfect on a chilly night, and what I love most is that it's a complete meal in a bowl.

When I feel like splurging, I will make us the large ramen bowls at home (think pork shoulder, soft-cooked eggs, and greens), but when I'm in a rush, I've started to utilize ramen noodles themselves. In full disclosure, I discard the sodium-laden packet if I buy the packaged noodles from the store. I simply boil the noodles, which takes just a few minutes, and then I add my own flavors in, making this such a quick and easy (and healthier) meal.

Sesame noodles are one of those meals that I make on nights when my husband isn't home or on days when I have the house to myself. It's not a dish that he loves, and he would definitely request chicken or steak with the noodles, while I like them alone. They're fast, comforting, and delicious, and they even make leftovers! I can usually stretch one serving of this over two or three meals, depending on how hungry I am.

In the past, I'd always use soba noodles or even whole wheat spaghetti noodles, but now I love the quick-cooking, delicate, twirly ramen noodles the most. When they're drizzled with toasted sesame oil and thinly sliced scallions, the flavor is so fantastic. You can also add chicken if you need a bit more satiety. Hot or cold, this meal is tops.   MAKES 2 SERVINGS

1   package ramen noodles,
     flavor packet discarded

1   tablespoon coconut oil

2   cloves garlic, minced

½   teaspoon grated fresh ginger

1   tablespoon brown sugar

2   tablespoons low-sodium soy sauce

1   tablespoon rice vinegar

1   teaspoon chili garlic paste

2   tablespoons toasted sesame oil

2   scallions, thinly sliced

Toasted sesame seeds, for sprinkling

Cook the ramen noodles according to the directions on the package.

While the noodles are cooking, in a large skillet, melt the coconut oil over medium-low heat. Stir in the garlic and ginger. Cook for 1 minute, then stir in the sugar, soy sauce, vinegar, and chili garlic paste. Turn off the heat and stir in the sesame oil. Add the cooked noodles to the skillet and toss well to coat.

Serve the noodles with lots of scallions and sesame seeds on top.

charred tomato and bacon fettuccine

Traditional tomato sauce has never been one of my favorite meals, mostly due to the fact that I have zero Italian blood and didn't grow up on "the good stuff." But I do love any version of fresh tomato sauce. And while we can't exactly call this a sauce, when hot pasta is twirled with the burst tomatoes, bacon, and a bunch of Parmesan cheese, it is pure summer heaven. Except you can make it any time of year!

I find that cherry and grape tomatoes are usually available year-round. I avoid the large orange rocks at the grocery store that masquerade as tomatoes; instead, I opt for the small cherry tomatoes that taste like juicy fruit. If they aren't in perfect condition, though, roasting them until they pop and burst is a key way to impart tons of sweet and juicy flavor. **MAKES 2 SERVINGS**

1   pint cherry tomatoes, halved
2   tablespoons olive oil
¼   teaspoon salt
¼   teaspoon ground black pepper
1   pound whole wheat fettuccine
8   slices bacon, chopped
⅓   cup finely grated Parmesan cheese, plus extra for sprinkling
Fresh herbs, such as basil and oregano, for topping

Bring a large pot of salted water to a boil.

Meanwhile, place the tomatoes on a baking sheet and drizzle with the olive oil. Sprinkle with ¼ teaspoon each of the salt and pepper. Roast for 15 to 20 minutes, or until charred and caramelly. This will depend on the size of your tomatoes, so keep an eye on them after 15 minutes. At this point, I like to add the fettuccini to the water to cook.

While the tomatoes are roasting, heat a large skillet over medium heat and add the bacon. Cook until crispy and the fat is rendered. Remove the bacon with a slotted spoon and place it on a paper towel–lined plate to drain any excess grease. Remove all but 2 tablespoons of the bacon grease from the skillet. Add the cooked fettuccine to the skillet and toss it with the bacon grease. Add the Parmesan and toss. Add the charred tomatoes and the bacon and toss to combine.

Serve, topped with extra Parmesan and fresh herbs.

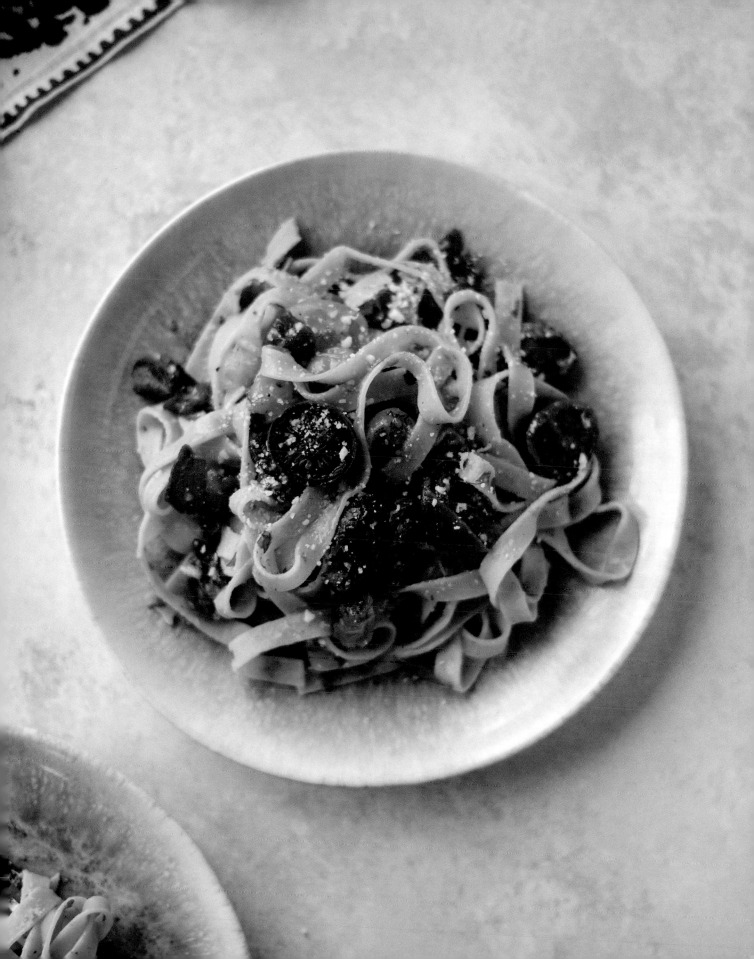

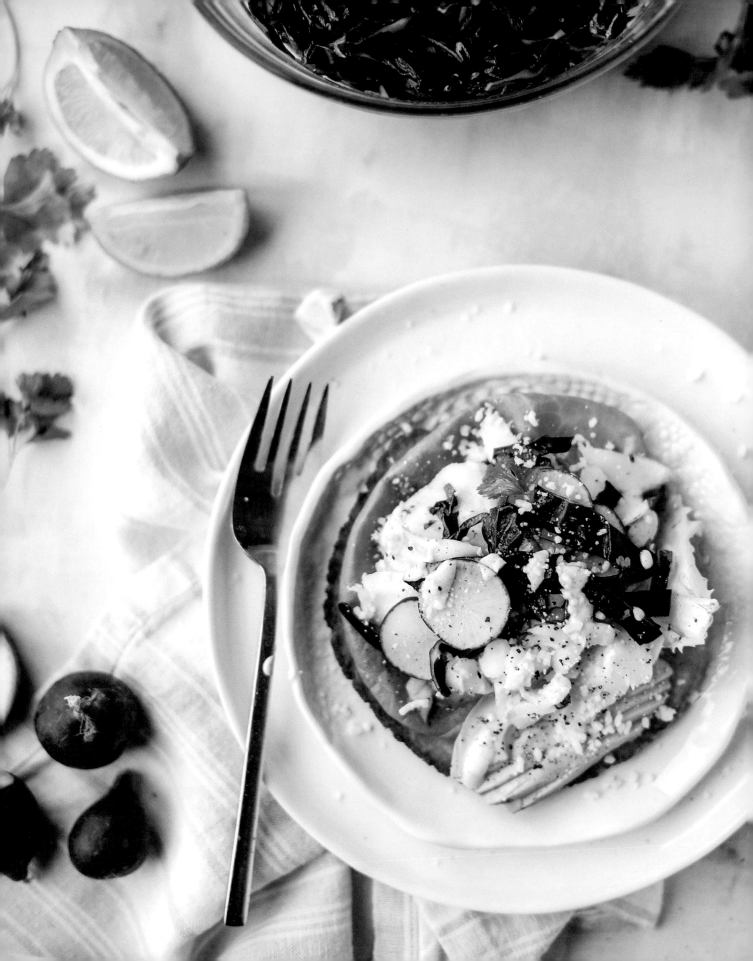

crispy fish tostadas

It wouldn't be an overstatement to say that tacos are a huge part of my life. Tacos make an appearance every single week, at least. Sometimes twice. Even three times! We eat an absurd number of tacos, and I'm not even mad about it. We search out tacos in new cities. We make taco bars at home. We have even had a taco truck at our house for parties!

But. Sometimes I want something . . . a little different. You know? I want that whole taco feel, the flavor, but a little variety in my dinner. Enter tostadas. For me, tostadas are satisfying because I'm all about the texture. And if you load them with veggies, they can even be good for you.

I choose a flaky fish here again because it's so delicate and light. Butter lettuce, avocado, cabbage, and queso fresco top the whole thing off. It's like a little flavor tower just for you.   MAKES 2 TO 4 SERVINGS

FISH

1   cup all-purpose flour
1   teaspoon garlic powder
½   teaspoon onion powder
½   teaspoon smoked paprika
½   teaspoon salt
¼   teaspoon chipotle chili pepper
10 ounces beer (your favorite variety)
¼   cup canola, vegetable, or olive oil
4   fillets (4 ounces each, at least) fresh or thawed cod

TORTILLAS AND TOPPINGS

1–2 tablespoons olive oil
1–2 tablespoons butter
6   corn tortillas
Fresh butter lettuce leaves
Sliced avocado
Sliced red cabbage
Thinly sliced jicama
Thinly sliced radishes
Chopped fresh cilantro
Crumbled queso fresco cheese

TO MAKE THE FISH

In a bowl, whisk together the flour, garlic powder, onion powder, paprika, salt, and chili pepper. Pour in the beer and whisk until a smooth batter forms.

In a large nonstick skillet, heat the oil over medium high heat. Working in batches, dip the fish in the batter and coat it completely, then drop it in the skillet to fry. Let each piece of fish fry for 6 to 8 minutes, turning once, or until golden and crispy and it flakes easily. Gently remove the pieces with a spatula and place them on a paper towel–lined plate to absorb any liquid. Repeat with all the fish, adding more oil if needed.

TO MAKE THE TORTILLAS

Heat a large skillet over medium heat and add about 1 teaspoon of olive oil and butter. Add a tortilla and cook for 4 minutes, turning once, or until golden and crisp on both sides. Remove the tortilla and set it on a paper towel to drain any excess oil and cool and crisp up slightly. Repeat with the remaining olive oil, butter, and tortillas.

Top the tortillas with the butter lettuce and avocado. Add on the fish and top with the cabbage, jicama, radishes, cilantro, and queso fresco.

winter rice bowls

"Bowl" meals seem to be a trend these days. But I've been eating bowl meals for years, as they're such a simple and hearty way to get dinner in and also a fantastic way to use everything in your fridge. Within reason, of course.

This rice bowl serves double duty. It could be a side dish for a dinner party, making just enough to serve smaller portions with an entrée and perhaps a salad. But personally, I love this bowl as a main meal. It's comforting. It's flavorful. It's extremely satisfying with the beans, kale, and sweet potatoes. It is balanced with flavor and even has a little punch from the pomegranate seeds!

The best part: It's topped with crispy shallots for some delicious crunch. Now just try to not eat those all by themselves. Completely addictive! **MAKES 2 SERVINGS**

1 large sweet potato, sliced into ¼" rounds

½ pound Brussels sprouts, stems removed, sliced

3 tablespoons olive oil, divided

½ teaspoon + a pinch salt

½ teaspoon + a pinch ground black pepper

½ teaspoon garlic powder

3 cups chopped green curly kale

2 cups cooked brown jasmine rice

1 can (15 ounces) cannellini beans, rinsed and drained

¼ cup pomegranate arils

CRISPY SHALLOTS

Vegetable or canola oil

2 large shallots, sliced

⅔ cup flour

½ teaspoon salt

½ teaspoon smoked paprika

½ teaspoon garlic powder

¼ teaspoon ground black pepper

Preheat the oven to 400°F. Line 2 baking sheets with parchment paper. On 1 sheet, place the sweet potato rounds. On the other sheet, place the sliced Brussels sprouts. Drizzle both the potato and sprouts with 2 tablespoons of the olive oil. Toss to coat. Sprinkle with ½ teaspoon each of the salt and pepper and the garlic powder.

Roast for 30 minutes, tossing once or twice.

While the vegetables are roasting, toss the kale with the remaining 1 tablespoon olive oil and pinch of salt and pepper. Massage the oil into the kale.

In a large bowl, toss together the rice, cannellini beans, and kale. Add in the Brussels sprouts and potato rounds.

TO MAKE THE CRISPY SHALLOTS

In a medium saucepan, heat about 2" of oil over medium-low heat. You want the oil to reach about 350°F, but after a few minutes of heating, I'll test it out by throwing a shallot slice in. While the oil is heating, in a small bowl, stir together the flour, salt, paprika, garlic powder, and pepper. Dredge the shallot slices in the flour mixture. Add them in batches to the oil. Fry until just golden and crispy, then remove with tongs or a slotted spoon and place on a paper towel to drain excess grease. Repeat with the remaining shallot slices.

Top the rice bowl with the crispy shallots and gently toss. Top with a sprinkling of pomegranate arils and serve.

TIP: To store the crispy shallots, toss them in a glass or plastic container and lightly tent with foil. They are best right after they're cooked, but storing them this way gives them a little extra life for leftovers the next day.

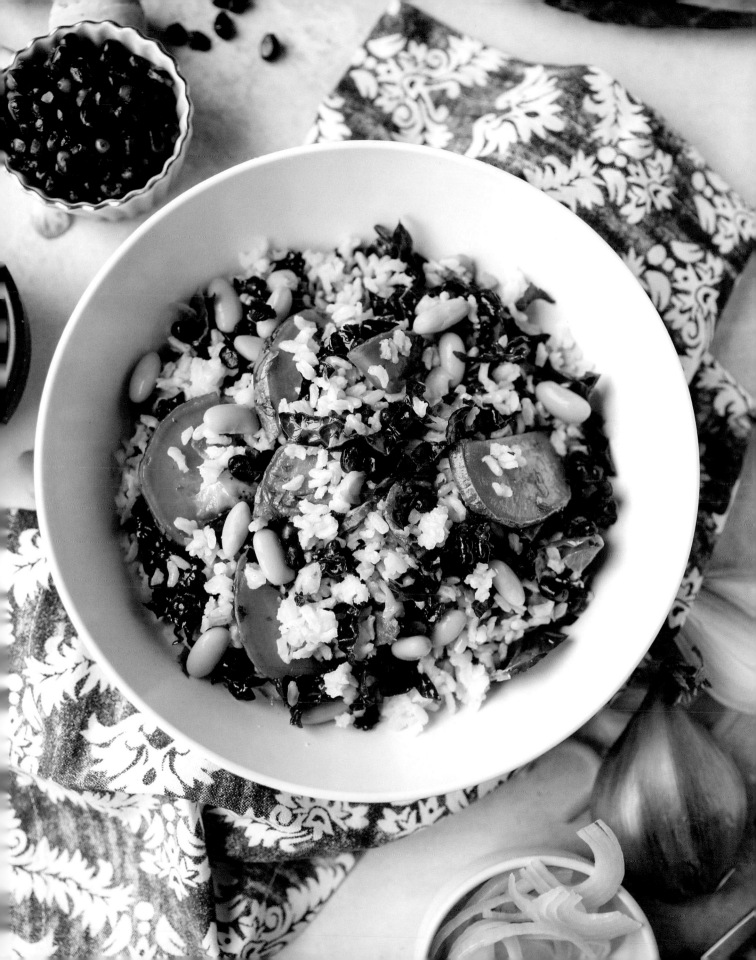

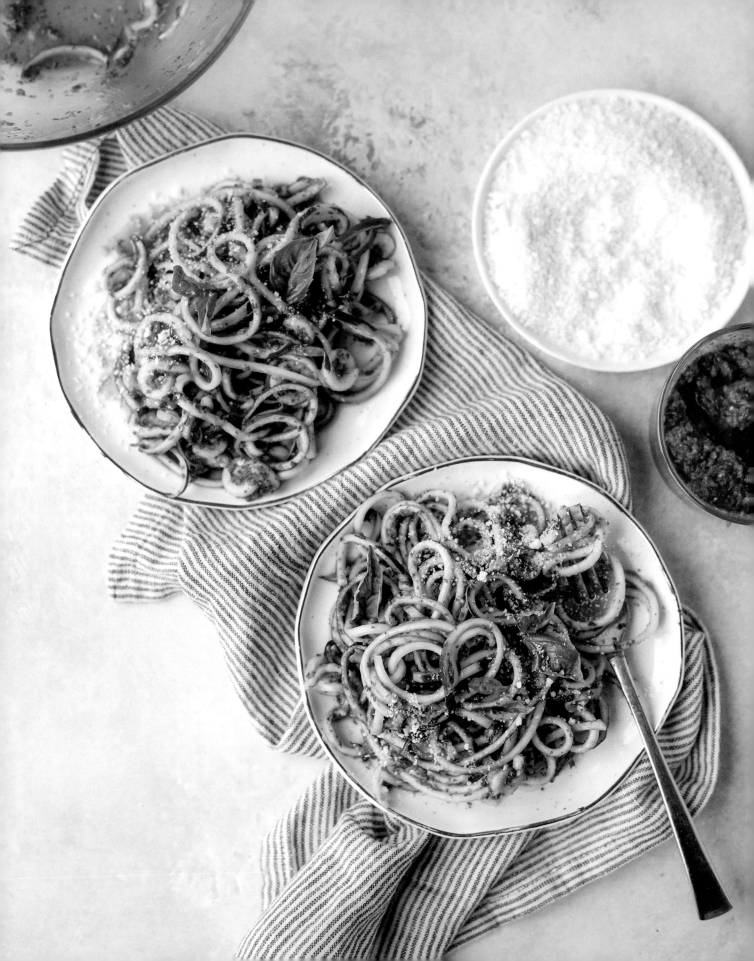

poblano pesto zoodles

Vegetable spiralizers have changed my life. I know that's a dramatic statement, but as someone who has never enjoyed eating vegetables and always struggles with new ways to serve them, I've found that this kitchen tool is a game changer for me. It's also another way to make eating vegetables fun, and Max loves it.

Now, first. I do not think that zucchini noodles (or, as I so lovingly refer to them, zoodles!) taste like traditional pasta noodles. As long as you don't expect them to, they can be enjoyed. I really love them for what they are, though. They take on the flavor of whatever you pair them with. And I even prefer them a bit crunchy, for that whole texture thing I'm into.

This pesto has a little heat from the poblanos and truly reminds me of a summer garden because that summer pepper flavor is strong. I like to toss the warm noodles with lots of pesto and add tons of Parmesan, because cheese will always be my one true love. **MAKES 2 TO 4 SERVINGS**

POBLANO PESTO

2 poblano peppers
½ cup fresh arugula
½ cup fresh basil
¼ cup fresh cilantro
¼ cup grated Parmesan cheese
¼ teaspoon salt
¼ teaspoon ground black pepper
3 tablespoons olive oil

ZOODLES

2 medium zucchini squash
2 tablespoons olive oil
1 tablespoon unsalted butter
2 cloves garlic, minced
Pinch of crushed red-pepper flakes
Juice of ½ lemon
Torn fresh basil, for topping
Grated Parmesan cheese,
    for topping

TO MAKE THE POBLANO PESTO

To roast the poblano peppers, preheat the broiler. Remove the core and seeds from the peppers and slice into pieces. Lay the pieces on a baking sheet. Broil skin side up for about 10 minutes, or until the skins are completely charred and black. Broiling time can vary, so check every 2 minutes or so. Immediately remove the peppers from the oven and use kitchen tongs to quickly place them in a resealable plastic bag. Seal the bag and set aside for 20 to 30 minutes, or until softened.

Remove the peppers from the bag. Peel off and discard the skins. It's okay if a little bit of char remains as it adds to the flavor.

In a food processor, combine the peppers, arugula, basil, cilantro, Parmesan, salt, and black pepper. Process until the mixture is combined, then stream in the olive oil with the processor running.

TO MAKE THE ZOODLES

Spiralize the zucchini into noodles. In a large skillet, heat the olive oil and butter over medium-low heat. Add the garlic and red-pepper flakes and cook for 1 minute, then stir in the lemon juice. Add the zoodles and toss well to coat. Cook, tossing often, for 5 to 6 minutes, or until the zoodles soften slightly. Add in the poblano pesto and toss well. Cook for 5 minutes, or until warmed. Serve immediately with basil and Parmesan.

TIP: If you're just getting into zucchini noodles, try combining them with pasta. Use half regular pasta, half zucchini noodles, and toss. It's a great way to incorporate more veggies and lighten up the meal.

blackened barbecue salmon

WITH MANGO SALSA

We have salmon weekly at our house, if only because it is such a powerhouse of nutrition. I've also perfected the way we love to eat it, and we make it super fast—broiled in the oven until buttery and flaky with a slightly crispy top.

This method allows for so many different flavors to be added. This is a basic, please-everyone type of salmon that is mild enough to enjoy with other side dishes. And it really allows the mango salsa to shine.

Fruit salsas are a staple in our summer meals. Not that this salsa can be made only in the summer, but when the fruit is fresh and sweet, I love using it in a savory component to our main dish. If mango isn't available, you can swap it for pineapple or even peaches. Whatever your little heart desires. **MAKES 2 TO 4 SERVINGS**

MANGO SALSA

1   mango, chopped

½   onion, diced

1   jalapeño chile pepper, seeded and diced

¼   cup chopped fresh cilantro

Grated zest and juice of 1 lime

1½   teaspoons silver tequila

¼   teaspoon salt

BARBECUE SALMON

2   tablespoons firmly packed brown sugar

2   teaspoons smoked paprika

2   teaspoons onion powder

1   teaspoon garlic powder

½   teaspoon chili powder

½   teaspoon salt

¼   teaspoon ground black pepper

2   pounds salmon fillet

2   tablespoons barbecue sauce

LIME BUTTER

4   tablespoons unsalted butter, at room temperature

Grated zest of ½ lime

⅛   teaspoon coarse sea salt

TO MAKE THE MANGO SALSA

In a bowl, combine the mango, onion, jalapeño pepper, cilantro, lime zest and juice, tequila, and salt. Toss well. Let sit at room temperature for 20 minutes before serving.

TO MAKE THE BARBECUE SALMON

Preheat the broiler to high and set the oven rack about 6" below it. In a small bowl, whisk together the sugar, paprika, onion powder, garlic powder, chili powder, salt, and pepper. Rub the mixture all over the salmon fillet. Brush with the barbecue sauce.

Broil the salmon for 6 to 8 minutes, or until just opaque and flaky.

TO MAKE THE LIME BUTTER

In a bowl, stir together the butter, lime zest, and salt until combined.

While the salmon is still hot, pat the lime butter over top and let it melt. Top with the mango salsa and serve.

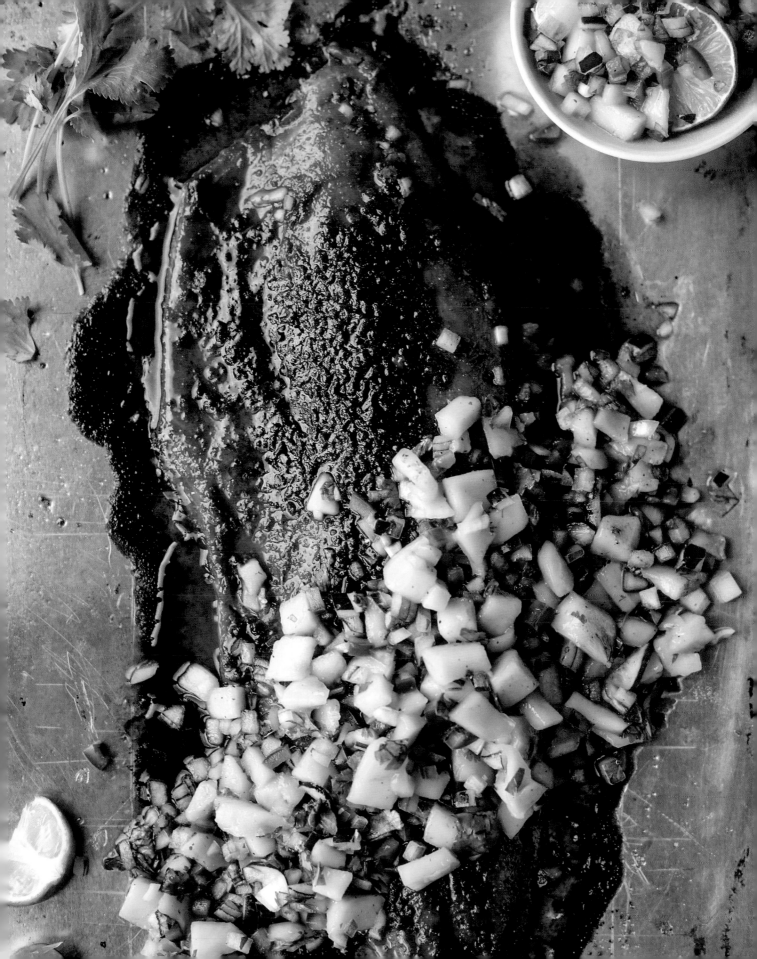

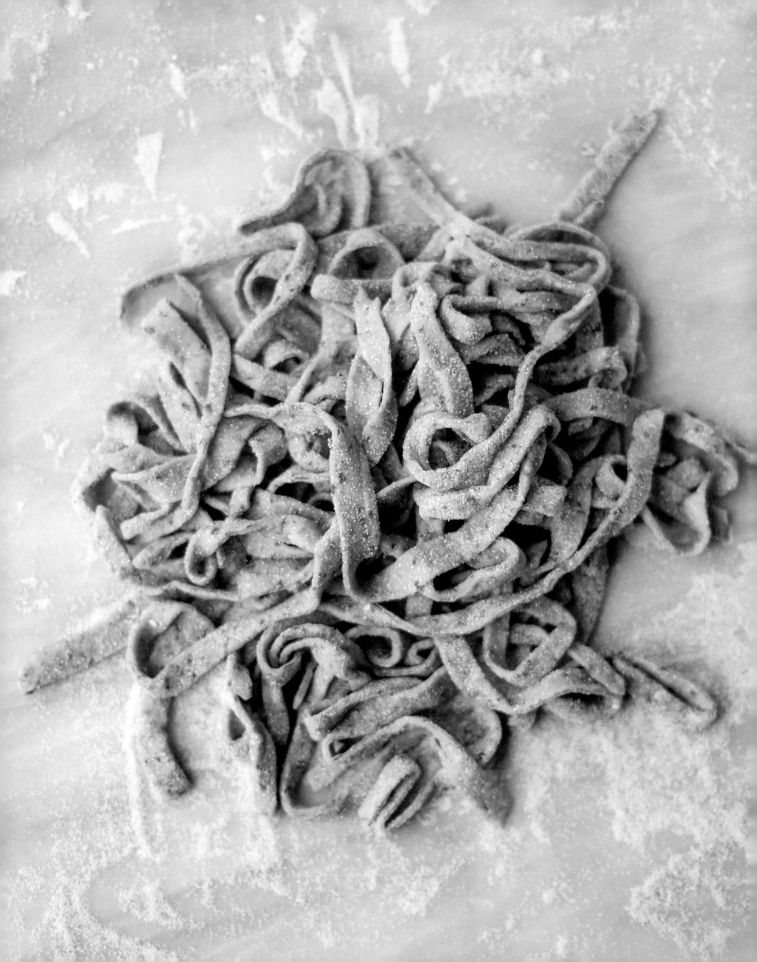

fresh hand-cut spinach pasta

Oh hello! Did you know that you can make your own green pasta and cut it by hand? No need for a pasta maker! I'm here to show you how ridiculously simple this can be—and make sure you know just how fabulous it tastes.

The dough comes together like a piece of cake—right on your countertop! Freshly minced spinach (best done in the food processor for the tiniest pieces) gets mixed in with flour, egg, and a touch of water for a delicate, homemade pasta. Use your pizza cutter or a sharp knife to cut it into strips once it's rolled thin, and then boil it for just a moment until it floats.

Drench it with melty, salted butter, freshly grated Parmesan, and a touch of basil. This is what dreams are made of!

Plus, do you see how green that is? Helllllllo health food. MAKES 2 TO 4 SERVINGS

8   ounces fresh spinach

3   whole eggs, divided

1   tablespoon water

4   cups all-purpose flour

Semolina flour, for sprinkling

2-4   tablespoons butter

Finely grated Parmesan cheese

Chopped fresh basil, for topping

Lots of white wine, to accompany the pasta!

Place the spinach in a food processor and pulse until just small crumbs remain. Add 1 of the eggs and the water. Blend until combined.

Place the all-purpose flour on your work surface and create a well in the middle. Add the spinach mixture and the remaining 2 eggs in the well. Use a fork to begin whisking the flour and egg mixture together. If needed, you can add more flour a few tablespoons at a time. You don't want the dough to be wet.

On a surface coated with semolina flour, roll out the dough as flat as you can into a very thin layer. Use a pizza cutter or sharp knife to cut long, thin noodles. Toss with a bit of semolina flour.

Bring a pot of salted water to a boil. Add the noodles (most likely in batches so as not to crowd the pan) and cook until they just float. With a slotted spoon, transfer the noodles to a serving bowl. Repeat with the remaining pasta. Add the butter and Parmesan and toss with the noodles. Sprinkle with the basil. Serve immediately, along with a glass of white wine.

our favorite

The fact that I am calling this "our" favorite Bolognese is huge.

My mom made pasta with tomato sauce every Thursday night when I was growing up, and being the brat that I was, I pitched a huge fit because I didn't love it. On those nights, I often ate cereal or buttered noodles with Parmesan for dinner, and it wasn't until I worked on this recipe for the last few years that I finally fell in love with a meat sauce.

Eddie, on the other hand? This is one of his dream meals. He is so excited on nights when I make this and even more pumped for leftovers the week after.

If you're serving only two-ish people, this also freezes great! **MAKES 6 TO 8 SERVINGS**

2 tablespoons unsalted butter

1 sweet onion, diced

4 cloves garlic, minced

Pinch + 1 teaspoon salt

12 ounces cremini mushrooms, chopped

1 pound ground beef

1 pound ground pork

1 teaspoon ground black pepper

2 teaspoons dried basil

2 teaspoons dried oregano

¼ teaspoon crushed red-pepper flakes

2 tablespoons brown sugar

½ cup half-and-half

1 cup dry red wine

2 cans (14 ounces each) fire-roasted diced tomatoes

1 can (28 ounces) crushed tomatoes

½ cup tomato paste

⅓ cup finely grated Parmesan cheese

In a large pot, melt the butter over medium-low heat. Add the onion and garlic with a pinch of salt. Cook for 5 minutes, or until slightly softened. Add the mushrooms and stir. Cook for 6 to 8 minutes, stirring occasionally, or until the mushrooms soften. Increase the heat to medium and add the beef and pork, pushing the vegetables to the sides and breaking apart the meat with a wooden spoon. Stir in the remaining 1 teaspoon salt, the pepper, basil, oregano, and red-pepper flakes. Cook for 8 to 10 minutes, stirring occasionally and breaking the meat into small pieces, or until the meat is browned.

Add the sugar, half-and-half, wine, diced tomatoes, crushed tomatoes, tomato paste, and Parmesan. Stir well. Bring the mixture to a simmer and cook for 10 minutes. Reduce the heat to low, cover, and cook for 20 minutes. Taste and season with additional salt if pepper, if desired.

Serve over your favorite pasta!

TIP: This sauce can also be made in the slow cooker, for extra, extra flavor! Brown the beef and the pork, then throw the whole thing in the slow cooker first thing in the morning and cook it all day on low.

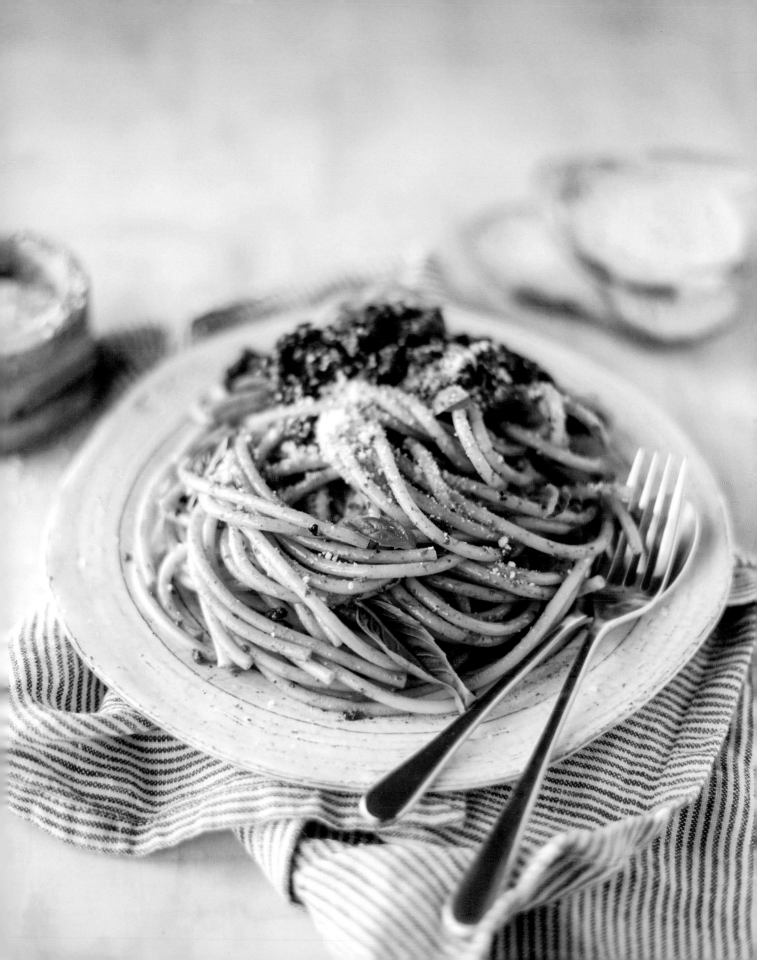

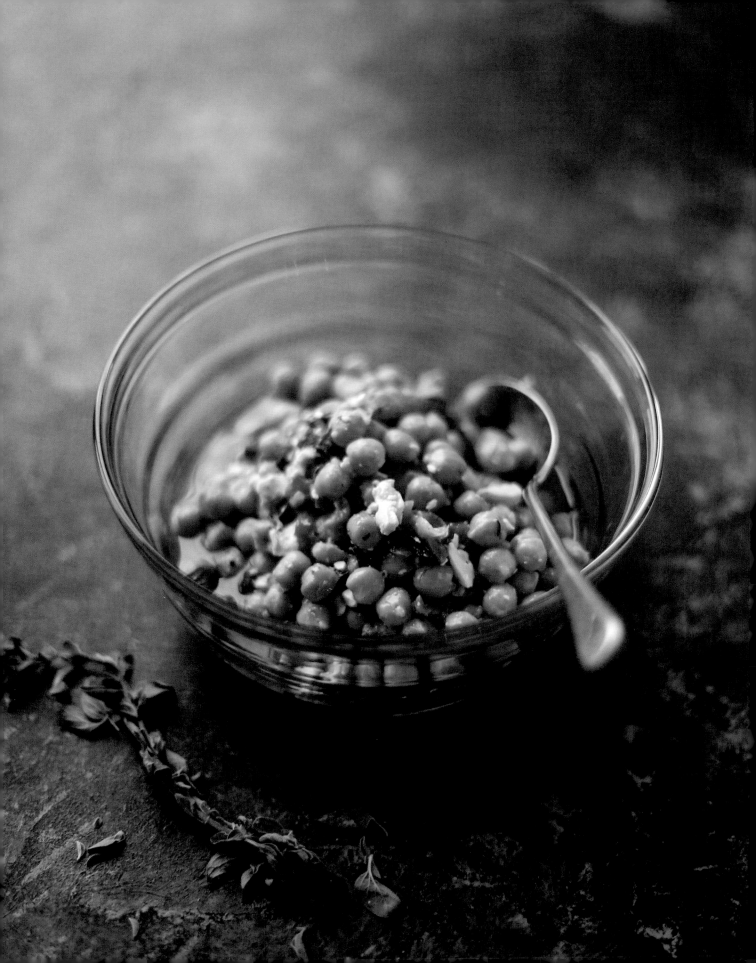

marinated chickpeas

I can easily fall into lunch ruts, especially since most days involve my working in the kitchen, which means a bit of this and a taste of that, and before I know it, I've had four pita chips with hummus and two brownies for lunch. Marinated chickpeas are one of the delicacies I discovered a few years ago in a desperate attempt to find new lunch options.

And I guess that we should use the term marinated here loosely, because technically you can eat these right after preparing them. But if they sit for a bit, they become more flavorful and a perfect addition to salads. Or pitas. Or your spoon! **MAKES 2 TO 4 SERVINGS**

1   can (15 ounces) chickpeas, rinsed and drained

⅓   cup chopped roasted red peppers

⅓   cup crumbled feta cheese

3   tablespoons olive oil

2   tablespoons red wine vinegar

¼   cup chopped fresh basil

2   teaspoons honey

2   cloves garlic, minced

¼   teaspoon dried oregano

¼   teaspoon salt

¼   teaspoon ground black pepper

¼   teaspoon crushed red-pepper flakes

In a large bowl, combine the chickpeas, red peppers, and feta.

In a small bowl, whisk together the oil, vinegar, basil, honey, garlic, oregano, salt, black pepper, and red-pepper flakes. Pour over the chickpeas and stir. Cover the bowl in plastic wrap and stick it in the fridge for at least 30 minutes.

TIP: Don't be afraid to switch up your beans! Using cannellini or great Northern beans is my second favorite way to use this dressing.

asparagus

Asparagus is one of the few veggies I can take to a party or gathering and know that it will be eaten with gusto. It's one of the vegetables that my entire family can agree on, and when there is bacon involved, how can you not be on board? **MAKES 2 TO 4 SERVINGS**

3 slices bacon, chopped

1 pound asparagus, woody stems removed

¼ teaspoon salt

¼ teaspoon ground black pepper

2 tablespoons olive oil

1 small shallot, finely chopped

4 tablespoons finely grated Parmesan cheese, divided

Preheat the oven to 400°F.

Heat a skillet over medium heat and add the bacon. Cook until some of the fat is rendered and the bacon just begins to crisp, but does not get very brown and crunchy. Remove it with a slotted spoon and place it on a paper towel–lined plate to drain.

Place the asparagus on a baking sheet. Sprinkle with the salt and pepper and drizzle with the olive oil. Toss to coat. Sprinkle the shallot over the top. Sprinkle on 2 tablespoons of the Parmesan and add the bacon.

Roast for 20 to 25 minutes, or until the asparagus becomes a bit crispy. Sprinkle with the remaining 2 tablespoons Parmesan before serving.

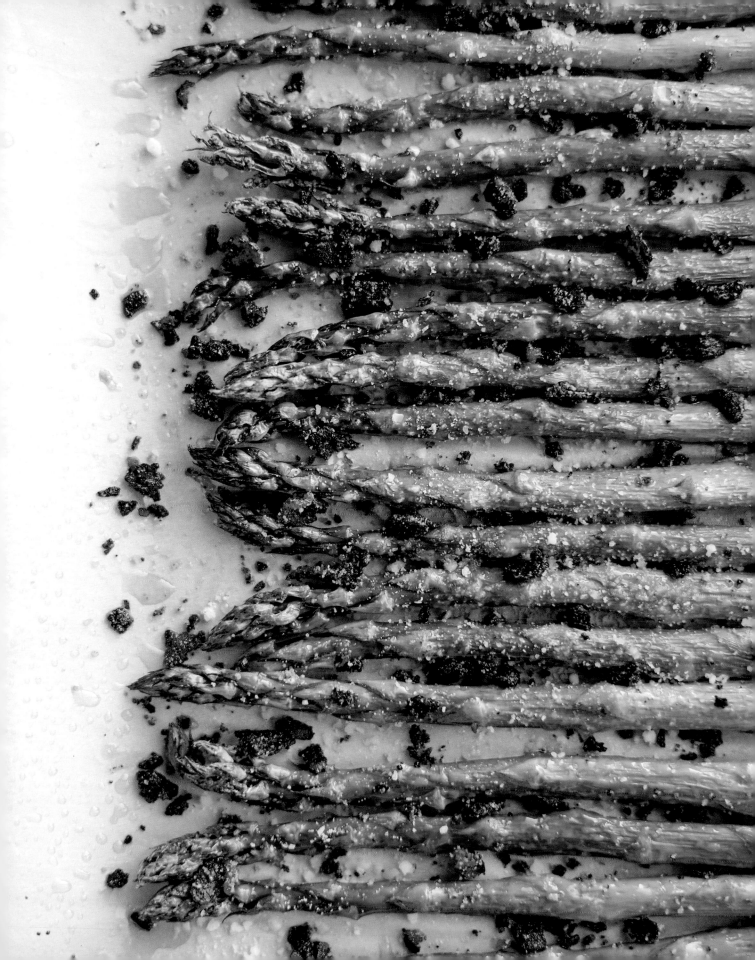

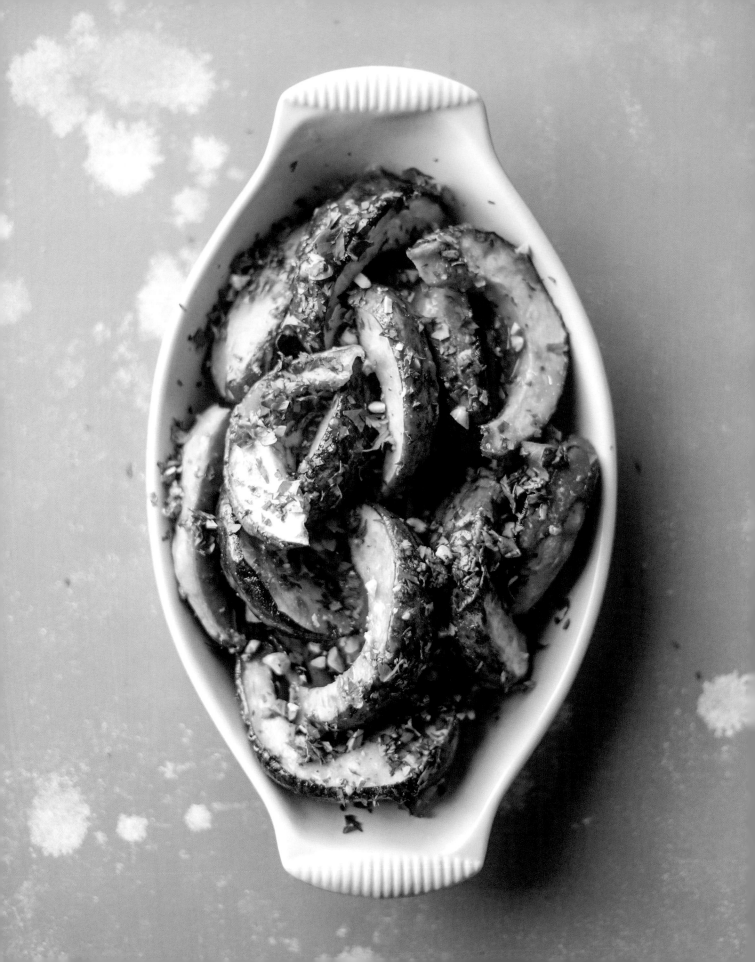

thai peanut acorn squash

Two of my all-time flavor loves—Thai-inspired cuisine and anything squash—come together in this dish to pack one heck of a flavor punch. Think creamy peanut butter, sweet chili sauce, lime, and cilantro all on top of caramelly roasted acorn squash.

I love to keep the skin on my acorn squash; it's a bit of chew and texture that I really enjoy. But feel free to peel it before roasting or discard it after. Just don't forget: lots of sauce! MAKES 4 TO 6 SERVINGS

2 acorn squash, sliced into rounds and seeds removed

½ cup sweet chili sauce

¼ cup rice vinegar

¼ cup lite canned coconut milk

3 tablespoons firmly packed brown sugar

1 tablespoon creamy peanut butter

3 cloves garlic, pressed or finely minced

1 teaspoon grated fresh ginger

Juice of 1 lime

½ tablespoon soy sauce

¼ cup chopped peanuts, for topping

½ cup chopped fresh cilantro, for topping

Preheat the oven to 400°F. Line a baking sheet with parchment paper and place the squash on the sheet.

In a bowl, combine the chili sauce, vinegar, coconut milk, sugar, peanut butter, garlic, ginger, lime juice, and soy sauce. Mix with a fork. Pour three-quarters of the sauce over the squash and toss well.

Roast the squash for 20 minutes, or until caramelly, golden, and fork-tender.

Top with the peanuts and cilantro. Use the reserved sauce for extra drizzle!

baked sweet potato fries
WITH DIP TRIO

By the third sweet potato recipe in the book, there is no need to explain our infatuation with them. In this case, it's all about the dips. Toppings and dips make everything better.

We have:

Basil Mayo, which needs no other introductions, other than that it tastes like fresh summer on your fries.

Chipotle Ketchup, a spicy take on the otherwise overly sweet stuff.

Our House Sauce, a creamy, barbecue-like, Dijon-tinged mayo.   MAKES 4 SERVINGS

3   pounds sweet potatoes, cut into wedges

3   tablespoons grapeseed or canola oil

1   teaspoon salt

1   teaspoon ground black pepper

Preheat the oven to 450°F.

Place the potato wedges in a large stockpot and cover with cold water. Bring to a boil. Once boiling, boil for 5 minutes. You have to keep an eye on it! After 5 minutes, drain the potatoes. Place them in a large bowl and drizzle with the oil, salt, and pepper. Gently toss with your hands or 2 spatulas to evenly coat.

Spread the potatoes on a baking sheet in 1 layer. Roast for 50 to 60 minutes, turning halfway through the cooking time. You want the potatoes to be deeply golden and crunchy on the outsides!

BASIL MAYO

½ cup mayonnaise

1 teaspoon Dijon mustard

¼ cup finely chopped fresh basil

In a bowl, whisk together the mayonnaise, mustard, and basil until combined.

CHIPOTLE KETCHUP

½ cup tomato ketchup

1 tablespoon adobo sauce from a can of chipotles in adobo

¼ teaspoon chipotle chili powder

In a bowl, whisk together the ketchup, adobo sauce, and chili powder until combined.

HOUSE SAUCE

½ cup mayonnaise

2 tablespoons Dijon mustard

1 tablespoon yellow mustard

1 tablespoon honey

1 tablespoon barbecue sauce

In a bowl, whisk together the mayonnaise, mustards, honey, and barbecue sauce until combined.

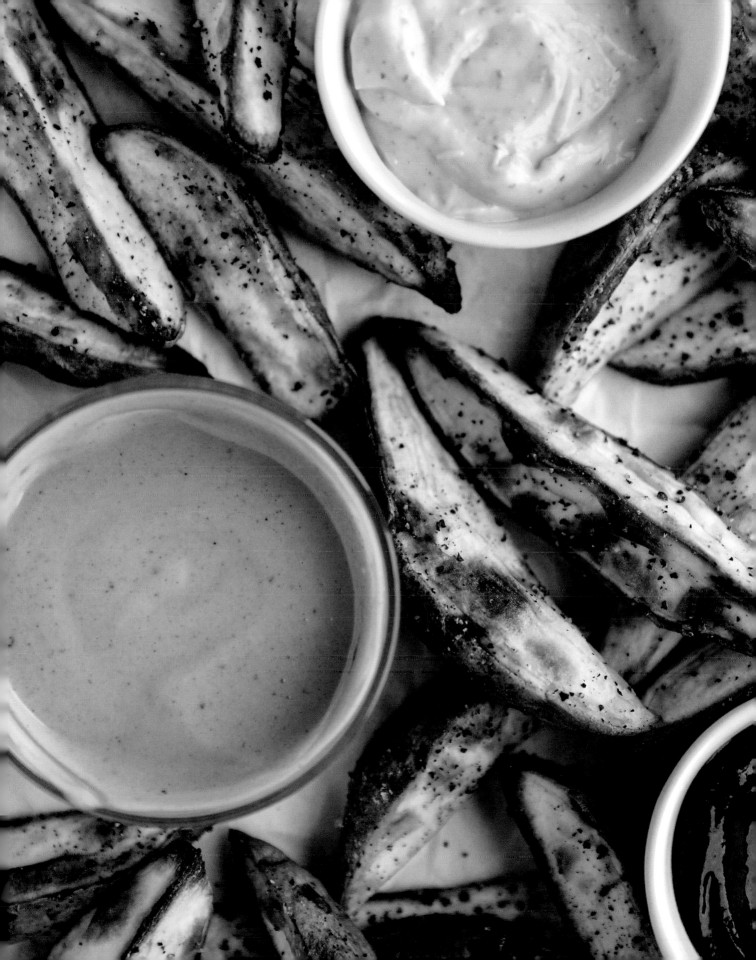

we're watching a ryan gosling movie tonight: comfort food

AKA, we need all the comfort food we can get, so we consume more than our own tears. In this section, you'll find all of my favorite soups, tacos, pizzas, and burgers! Only the best for us, of course.

compound butters

Flavored butters make my life complete. A bold statement, but tell me—isn't it so exciting when you order pancakes in a brunch spot and they come with a side of cinnamon vanilla butter? Instead of just plain butter?

See? Life changing. It can turn the entire day around before you know it.

These butters are ridiculously simple to make. If you want them to be in solid form (so they, say, melt lovingly over your grilled fillet or can be cut into adorable pats on your pretty butter dish), they will take a bit of prep work. That really just means that the night before, you should make the butter and shape it into a cute log or round ball so it can firm up in the fridge. Easy as pie.

But for those of us who are more fly-by-the-seat-of-our-pants planners, you can make these right before serving, as long as you don't mind softened butter.

Wait. Who would mind softened butter?

You can also package these in a sweet way for hostess gifts or holidays. I mean, I certainly would love if you showed up at my door with a jar of basil bacon butter. Just saying.

LEMON PISTACHIO COMPOUND BUTTER

½ cup unsalted butter, softened

¼ cup roasted and salted pistachios, chopped

Grated zest of 1 lemon

In a bowl, combine the butter, pistachios, and lemon zest and stir until mixed.

BASIL BACON COMPOUND BUTTER

½ cup unsalted butter, softened

¼ cup crumbled cooked bacon

3 tablespoons chopped fresh basil

In a bowl, combine the butter, bacon, and basil and stir until mixed.

BUTTERNUT SQUASH SAGE COMPOUND BUTTER

½ tablespoon unsalted butter

15 fresh sage leaves

½ cup unsalted butter, softened

2 tablespoons butternut squash puree

In a saucepan, melt the ½ tablespoon butter over medium heat. Add the sage leaves and cook for 1 to 2 minutes, or until the leaves are crisp. Transfer them to a paper towel to cool.

In a bowl, crumble the sage into the softened butter. Add the squash and stir until mixed.

BLUE CHEESE CHIVE COMPOUND BUTTER

½ cup unsalted butter, softened

3 tablespoons crumbled blue cheese

2 tablespoons snipped fresh chives

In a bowl, combine the butter, blue cheese, and chives and stir until mix

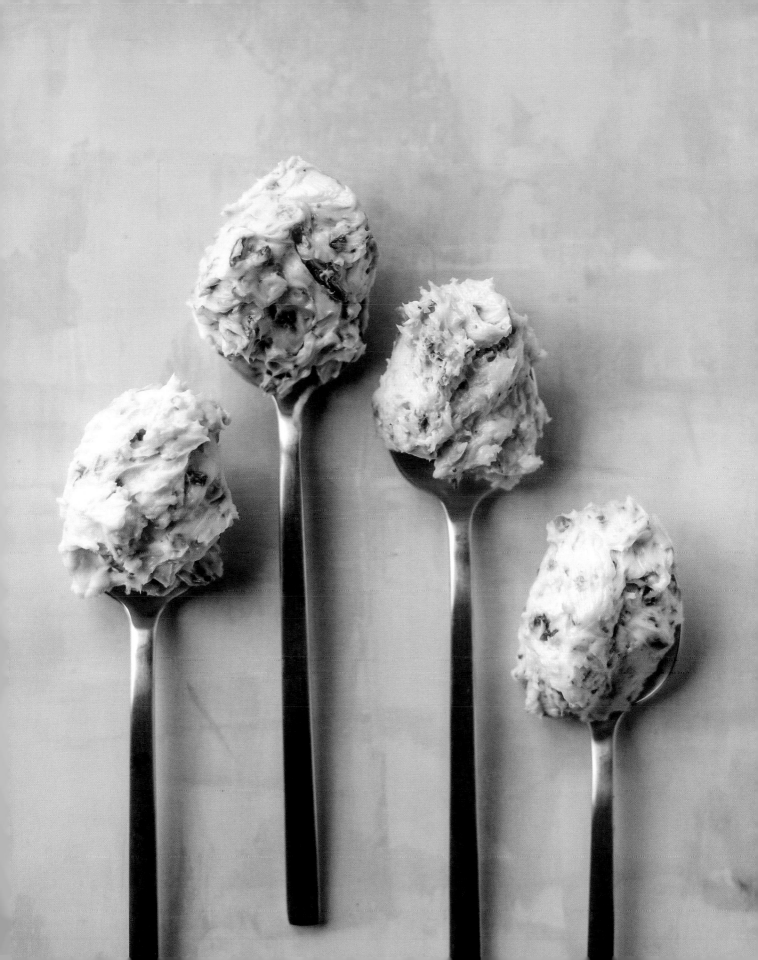

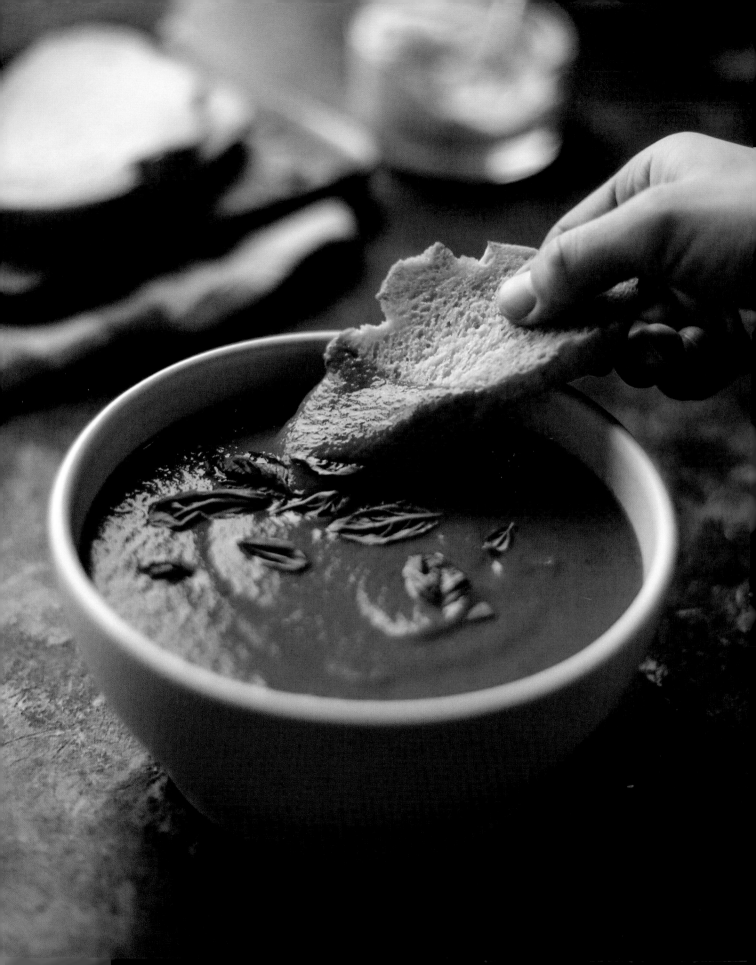

toasted garlic tomato bisque

I like to tease my mom that this is another deprivation of my childhood: I never had tomato soup as a kid. Never. There is a good reason for it. My maternal grandmother, who didn't have 1 ounce of Italian blood anywhere near her, would use cans of Campbell's tomato soup for marinara sauce when my mom was a child. Yes. I know. I hear the collective gasp, and I'm totally joining it. That sauce turned my mom off tomato soup forever. It wasn't until I learned the deliciousness of dipping grilled cheese into tomato soup and developed a few of my own recipes that I really fell in love with it. It might be the eternal shopper in me, but I hold the standard of tomato soup against the tomato basil version from Nordstrom Café. I have a similar recipe on my blog, but I switched it up a little bit here to add a bit more garlicky flavor. It's divine for bread dipping and the ideal comfort food.

Since I now have a child, and in the spirit of starting new traditions, we now serve tomato soup on Halloween. Hot tomato soup with grilled cheese sticks before trick-or-treating is perfect sustenance. And while I have a delicious grilled cheese sandwich you can throw in with this recipe (see the Gruyère French Onion Grilled Cheese with Thyme Butter recipe on page 140), the flavor can stand on its own.

All you need is some bread for the almighty dipping process. MAKES 2 TO 4 SERVINGS

2 tablespoons unsalted butter

4 cloves garlic, thinly sliced

2 shallots, sliced

1½ tablespoons tomato paste

1 can (28 ounces) fire-roasted diced tomatoes

⅔ cup sherry

⅓ cup chicken stock

3 tablespoons brown sugar

½ teaspoon dried basil

¼ teaspoon salt

¼ teaspoon ground black pepper

¾ cup heavy cream, plus extra for drizzling

Chopped fresh basil and oregano, for topping

In a medium saucepan, melt the butter over medium-low heat. Add the garlic and cook, stirring often, until it is golden brown and toasty. With a slotted spoon, transfer it to a plate. Add the shallots to the pan and cook, stirring occasionally, for 8 to 10 minutes, or until soft and slightly golden. Stir in the tomato paste and cook for 5 minutes. Return the garlic to the pan, along with the tomatoes, sherry, stock, sugar, basil, salt, and pepper. Bring the mixture to a boil. Reduce to a simmer and cook for 20 minutes.

Transfer the soup to a high-powered blender and carefully blend until pureed. Return the soup to the pot and heat over low heat. Right before serving, stir in the cream. Taste and season with additional salt and pepper if needed. To serve, drizzle the soup with the extra cream and top with basil and oregano.

coconut carrot soup

Behold! This is the only way that I thoroughly enjoy carrots.

To continue my weird childhood behavior, I was never a fan of carrots. Which is crazy, since I love crunchy stuff.

It's more of a texture thing than a flavor thing, so roasted carrots are okay, as well as carrot soup!

In this case, I used two of my favorite ingredients, coconut oil and coconut milk, to bring a richness to the soup without cream. It's fantastic. My favorite way to enjoy this is for lunch—any time of year. It's filling but light at the same time, and it pairs well with most lunch and dinner options.

MAKES 4 SERVINGS

3 tablespoons coconut oil

1 sweet onion, chopped

4 cloves garlic, minced

A pinch + ½ teaspoon salt

¼ teaspoon grated fresh ginger

1 pound carrots, chopped into
   1" pieces

2 cups low-sodium vegetable stock

1 can (14 ounces) coconut milk,
   plus extra for drizzling

Juice of 1 lime

½ teaspoon ground black pepper

Chopped fresh herbs, such as basil,
   oregano, or cilantro

Toast or baguettes, for serving

In a large pot, melt the coconut oil over medium-low heat. Add the onion and garlic with a pinch of salt and stir. Cook for 5 minutes, or until the onion is soft and translucent. Add the ginger and stir until it is incorporated. Add the carrots and stock. Cover the pot and increase the heat to medium. Cook for 20 minutes, or until the carrots are soft.

Turn off the heat and very carefully transfer the mixture to a blender. Blend until the soup is pureed and smooth. Return the soup to the pot and place over medium-low heat. Stir in almost the entire can of the coconut milk (reserving a few tablespoons for drizzling), lime juice, remaining ½ teaspoon salt, and the pepper. Cover and cook for 10 minutes, or until warmed. Taste and season with additional salt and pepper if desired. Serve the soup with a drizzle of coconut milk and garnished with fresh herbs, along with toast or baguettes on the side.

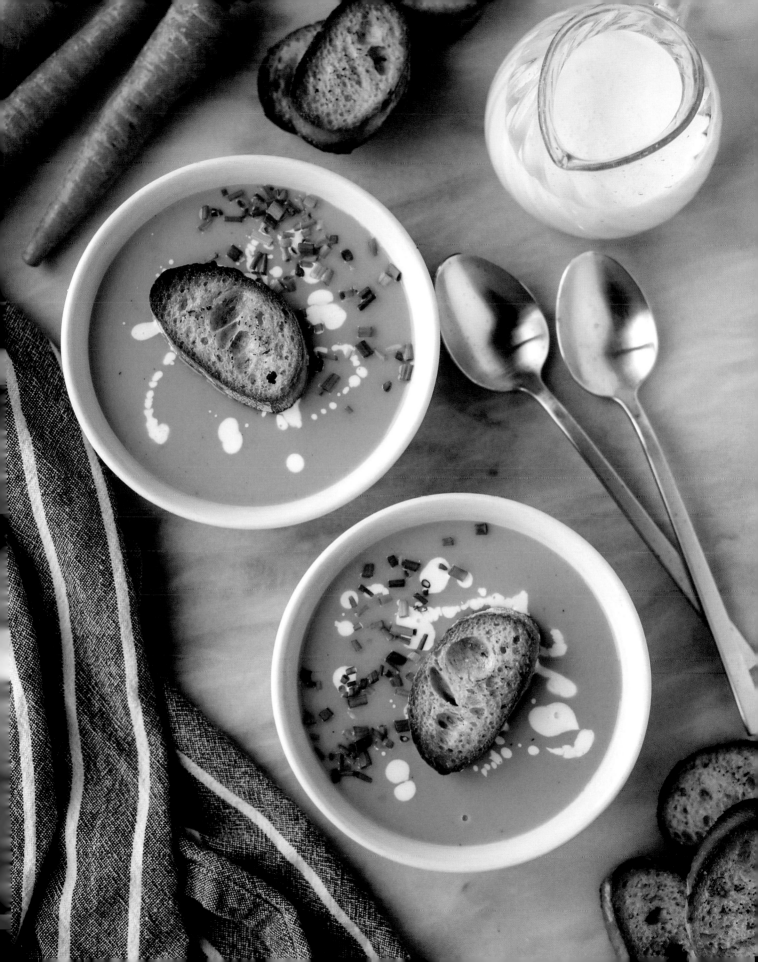

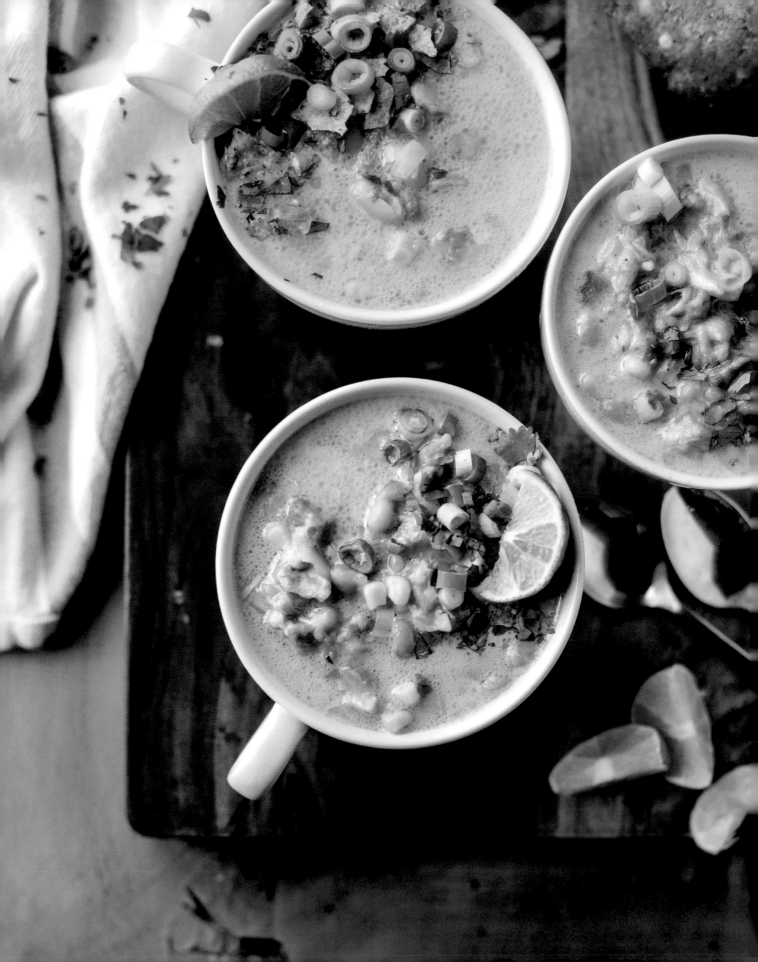

roasted corn and white chicken chili

Hearty, white chilis like these are the most requested form of soup in our house. Eddie goes crazy over this chili, and given my long-standing love for corn, I find this combination to be fantastic. It's corn chowder meets chili, in the most delicious way.

The best time to serve this is when the corn is super sweet and fresh, right around late August and September. In a pinch, frozen corn will work, too. I love to make a large batch near the end of summer and freeze portions that we can use throughout the beginning of fall.

I will pick white chili over red chili any day, most likely because of the creamy, cheesy vibe. And don't forget the best part: the toppings!

Life really is all about toppings, isn't it? Toppings can take a rather boring meal or a slightly plain bowl of soup and liven it up beyond belief. Cheese is necessary, as is some crunch from tortilla chips or strips. Extra heat in the form of jalapeños works (I love the pickled version!), and a sprinkle of cilantro adds the best freshness. MAKES 4 TO 6 SERVINGS

2   boneless, skinless chicken breasts, cut into 1– 2" pieces

1½ teaspoons ground cumin

½   teaspoon smoked paprika

½   teaspoon salt

½   teaspoon ground black pepper

2   tablespoons olive oil

2   tablespoons unsalted butter

1   sweet onion, chopped

1   can (4 ounces) diced green chiles

2   cloves garlic, minced

½   teaspoon crushed red-pepper flakes

2   cans (14 ounces each) cannellini beans, rinsed and drained

1   cup roasted or grilled corn

4   cups low-sodium chicken stock

8   ounces Monterey Jack cheese, freshly grated

⅓   cup sour cream

TOPPINGS

Tortilla strips

Chopped fresh cilantro

Sliced jalapeño chile peppers

Queso fresco cheese

Season the chicken with the cumin, paprika, salt, and black pepper and toss well. In a large pot, heat the olive oil and butter over medium heat. Add the chicken and cook for 6 to 8 minutes, or until browned on all sides. With a slotted spoon, transfer the chicken to a plate.

Add the onion to the pot and stir to scrape up some of those brown bits on the bottom. Stir in the green chiles and garlic. Cook for 5 minutes, or until the onion softens. Stir in the red-pepper flakes.

Add the beans, corn, stock, and chicken to the pot. Stir well. Bring the mixture to a boil. Reduce the heat to a simmer, cover the pot, and cook for 20 minutes.

Stir in the Monterey Jack in small handfuls until melted. Stir in the sour cream.

Serve with tortilla strips, cilantro, jalapeño peppers, and queso fresco on top!

NOTE: To roast or grill the corn, rub the ears with olive oil and sprinkle with salt and pepper. Place them on a high-heat grill or under the broiler in your oven. Cook until the kernels become golden and caramelly, turning often. Once the corn has cooled slightly, slice it off the cob.

cream of spinach soup
WITH SHOESTRING FRIES

This lovely soup is oh so good for you, packed with vitamins and nutrients from the fresh spinach and creamed up with some plain Greek yogurt, that I just had to go and ruin it by adding some shoestring fries on top.

It's basically the equivalent of when you go to lunch with your girlfriends and you all order salads . . . with a side of french fries to split. Who can resist the fries? Plus, when you share that kind of decadence with friends, calories don't count. I'm pretty sure of it.

The way you utilize these fabulous fries is up to you. I love some piled on top of my soup, but eating them on the side is just as great of an idea. I achieved the whole "shoestring" look from using my vegetable spiralizer, a product that I find is absolutely worth the small space it takes up in your kitchen. We use our spiralizer all the time (see the Poblano Pesto Zoodles on page 107!), and it's such a fun way to incorporate vegetables into meals in different ways.

Or you could always be like me and use it for french fries as your main priority in life. **MAKES 4 SERVINGS**

1 tablespoon olive oil

1 tablespoon unsalted butter

2 shallots, chopped

2 cloves garlic, minced

½ teaspoon salt

½ teaspoon ground black pepper

Pinch of crushed red-pepper flakes

16 ounces baby spinach, chopped

4 cups low-sodium vegetable stock

½ cup full-fat Greek yogurt

In a large pot, heat the olive oil and butter over medium heat. Add the shallots, garlic, salt, black pepper, and red-pepper flakes and stir. Cook for 5 minutes, or until the shallots are softened. Stir in the spinach. Add the stock and bring the mixture to a boil. Reduce the heat to a simmer and cook for 10 minutes.

Very carefully transfer the mixture to a high-powdered blender and blend until smooth. (You can also use an immersion blender here!) Return the soup to the pot and heat it over low heat. Stir in the yogurt right before serving. Top with the shoestring fries.

SHOESTRING FRIES

1 quart vegetable or canola oil

2 russet potatoes, peeled

Salt and ground black pepper

In a large pot fitted with a candy thermometer, heat the oil over medium heat. You want the oil to reach 350°F.

Use a spiralizer to slice the potatoes into shoestring shapes. Once the oil is hot, add the potatoes 1 handful at a time. Fry until golden. Remove with a slotted spoon and place on a paper towel–lined plate to drain any excess grease. Hit them with a pinch of salt and pepper. Repeat with the remaining potatoes.

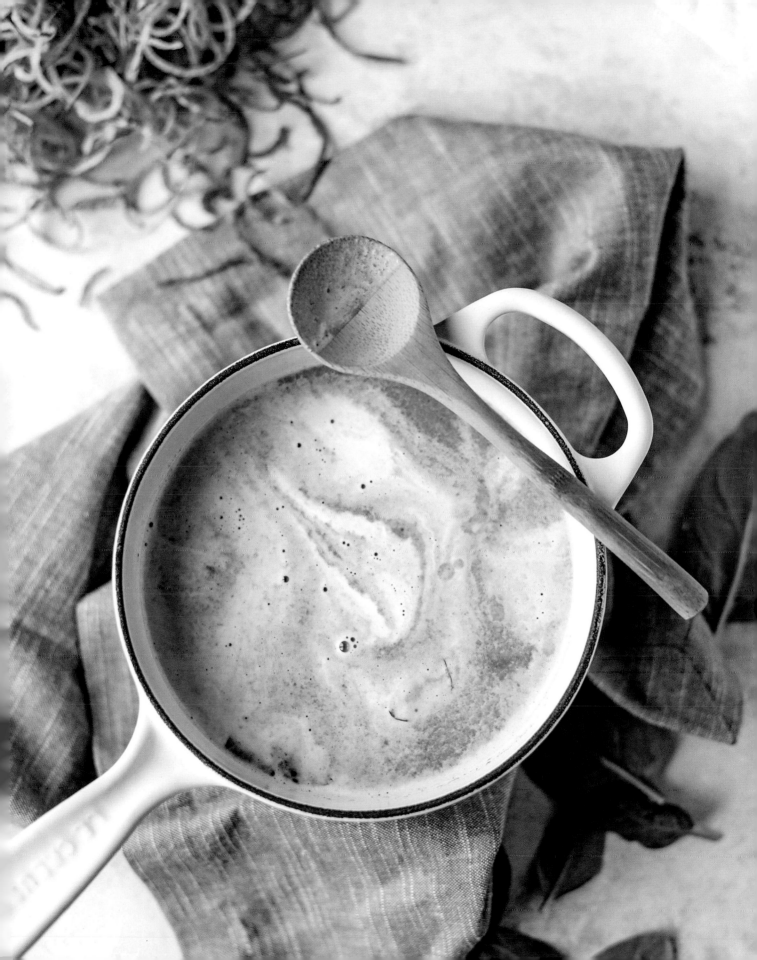

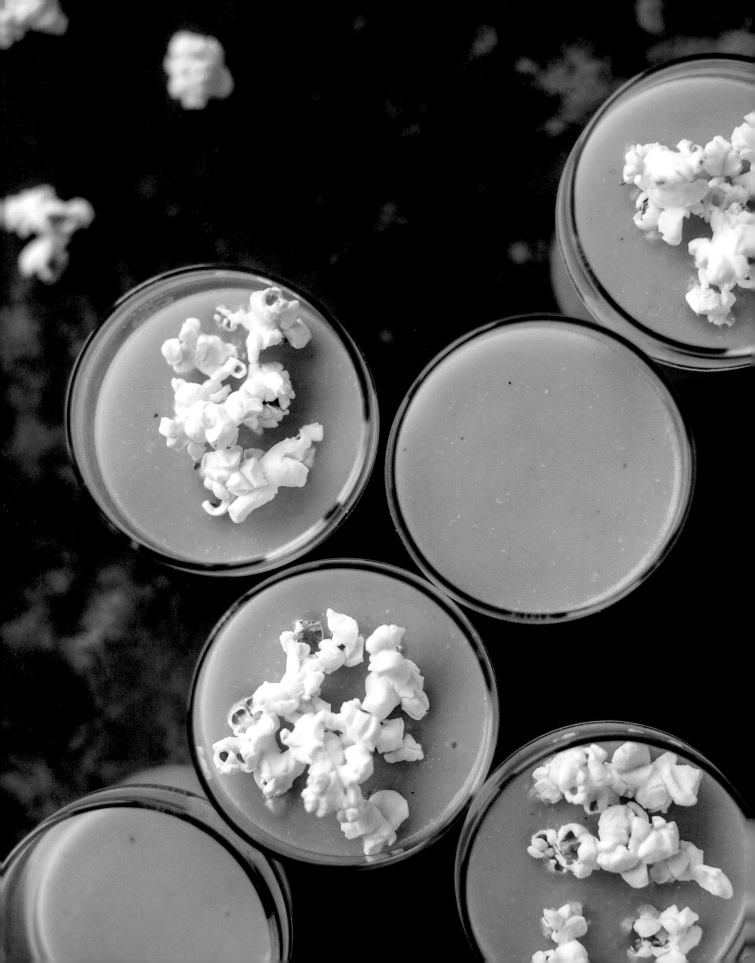

any-squash-you-choose shooters
WITH BUTTERED POPCORN

Squash soup will never go out of style!

I've made many a version of squash soup in the last few years. I almost always utilize butternut squash because that's what I usually have on hand, but I wanted to be sure to develop a soup recipe where you could use any kind of squash you happen to have.

The recipe for these little shooters was born a few years ago when I hosted my first Thanksgiving dinner. Our families are very into the traditional Thanksgiving spread, so I didn't want to mess with that. Instead, I created these little soup appetizers and made sure to tell no one before the day came. I didn't need any preconceived notions of how I was slightly trashing up our otherwise very traditional meal.

As soon as our guests walked in the door, I served these shooters with buttered popcorn on top, along with a cheese and vegetable plate. They were such a hit! The portion was small enough that everyone was still hungry for dinner, and it was also tiny enough that it didn't intimidate them into trying new things. Wins all around! To serve this, you can use a shot glass or even a smaller drinking glass and fill it only halfway. Super fun! MAKES 8+

1   tablespoon olive oil

2   tablespoons unsalted butter

1   shallot, chopped

2   cloves garlic, minced

½   teaspoon salt

½   teaspoon ground black pepper

4   cups cubed squash

¼   teaspoon freshly grated nutmeg

Pinch of crushed red-pepper flakes

4–6   cups chicken or vegetable stock

Freshly popped, buttered popcorn,
        for topping

In a large pot, melt the olive oil and butter over medium-low heat. Add the shallot, garlic, salt, and black pepper and stir. Cook for 5 minutes, or until the shallot is soft and translucent. Add the squash, nutmeg, and red-pepper flakes and stir.

Cook for 2 to 3 minutes, stirring often. Pour in the stock. Bring the mixture to a boil, cover, and reduce the heat to a simmer. Cook for 20 minutes, or until the squash is soft.

Turn off the heat and very carefully transfer the mixture to a blender. Blend until the soup is smooth and pureed. Return it to the pot and place over medium-low heat to heat through.

Meanwhile, pop your popcorn! Use whichever way is most convenient for you—microwave, stovetop, or air pop. Just drizzle a few tablespoons of melted butter over top before hitting it with a sprinkle of salt.

Pour the soup into shot glasses or small drinking glasses and top with popcorn.

NOTE: Did you know you can make healthy microwave popcorn at home? Throw ⅓ cup of kernels in a brown paper bag (add some coconut oil or canola oil if you wish!) and fold the top of the bag down. Microwave for about 2 minutes and 30 seconds (give or take a few, depending on your appliance) and voilà! Home-made microwave popcorn!

short rib chili

I present to you . . . Eddie's most favorite chili, ever. Ever ever.

We love using short ribs in recipes, though they are somewhat of a splurge. This chili is best made in your slow cooker, but your prep time should still be under an hour! The ribs are deglazed with Cabernet, which makes the flavor so deep.

I also really love to use fire-roasted tomatoes in my chili, as I find they add a little bit of extra something to the recipe that can be difficult to pinpoint.

This recipe is great for a crowd! For my son's 2nd birthday party, we set up a chili bar with two versions of chili in slow cookers, loads of toppings, some homemade queso, and lots of tortilla chips. It was a huge hit, and everyone could have a plate or bowl of exactly what they wanted! **MAKES 4 TO 6 GENEROUS SERVINGS**

10–12 beef short ribs

1   teaspoon salt

1   teaspoon ground black pepper

3   tablespoons flour

2   tablespoons canola or vegetable oil

⅓   cup Cabernet (your favorite variety)

2   cloves garlic, minced

1   shallot, chopped

1   red bell pepper, chopped

1   green bell pepper, chopped

¼   cup chili powder

2½ tablespoons ground cumin

2   tablespoons brown sugar

1   tablespoon ground chipotle chile pepper

1   tablespoon smoked paprika

3   tablespoons tomato paste

1   can (28 ounces) crushed tomatoes

1   can (14 ounces) fire-roasted diced tomatoes

1   can (14 ounces) kidney beans, rinsed and drained

1   can (14 ounces) pinto beans, rinsed and drained

⅔   cup red wine

Sour cream or Greek yogurt, grated cheese, sliced green onions or chives, chopped fresh cilantro, and/or tortilla chips, for serving

Sprinkle the short ribs with the salt, pepper, and flour. In a large skillet, heat the oil over medium-high heat. Add the short ribs in batches and sear until golden brown on all sides. Transfer the seared ribs to a slow cooker. Deglaze the pan with the Cabernet. Transfer the liquid in the pan to the slow cooker.

Cover and cook on low for 8 to 10 hours. Remove the meat from the ribs and discard the bones. Drain any liquid in the slow cooker.

Add the garlic, shallot, and bell peppers to the slow cooker. Stir in the chili powder, cumin, sugar, chipotle pepper, paprika, and tomato paste, stirring well to coat. Add the crushed tomatoes, diced tomatoes, beans, and red wine. Stir in the beef. Mix well to evenly distribute the ingredients. Cover and cook on low for at least 4 hours, but up to another 8. If you're home, taste the chili halfway through and add more seasoning, salt, and pepper if desired. This is normal—everyone likes their chili a little differently! Before serving, taste again. Serve with your toppings of choice.

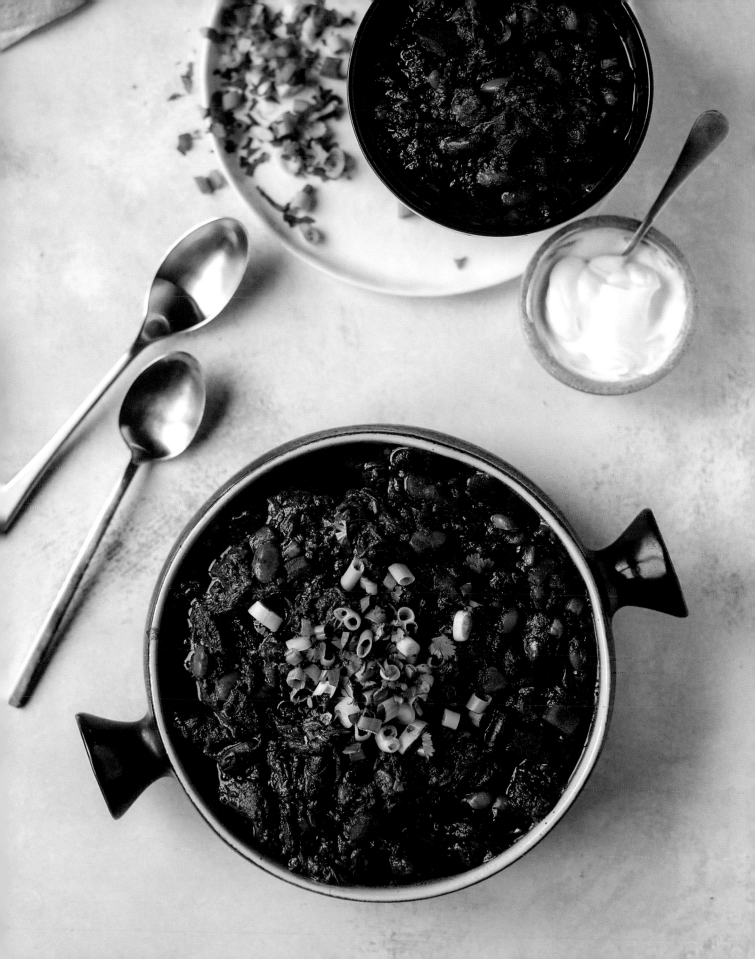

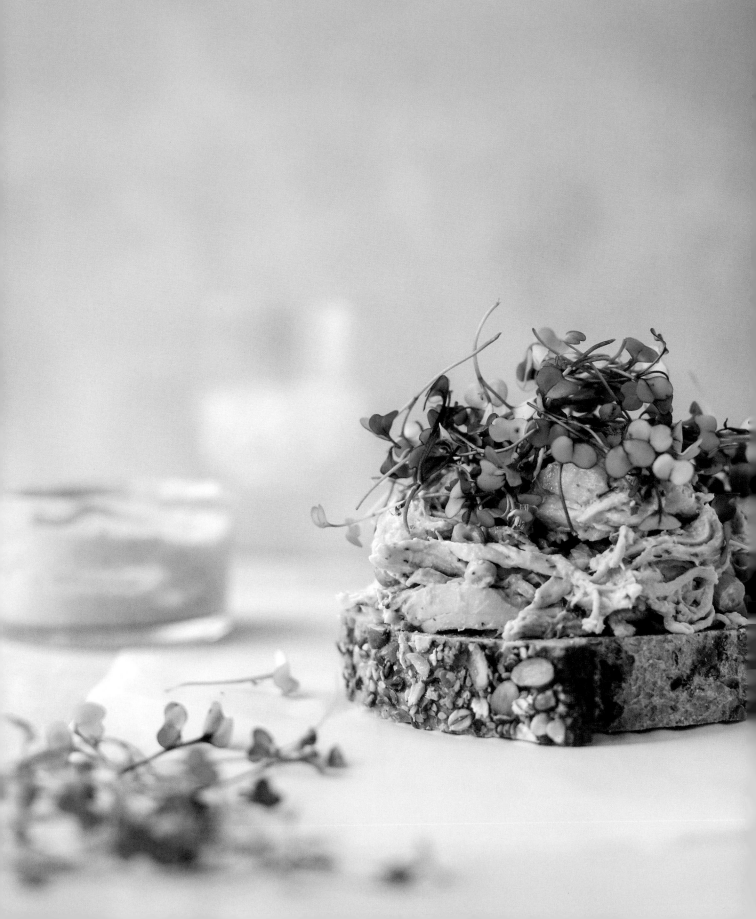

green goddess chicken salad sandwich

Chicken salad is one of my go-to make-ahead lunches. It's so versatile, with the options of a sandwich, cracker and cheese plate, or greens salad for lunch.

This green goddess dressing is packed with avocado, spinach, and basil. It has lots of flavor and even better-for-you ingredients. I like to use only a touch of mayo with a lot of yogurt for a tangy creaminess that pairs wonderfully with toast.

Top it off with some rainbow microgreens, and you've got one pretty open-faced sandwich!

MAKES 2 SERVINGS

GREEN GODDESS DRESSING

1   avocado, pitted and peeled

1   cup fresh spinach

⅔   cup plain Greek yogurt (I like full fat or 2%)

⅓   cup mayonnaise

¼   cup chopped fresh parsley

¼   cup chopped fresh basil

2   tablespoons snipped fresh chives

2   cloves garlic

Juice of ½ lemon

Salt and ground black pepper

CHICKEN AND SANDWICH

1   cup shredded chicken breast

2   slices bread, toasted if desired

Fresh microgreens or arugula, for topping+

TO MAKE THE GREEN GODDESS DRESSING

In a food processor, combine the avocado, spinach, yogurt, mayonnaise, parsley, basil, chives, garlic, lemon juice, and salt and pepper to taste. Blend until smooth.

To make the chicken salad, in a bowl, toss the chicken with a few tablespoons of the green goddess dressing. I like to toss in some extra chives or scallions, too. The amount of sauce that you use will depend on how "wet" you like your chicken salad to be!

To serve, scoop the salad on top of the bread or toast and top it with some fresh microgreens or arugula.

gruyère french onion grilled cheese

WITH THYME BUTTER

Even before I enjoyed eating onions, I had an obsession with French onion soup. I would convince my mom to let me order it in a restaurant when I was a kid, only for the gooey, melty cheese on top and the crunchy yet soup-soaked chunk of bread that would float in the broth. Every time she would tell me that I must "eat the whole bowl!" if I wanted to order it, and every time I would still eat only the cheese and the bread.

Every. Single. Time.

As I grew up and learned just exactly how wonderful caramelized onions are, I began consuming the actual soup underneath all the cheese and the bread. I would be lying, however, if I said that the onions are my favorite part. It's still the cheese and the bread, of course.

So it only seems natural that I would take those ingredients and make them into a grilled cheese! Lots of caramelly onions, the meltiest Gruyère cheese, some fresh thyme, and soft butter. This is pure decadence. Perhaps we should dip it in soup? **MAKES 2 SERVINGS**

THYME BUTTER
¼ cup unsalted butter, softened
1½ teaspoons chopped fresh thyme
Pinch of salt

SANDWICHES
¼ cup unsalted butter
1 sweet onion, very thinly sliced
¼ teaspoon dried thyme
¼ teaspoon salt
4 slices bread
6 ounces Gruyère cheese, freshly grated

TO MAKE THE THYME BUTTER
In a small bowl, stir together the butter, thyme, and salt. Set aside.

TO MAKE THE SANDWICHES
In a large pot, melt the butter over low heat. Add the onion, thyme, and salt and stir well. Cook, stirring occasionally, until the onion is golden and caramelized. This will take a full 30 to 40 minutes!

Heat a large skillet over medium heat. Spread 1 side of each bread slice with the thyme butter. Turn the slices over and top 2 slices with a quarter of the cheese each, then a spoonful of the caramelized onions. Top with the rest of the cheese and the other slices of bread.

Cook the sandwiches in the skillet until the cheese is melted and bubbly and the bread is golden brown. Serve immediately!

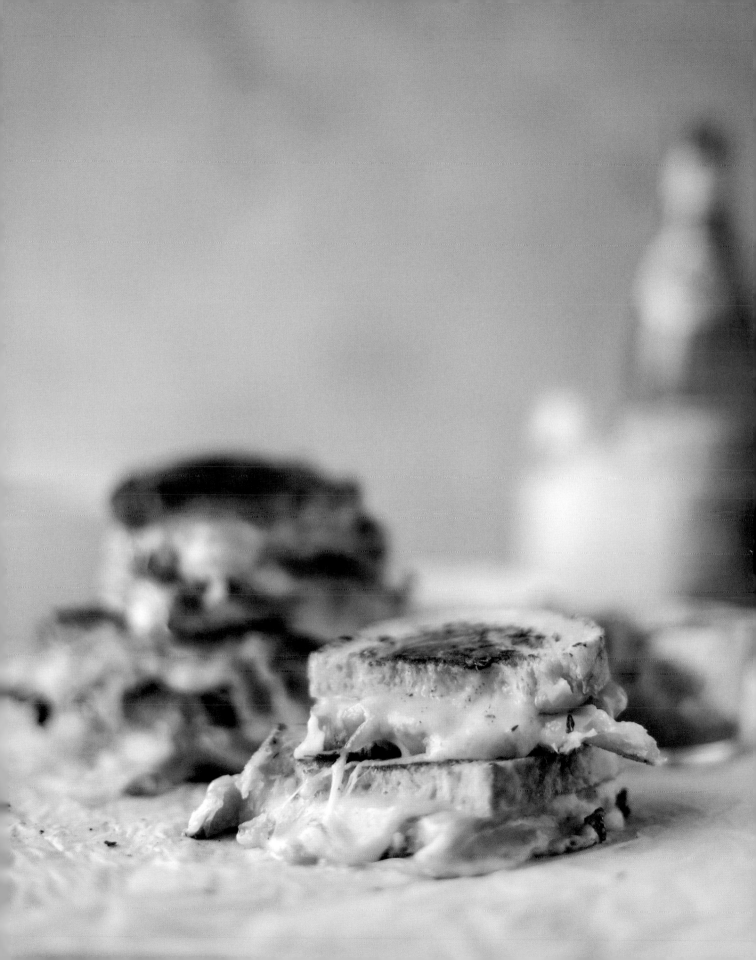

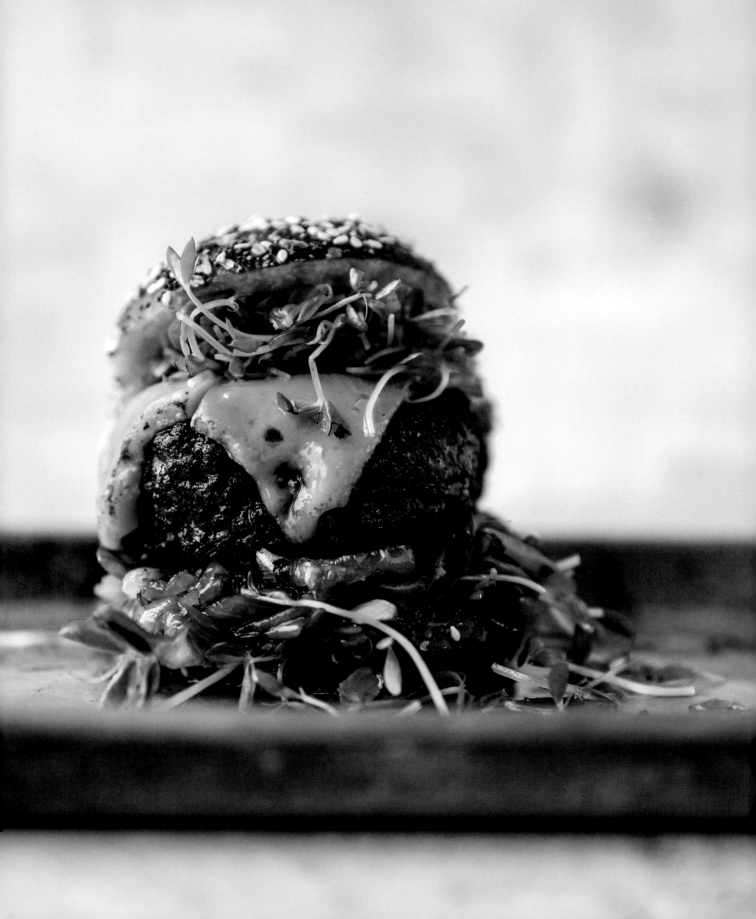

barbecue bourbon burgers

We grill a lot of burgers in our house since they are a family favorite. And with all of the gourmet burger restaurants around the area now, we're always aiming to create our own fancy version at home.

These ones . . . oh, let me tell you. They have bourbon caramelized onions. Yes, onions caramelized with bourbon. And lots of cheese and lots of greens on top. We love a chipotle barbecue ketchup spread for a bit of heat. And for a real splurge? We serve them on brioche or pretzel buns. You won't ever need to order another burger out again. MAKES 4 SERVINGS

BARBECUE KETCHUP

½ cup tomato ketchup

3 tablespoons barbecue sauce (your favorite variety)

1 tablespoon adobo sauce from a can of chipotle peppers in adobo

BOURBON CARAMELIZED ONIONS

¼ cup butter

1 sweet onion, thinly sliced

Pinch of salt

3 tablespoons bourbon

BURGERS

1 pound 85% lean ground chuck

1 teaspoon salt

1 teaspoon ground black pepper

2 cloves garlic, minced

⅓ cup finely grated sharp Cheddar cheese

1 tablespoon barbecue sauce

2 tablespoons butter

4 slices Cheddar cheese

Kale micro greens, for serving

4 buns, such as brioche or pretzel

TO MAKE THE BARBECUE KETCHUP
In a small bowl, stir together the ketchup, barbecue sauce, and adobo sauce until mixed. Set aside.

TO MAKE THE CARAMELIZED ONIONS
Heat a large pot over low heat and add the butter and onion. Add the salt and stir. Cook, stirring occasionally, until the onion starts to become golden. Stir in the bourbon and cook until there is no liquid left and the onion darkens in color. This process will take about 30 to 40 minutes.

TO MAKE THE BURGERS
In a bowl, combine the beef with the salt, pepper, garlic, Cheddar, and barbecue sauce. Gently mix with your hands a few times until the ingredients are evenly spread throughout the beef. Form the mixture into 4 equal-size patties.

You can grill these burgers, but I also love to cook mine in a buttery skillet. To do so, heat the skillet over medium-high heat and add the butter. When the butter has melted, place the patties in the skillet. Cook until a thermometer inserted in the center of a burger registers 160°F and the meat is no longer pink. About 1 to 2 minutes before the burger is finished, place a slice of cheese on top and cover the skillet with a lid. Let the cheese melt until the point when it's about to drip down the burger.

Assemble by placing the caramelized onions on the bottom half of the bun with a few greens. Top with the burger. Add more greens on top and finish off with the top half of the bun. Serve with the barbecue ketchup.

rainbow veggie sandwich

So how do I force myself to eat veggies? Make them into a rainbow. Sure, you might be thinking that this is a trick that we use on kids. On toddlers. Maybe even tweens. But if you're someone who always chooses cheese over veggies when it comes to your sandwich insides, I have news for you.

You can make a veggie sandwich look pretty. You can combine a few pickled veggies for that briny, tart flavor along with some roasted ones for sweetness. And if you're anything like me, potato chips on your sandwich are a delicacy. They add a special kind of crunch that cannot be beat.

Plus, we are eating all these veggies. So a few chips are okay. Life is alllll about balance.

The pickled veggies here take a bit longer to make—they are best if they sit in the brine for 60 minutes or so. You can make them the night before or even a few days ahead of time and just keep them in the fridge! MAKES 2 BIG SANDWICHES!

PICKLED RADISHES
½ cup thinly sliced radishes
½ cup apple cider vinegar
1½ tablespoons sugar
1 teaspoon coarse salt

ROASTED PURPLE POTATO
1 purple sweet potato, sliced
1 tablespoon olive oil
Salt and ground black pepper

ROASTED PEPPERS
1 red bell pepper, seeded and sliced
1 yellow bell pepper, seeded and sliced
1 tablespoon olive oil

HERB GOAT CHEESE SPREAD
6 ounces goat cheese, softened
½ teaspoon olive oil
1 tablespoon chopped fresh basil
1 teaspoon chopped fresh oregano

SANDWICHES
4 slices bread
1 avocado, thinly sliced
Butter lettuce leaves
Handful of rainbow micro greens
¼ red onion, thinly sliced

TO MAKE THE PICKLED RADISHES
Place the radish slices in a jar or cup. In a bowl, whisk together the vinegar, sugar, and salt until the sugar and salt dissolve. Pour over the sliced radishes. Let sit at room temperature for an hour. You can make this a day or 2 ahead of time and store it in the fridge in a sealed container or jar.

TO MAKE THE ROASTED PURPLE POTATO
Preheat the oven to 400°F. Place the potato slices on a baking sheet and drizzle with the olive oil. Season with salt and pepper to taste. Roast for 30 minutes, or until fork-tender.

TO MAKE THE ROASTED PEPPERS
Preheat the broiler to high. Rub the pepper slices with the olive oil and place them on a baking sheet, skin side up. Broil the peppers until the skin becomes blackened and charred.

Remove the peppers and place them in a resealable plastic bag for 30 minutes to steam. Peel the skin off the peppers.

TO MAKE THE HERB GOAT CHEESE SPREAD
In a bowl, stir together the goat cheese, olive oil, basil, and oregano until combined.

TO ASSEMBLE THE SANDWICHES
Spread 2 slices of the bread with the goat cheese mixture. Begin by adding a few of the pickled radishes, the red peppers, the yellow peppers, and then the avocado, lettuce, and micro greens. Add the onion and purple potato. Serve with lots of potato chips!

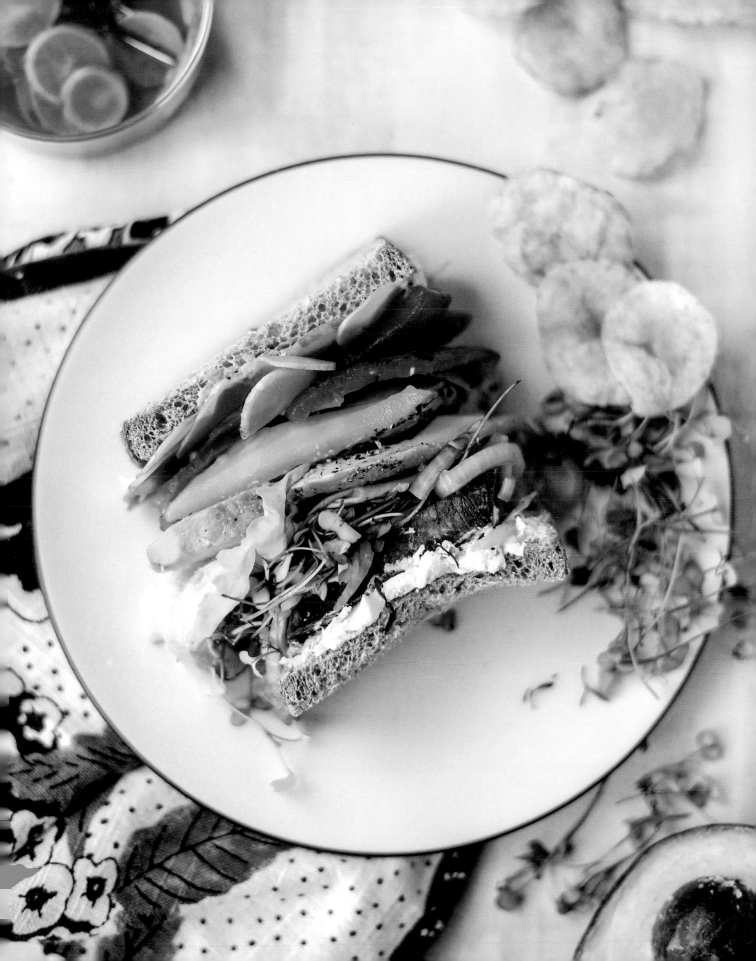

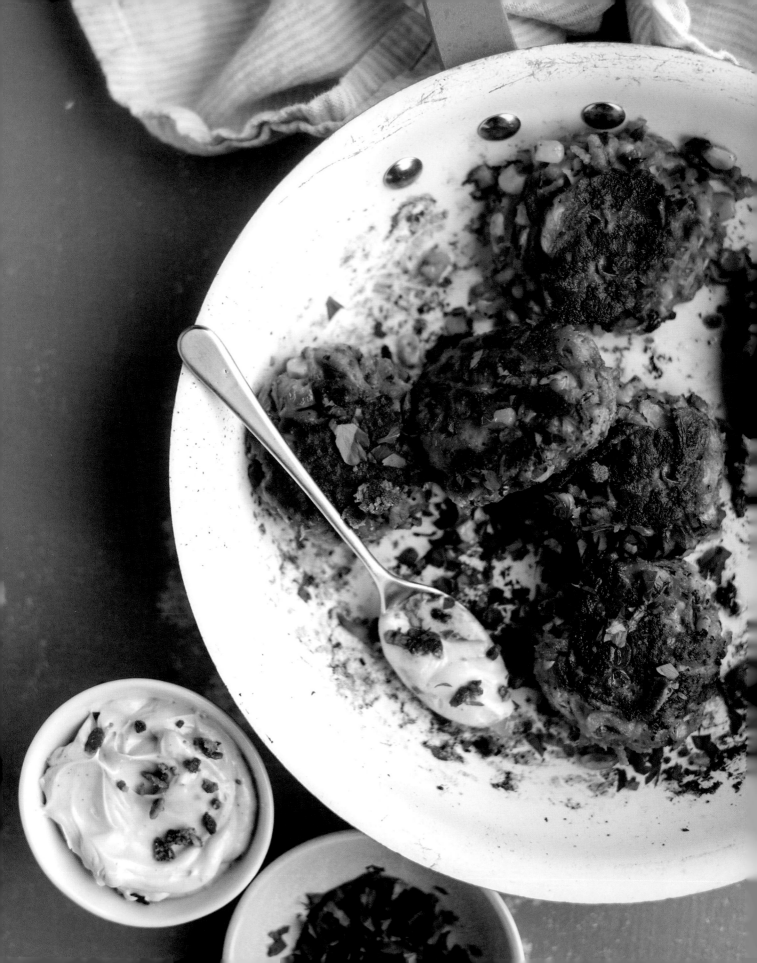

sweet potato corn fritters

These fritters can work triple duty for you. They can be a side dish, an appetizer, or, heck, a main meal if you're asking me. Add a green salad and I'd be thrilled if this was on my plate for dinner.

We absolutely adore sweet potatoes in this house—much more than red or white potatoes—so they are something we have multiple times per week. These crunchy, savory-and-sweet fritters are perfect for any season. They are lovely in the summer if you have farm-fresh corn, but they're fantastic in the winter as well because you can use the frozen stuff in a pinch. MAKES 2 TO 4 SERVINGS

1   sweet potato, freshly grated

⅔   cup sweet corn kernels

8   saltine crackers, crushed (I use multigrain)

1   large egg, lightly beaten

1   tablespoon Dijon mustard

1   tablespoon full-fat or 2% plain Greek yogurt

1   tablespoon Homemade Bacon Mayo, plus additional for serving (page 148)

1   tablespoon chopped fresh chives

2   cloves garlic, minced

¼   teaspoon salt

¼   teaspoon ground black pepper

Pinch of crushed red-pepper flakes

3   tablespoons olive oil

Place the sweet potatoes in a large bowl. Add the corn, crackers, egg, mustard, yogurt, mayo, chives, garlic, salt, black pepper, and red-pepper flakes. Stir until combined (use your hands to mix if necessary). Form the mixture into 1"-thick cakes that are about 2" in diameter. You can obviously make whatever size you'd like!

In a large skillet, heat the olive oil over medium heat. Add the fritters and cook for 6 to 8 minutes, turning once, or until deeply golden on both sides. Transfer the fritters to a paper towel–lined plate to drain. Serve hot with additional bacon mayo.

homemade bacon mayo

It took me a few years to discover my love for mayo. I'm pretty sure that I enjoyed it as a kid, as my mom was often preparing chicken, egg, or tuna salads on toast for lunches. I didn't mind it back then.

But then in my tween years, something changed. It must have been too much exposure to horrible, sat-in-the-sun potato and pasta salads, or a way-too-thick layer on a sandwich that completely turned me off. And I joined the mayo-haters club for many, many years.

As a pretty big fan of yogurt, especially Greek yogurt, I started using that in most mayo-based recipes. However, there are just some instances and a handful of recipes where that doesn't work. Take the perfect BLT, for example. I love a good BLT, and the last thing I want is to slather it with tangy Greek yogurt. No, thanks.

But it needs some sort of spread, right? We can't have a BLT with no spread!

This was when my stance on mayo changed greatly. It often gets such a terrible rap, but the ingredients are simple and things I love: egg yolks, olive or vegetable oil, and vinegar. Sometimes lemon juice or mustard. All things I adore. So I started making my own in order to fall back in love. I have used this trick over the years to learn to love certain veggies, so I figured, why not mayo?

Which then turned into . . . bacon mayo. Instead of oil, we use bacon grease and then add crispy bacon bits into the mayo. It is absolutely divine. And full of flavor. And perfect for dipping or spreads!

Just a note: Since we're using a raw egg in this recipe, finding the freshest (and pasteurized) egg that you can is best! **MAKES ABOUT ¾ CUP**

1   large egg

1   teaspoon white vinegar

Juice of ½ lemon

1   clove garlic, minced

½   cup bacon fat, melted

¼   cup crumbled cooked bacon

In a food processor, combine the egg, vinegar, lemon juice, and garlic. Process until smooth. With the processor on, very slowly stream in the bacon fat about 2 tablespoons at a time, letting the processor really blend the mixture together each time. Blend until smooth. Blend in the bacon. Store in a sealed jar in the fridge.

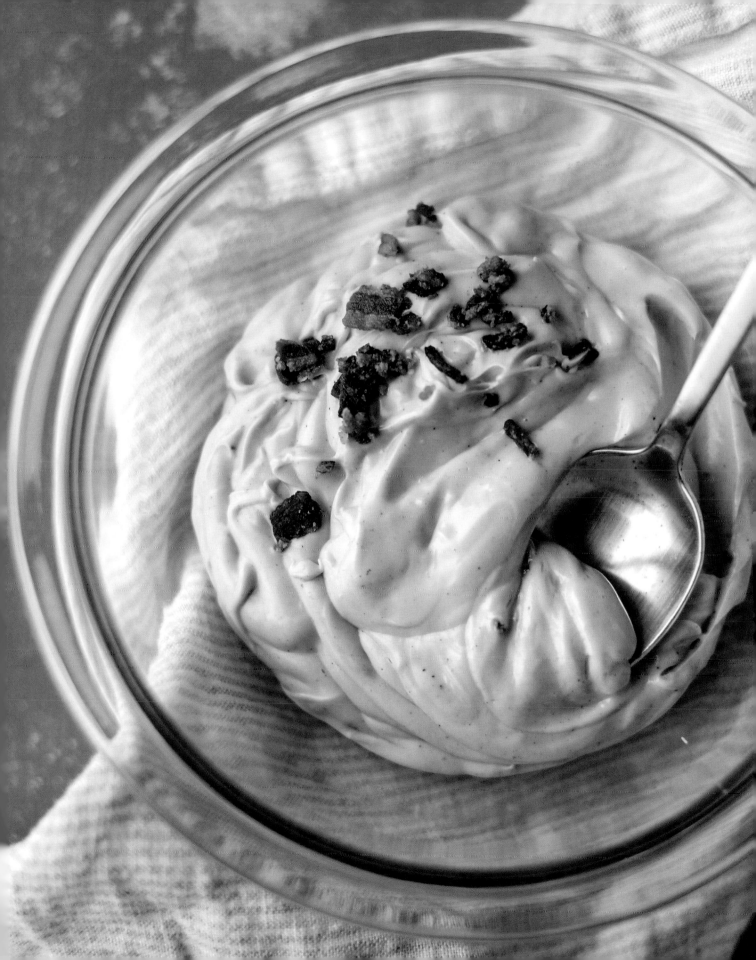

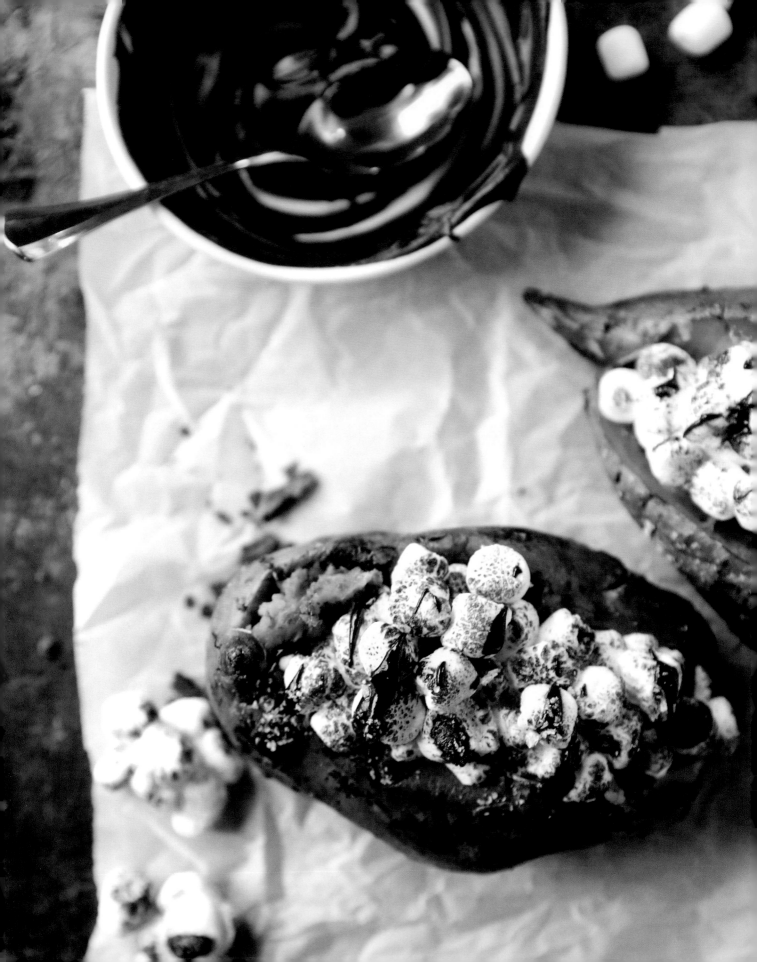

s'mores stuffed sweet potatoes

Oh yes. I really did do this. I did!

I stuffed slow-roasted sweet potatoes with marshmallows. And dark chocolate. And sprinkled graham cracker crumbs over the entire thing.

It's probably no surprise that I am not into camping. I'm not even into glamping. It's not necessarily something I'm proud of, but I know myself, and me and the great outdoors for a few days . . . with nothing else? No thanks.

But! I always wanted to camp when I was a kid. I always wanted to make those fun treats that families made while camping, like bananas stuffed with chocolate and mud pies or something with bread and cheese. You know, whatever those things were called.

My next-door neighbor and I once "camped" in her backyard in a big tent, while her dad slept on the porch since we were terrified. Scratch that—I was terrified. It was like, hello? Where are the s'mores and the shooting stars? I think I just saw a bear. I'm going home. Bye.

This is my semi-adult answer to all those fun campfire treats. And it can be whatever you'd like. A snack? A party treat? A dessert? Your dinner?

I will not judge. Just please do not ask me to go sleep in a tent in the woods with you. **MAKES 4 SERVINGS**

4   sweet potatoes

1   tablespoon olive oil

Salt and ground black pepper

4   ounces dark chocolate, chopped

2   cups mini marshmallows

⅓   cup graham cracker crumbs

CHOCOLATE GANACHE

6   ounces milk, dark, or semisweet chocolate, chopped

⅓   cup heavy cream

Preheat the oven to 300°F. Line a baking sheet with foil or parchment paper. Scrub the sweet potatoes and dry them completely. Rub the outsides with the olive oil and season them with salt and pepper to taste. Bake for 2 to 2½ hours, or until golden on the bottoms and super soft. Let them cool just slightly. Preheat the broiler to high.

While the potatoes are still warm, gently slice them open. Sprinkle them with the dark chocolate. Top with the marshmallows. Broil until the marshmallows toast.

TO MAKE THE CHOCOLATE GANACHE
Place the chocolate in a large bowl. In a saucepan, heat the cream over medium heat until it is hot but not boiling—just until bubbles form on the sides of the pan. Pour the cream over the chocolate. Allow it to sit for 1 to 2 minutes, then stir continuously until the chocolate is smooth and comes together as a ganache. This may take a full 5 minutes, but keep stirring! It will look like hot fudge.

Drizzle the potatoes with the chocolate ganache and sprinkle with the graham cracker crumbs.

herbed feta cornbread

When I married Eddie, he turned me on to cornbread. It wasn't ever something my mom made when I was growing up—never even with chili—so I ignorantly assumed that I wasn't really into it.

But given my severe lust for all things sweet corn, that was a very incorrect thought. Cornbread is the perfect side dish to so many things. With so many different soups and chilis in this book, I wanted to make sure that we had an adequate number of dippers and bread sides. Enter first: herb-loaded cornbread with lots of feta cheese. It's flavorful and cheesy, so you don't have to twist my arm on this one. It goes great with all sorts of soups and is even better toasted! Warm and golden, spread with a hint of butter. Ooooh my. MAKES 9 SERVINGS

½ cup all-purpose flour

½ cup whole wheat flour

1 cup finely ground yellow cornmeal

1 tablespoon baking powder

1 tablespoon sugar

½ teaspoon salt

2 large eggs

½ cup butter, melted

½ cup milk

¼ cup plain Greek yogurt

½ cup sweet corn

4 ounces feta cheese, crumbled

¼ cup chopped fresh herbs (such as basil, rosemary, thyme, sage, parsley)

Preheat the oven to 400°F. Spray an 8" x 8" baking dish with cooking spray.

In a large bowl, whisk together the flours, cornmeal, baking powder, sugar, and salt.

In a medium bowl, whisk together the eggs, butter, milk, and yogurt until smooth. Add to the dry ingredients and stir until just combined. Fold in the corn, feta, and herbs.

Pour the mixture into the baking dish. Bake for 30 to 35 minutes, or until set and golden on top.

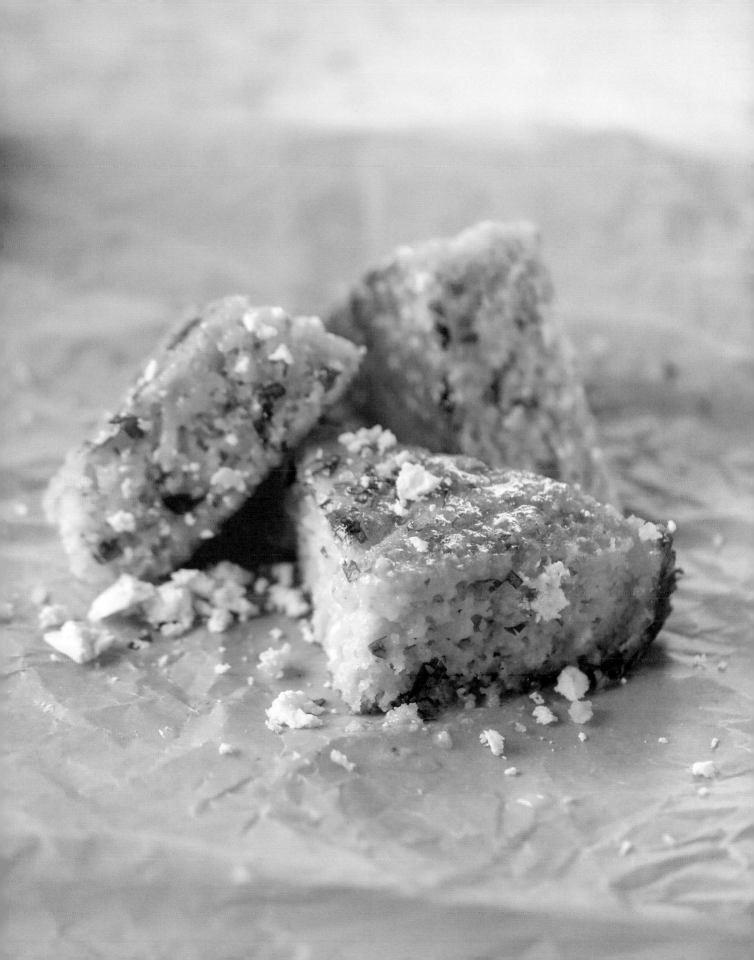

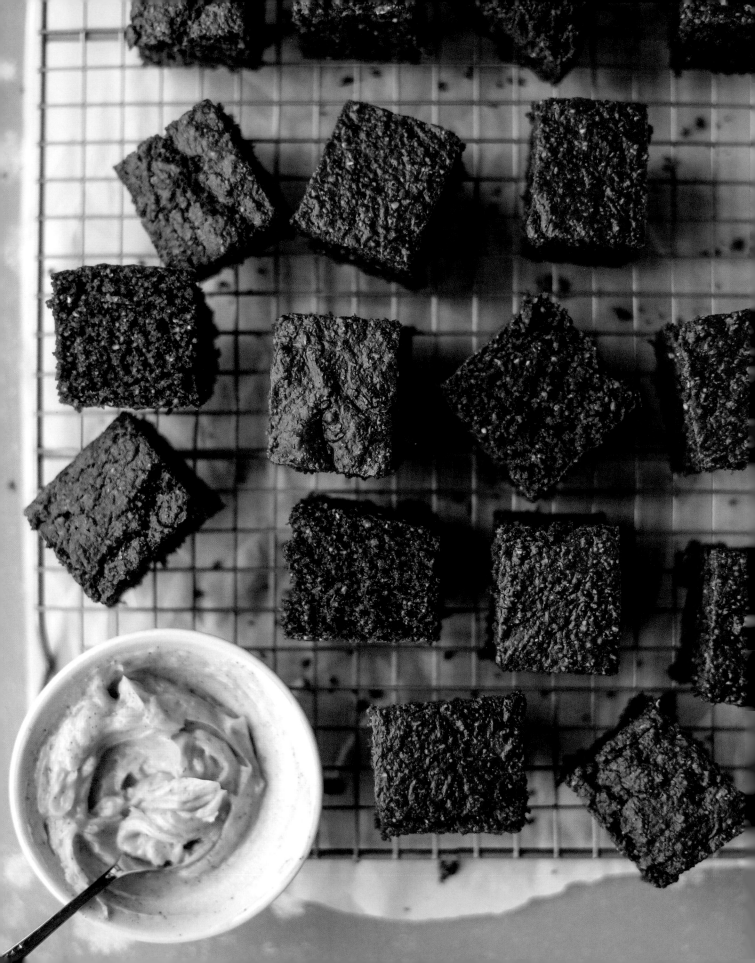

chocolate chili cornbread

Do not be afraid! While this cornbread is not for the faint of heart, it also doesn't taste like brownies. It's mildly flavored with cocoa for that chocolate hint (if you're like me, then you probably add a spoonful of cocoa into your chili!) and has a touch of heat from the cayenne.

In my personal opinion, this cornbread pairs best with red chili: a hearty, tomato-based chili with lots of beans and beef. Use the cornbread for dipping or simply sitting on the side of your bowl for bites in between spoonfuls. It's also excellent plain, of course!

And by "plain," I mean slathered in butter. MAKES 9 SERVINGS

1   cup all-purpose flour

1   cup finely ground cornmeal

⅓   cup unsweetened cocoa powder

1   tablespoon baking powder

1   tablespoon sugar

1   teaspoon chili powder

½   teaspoon salt

¼   teaspoon ground cayenne pepper

½   cup butter, melted

½   cup milk

½   cup heavy cream or half-and-half

2   eggs

Preheat the oven to 375°F. Spray an 8" x 8" baking dish with cooking spray.

In a large bowl, combine the flour, cornmeal, cocoa, baking powder, sugar, chili powder, salt, and cayenne pepper. In a smaller bowl, whisk together the butter, milk, cream or half-and-half, and eggs. Add the wet ingredients to the dry, mixing until just combined.

Pour the mixture into the baking dish. Bake for 20 to 25 minutes, or until set and the edges start to pull away from the sides of the pan. Let cool slightly before cutting.

cheesy pizza baked gnocchi

While I've never been a serious pasta lover, gnocchi have always had a space in my heart. Those adorable potato dumplings are so perfect with sauce and cheese. And wine on the side, of course.

Since we are serious pizza people, I occasionally make plans to "pizza-fy" everything in our fridge. What can be made into pizza? Zucchini boats? Grilled cheese? Chicken on the grill? There are always options when sauce, cheese, and pepperoni are involved.

Here, we have mini potato gnocchi (DeLallo Foods makes the best!) that are baked in warm sauce with tons of melty provolone and fontina. It's covered with extra cheese that gets golden and bubbly, along with mini pepperoni pieces that get a bit crispy in the oven. This is an indulgent side dish to serve, but one that kids and adults alike go crazy for. **MAKES 4 TO 6 SERVINGS**

1   pound mini potato gnocchi

2   cups marinara sauce

1   teaspoon dried Italian seasoning

6   ounces provolone cheese, freshly grated, divided

2   ounces fontina cheese, freshly grated, divided

¼   cup finely grated Parmesan cheese, divided

¼   cup mini pepperoni pieces

Chopped fresh basil and oregano, for topping

Preheat the oven to 350°F.

Cook the gnocchi according to the package directions. Pour the marinara sauce in an 8" x 8" baking dish. Stir in the Italian seasoning. Add the gnocchi to the marinara and toss to coat. Toss in almost all of the provolone and fontina, reserving some for the topping. Stir in half of the Parmesan. Spread the gnocchi evenly in the dish.

Top with the remaining provolone and fontina. Add the pepperoni on top. Bake for 25 to 30 minutes, or until the cheese is super bubbly and golden. Sprinkle on the basil and oregano, along with the remaining Parmesan. Serve immediately.

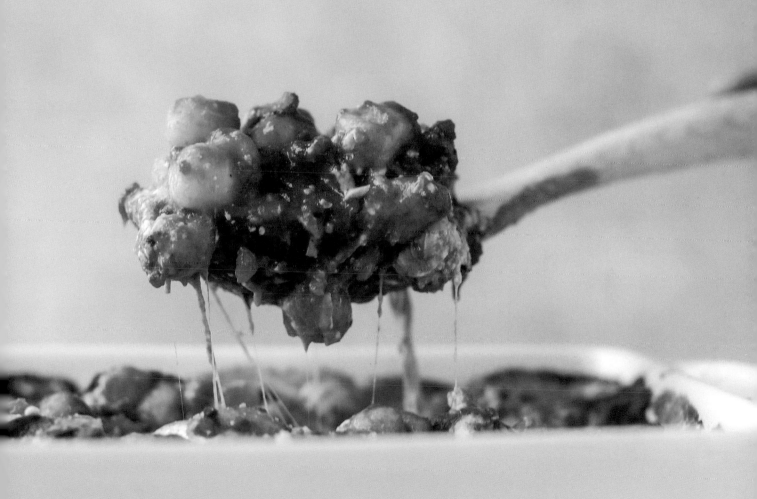

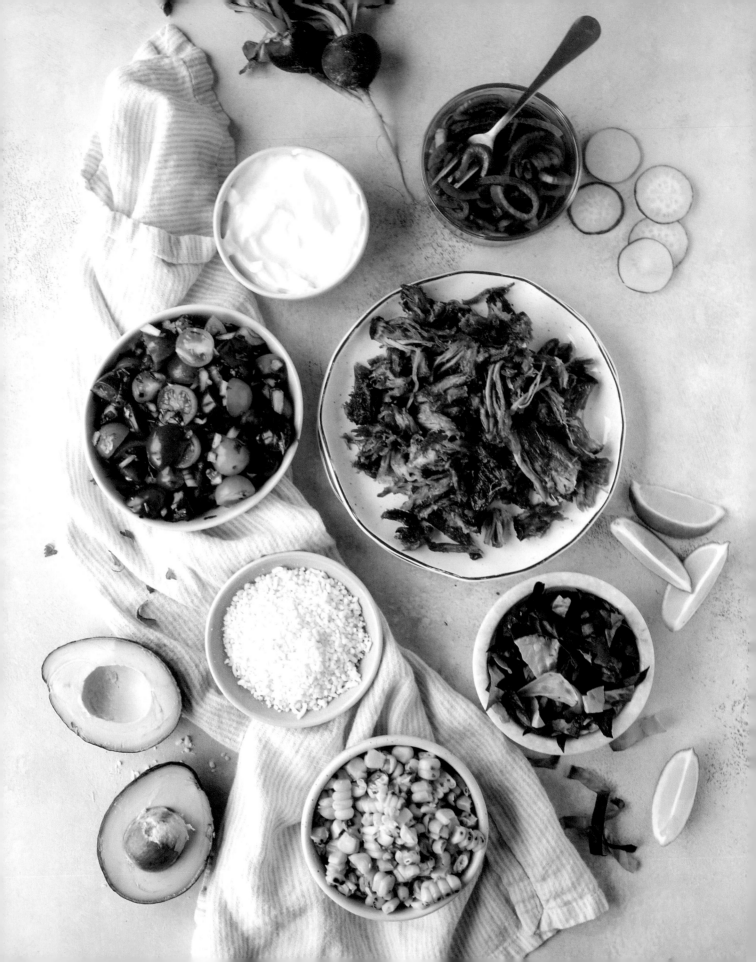

carnitas burrito bowls

I can turn anything Mexican-inspired into a meal, and that includes all forms of nachos and especially homemade guacamole. Give me a bowl of sliced avocado and a bag of chips, and I will be one happy girl. As I sit here pregnant with my second child, I can embarrassingly count the number of times that I considered guacamole and chips to be lunch, if only because nothing else sounded good.

Guac always sounds good.

The other thing that I'm always up for? Any and all forms of pulled pork, especially in a crispy carnitas bowl. This bowl is rice-less because when it comes to the bowls, the rice is my least favorite part. Don't get me wrong, I enjoy rice, but I love all the other aspects of the bowl so much more.

The pickled onions!

The corn salsa!

The quick pico!

The perfect sliced avocado!

Together, this makes what I can easily say is one of my favorite meals in this entire book. Leftovers can be stored for days, and you can have bowls on the fly! Just how I like it. Since this is a slow cooker meal, it will require a little more time to make, albeit mostly hands-off time. You can cook the pork overnight and place it in the fridge for the day or cook it while you are at work. **MAKES 4 SERVINGS (PLUS LEFTOVER PORK)**

PORK

1 tablespoon canola oil

1 pork shoulder roast (4 pounds)

1 teaspoon salt

1 teaspoon ground black pepper

6 ounces Mexican beer, such as Tecate or Corona

4 cloves garlic, minced

1 teaspoon smoked paprika

1 teaspoon chili powder

½ teaspoon ground cumin

CORN SALSA

1½ cups corn

½ red onion, diced

1 jalapeño chile pepper, diced

Juice of 1 lime

3 tablespoons chopped fresh cilantro

Salt and ground black pepper

TO MAKE THE PORK

In a large skillet, heat the oil over medium-high heat. Season the pork with the salt and black pepper and place it in the skillet, searing it on all sides. Transfer to a slower cooker and add the beer, garlic, paprika, chili powder, and cumin. Cover and cook on low for 8 to 10 hours.

TO MAKE THE CORN SALSA

In a bowl, combine the corn, onion, jalapeño pepper, lime juice, cilantro, and salt and black pepper to taste. Mix well.

TO MAKE THE QUICK PICO DE GALLO

In a bowl, combine the tomatoes, onion, cilantro, lime juice, and salt and black pepper to taste. Mix well.

TO MAKE THE PICKLED ONIONS

Place the onions in a jar or a cup. In a bowl, whisk together the vinegar, water, sugar, and salt until the sugar and salt dissolve. Pour over the sliced onions. Let sit at room temperature for an hour. You can make this ahead of time and once made, store it in the fridge in a sealed container or jar!

(continued)

QUICK PICO DE GALLO

1 cup cherry tomatoes, halved

½ red onion, diced

3 tablespoons chopped fresh cilantro

Juice of 1 lime

Salt and ground black pepper

PICKLED ONIONS

1 medium red onion, thinly sliced

¾ cup apple cider vinegar

⅓ cup water

1½ tablespoons sugar

1 teaspoon coarse salt

THE BASIC BOWL SETUP

2 cups shredded lettuce

2 avocados, thinly sliced

A few spoonfuls Pickled Onions

3 tablespoons cotija cheese

TOPPINGS (OPTIONAL)

Sliced scallions

Chopped fresh cilantro

Lime wedges

To assemble each bowl, place ½ cup of the lettuce on the bottom and top with 4 ounces or so of pork shoulder, about ⅓ cup pico de gallo, ⅓ cup corn salsa, one-quarter of the avocado, a few pickled onions, and a handful of cotija cheese. If desired, add scallions, cilantro, lime wedges, and sour cream or Greek yogurt.

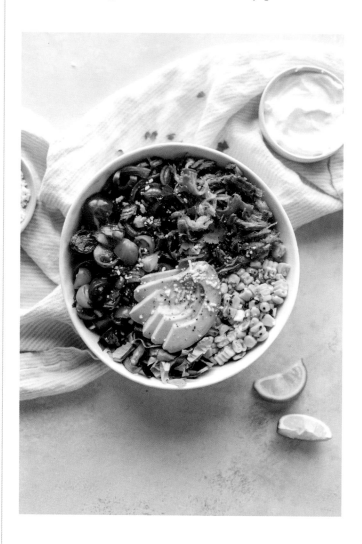

flank steak tacos

When it comes to using beef in my tacos, I'm partial to beef short ribs. They are my favorite cut; however, they can be difficult to find, it takes a good long while for them to cook, and it also requires a lot of ribs to feed a crowd.

So my go-to? Flank steak. Always.

That's probably because it's the cut of beef I grew up on. My dad would grill flank steak once or twice a month. In fact, he still does. We wouldn't eat it in tacos back then, but it's such an economical cut of beef and one that I find easy to cook, so it's what I use and slice for our soft tacos. When I was a kid, we'd eat it with potatoes or rice, and the next night, we'd have the leftovers on salads.

The key is the marinade! I like to marinate mine overnight, if possible. I broil it or grill it, which doesn't take long at all, and then let it rest for a good while. Slicing it against the grain yields a tender, easy-to-chew cut, and it's just lovely when piled high with Mexican corn.

Speaking of Mexican corn, this is my little take on elote (a Mexican street corn), in corn salad form. I season it with chili powder and toss it with a touch of queso fresco and some cilantro. This recipe is two of my favorite things combined: elote (well . . . sort of!) and steak tacos. Perfection.

MAKES 4 SERVINGS

(continued)

2 pounds flank steak (about 1" thick)

⅓ cup olive oil

1 teaspoon chili powder

½ teaspoon ground cumin

½ teaspoon salt

½ teaspoon ground black pepper

1 tablespoon brown sugar

Juice of 1 lime

4 cloves garlic, minced

Corn or flour tortillas

MEXICAN CORN

2 ears sweet corn

1 tablespoon olive oil

2 tablespoons unsalted butter, softened

½ teaspoon smoked paprika

½ teaspoon chili powder

¼ teaspoon salt

¼ teaspoon ground black pepper

⅓ cup crumbled queso fresco cheese

2 tablespoons finely chopped fresh cilantro

Place the flank steak in a large baking dish. In a bowl, whisk together the olive oil, chili powder, cumin, salt, pepper, brown sugar, lime juice, and garlic. Pour the marinade over the steak, turning to coat, and marinate in the fridge anywhere from 2 hours to overnight.

You can grill, broil, or pan sear the steak to your liking. I tend to broil it as I find that easiest. Preheat the broiler and move the oven rack as close as possible. Place the steak on a broiler pan or baking sheet and broil for 10 minutes, turning once, or until a thermometer inserted in the center registers 145°F for medium-rare.

Allow the steak to rest for 10 minutes before slicing it thinly against the grain.

TO MAKE THE MEXICAN CORN

Brush the ears with the olive oil. Place the ears on the grill and cook until the corn is golden or charred—whichever you prefer—turning the ears as you go. Remove them from the grill and let cool slightly. In a small bowl, stir together the butter, paprika, chili powder, salt, and pepper. Spread the mixture over the corn. Let it sit for a few more minutes before slicing the kernels from the cob into a bowl or plate. This helps keep the buttery flavor and seasonings with the corn. Toss the corn with the queso fresco and cilantro.

Assemble the tacos by charring the tortillas on the grill and adding the steak on top. Top with the Mexican corn and serve.

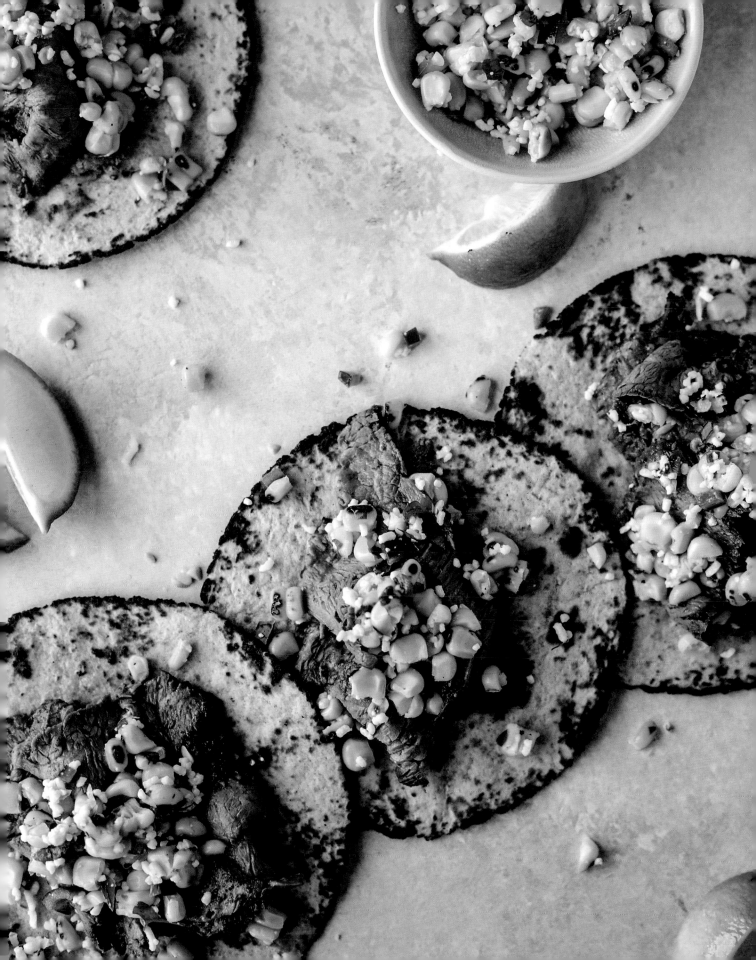

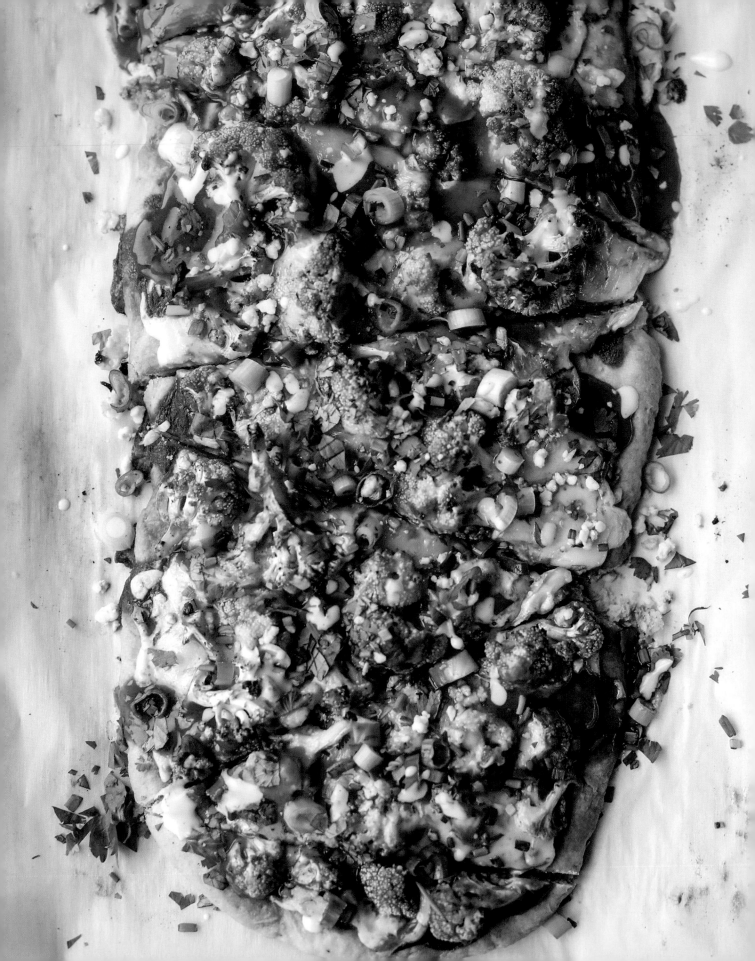

roasted buffalo cauliflower flatbread

If you're anything like Eddie, you're probably thinking, "But where is the chicken?!" Buffalo-inspired anything is not Buffalo to him unless it involves chicken. However, I am the weirdo who likes to order Buffalo chicken pizza, hold the chicken, and eat the dough that is covered is melty cheese and hot sauce.

So this is my answer to that. With cauliflower all the rage these days, I actually get excited about it. I enjoy cauliflower when it's roasted; I find that it almost takes on the flavor of popcorn. I don't even miss the chicken; heck, I don't even notice it isn't there.

For readers of my blog, you know how much we love Buffalo-inspired recipes. The combination of cheeses, sauce, chives, scallions, and cilantro here is what I feel makes the Buffalo flavor for me. If I don't have all of these things, the flavor is not complete. It's spicy but a bit refreshing with the herbs. Exactly how I want it! **MAKES 2 SERVINGS**

BUFFALO CAULIFLOWER

- 1 cup Buffalo wing sauce
- 3 tablespoons unsalted butter
- 1 head cauliflower, cut into florets
- 2 tablespoons olive oil
- ½ teaspoon salt
- ¼ teaspoon ground black pepper

FLATBREAD

- 2 cups all-purpose flour
- 1 teaspoon baking powder
- ½ teaspoon salt
- ⅔ cup water
- ⅓ cup olive oil + more for brushing

- 8 ounces fontina cheese, freshly grated, divided
- 4 ounces Gorgonzola cheese, crumbled, divided
- 3 tablespoons ranch dressing
- 2 scallions, thinly sliced
- 2 tablespoons chopped fresh chives
- 1 bunch fresh cilantro, chopped

TO MAKE THE BUFFALO CAULIFLOWER

In a saucepan, heat the wing sauce and butter over low heat until the butter is melted. Set aside.

Preheat the oven to 400°F. Line a baking sheet with foil and place the cauliflower florets on the sheet. Drizzle with the olive oil, salt, and pepper. Toss well. Toss with ½ cup of the wing sauce mixture. Roast for 20 to 25 minutes, or until golden.

Increase the heat to 450°F.

TO MAKE THE FLATBREAD

In a bowl, combine the flour, baking powder, and salt, stirring to mix. Add the water and olive oil and mix with a spoon until the dough comes together. Use your hands to finish bringing it together into a ball, then knead it a few times on a floured surface. Form the dough into your desired shape. Place it on a nonstick (or parchment-lined) baking sheet and brush with a bit of olive oil. Bake for 10 minutes, or until a few air bubbles form and the dough is golden.

Cover the flatbread with half of the cheeses. Drizzle with the ranch dressing. Add the cauliflower and top with the rest of the cheeses. Drizzle with the remaining wing sauce mixture. Bake for 10 to 15 minutes, or until the cheese is melted, bubbly, and golden. Let cool for a few minutes, then top with the scallions, chives, and cilantro.

korean beef bowls

Another day, another bowl! If you love Asian-inspired flavors like I do, this bowl will probably become your new favorite dinner. This time, the bowl features thinly sliced, tender and flavorful beef with fluffy rice and spiralized carrots.

Oh, and I should definitely mention that it's not like you need to eat these ingredients piled together in a bowl. You can absolutely plate them separately, especially if you're not into your food touching. I get it! I totally do. **MAKES 2 SERVINGS**

1   pound sirloin beef, thinly sliced

1   tablespoon all-purpose flour

2   tablespoons brown sugar

2   tablespoons low-sodium soy sauce

1   tablespoon toasted sesame oil

2   cloves garlic, minced

¼   teaspoon grated fresh ginger

Pinch of crushed red-pepper flakes

1   tablespoon vegetable oil

1½ cups cooked jasmine rice

2   large carrots, peeled and
    spiralized (see note)

1   scallion, thinly sliced

1   teaspoon toasted sesame seeds

Toss the beef with the flour. In a bowl, whisk together the sugar, soy sauce, sesame oil, garlic, ginger, and red-pepper flakes.

In a large skillet, heat the vegetable oil over high heat. Add the beef and cook for 1 minute, searing until golden brown. Turn the beef pieces and cook for 1 minute. Reduce the heat to medium and pour in the sauce. Cook, tossing constantly, for 1 to 2 minutes. Pour the beef and any extra sauce in a bowl.

To assemble the bowls, divide the rice and carrots between 2 bowls. Top with the beef, then add the scallion and a sprinkle of sesame seeds. If desired, you can add another drizzle of toasted sesame oil.

NOTE: If you don't have a spiralizer, you can use a vegetable peeler to peel large "ribbons" of carrot!

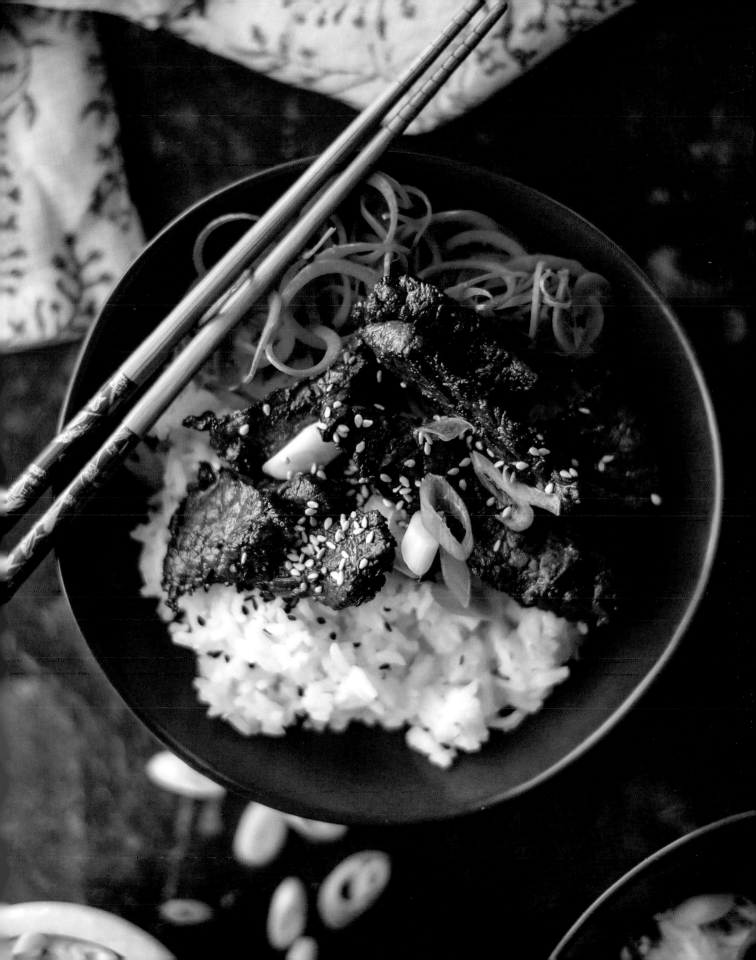

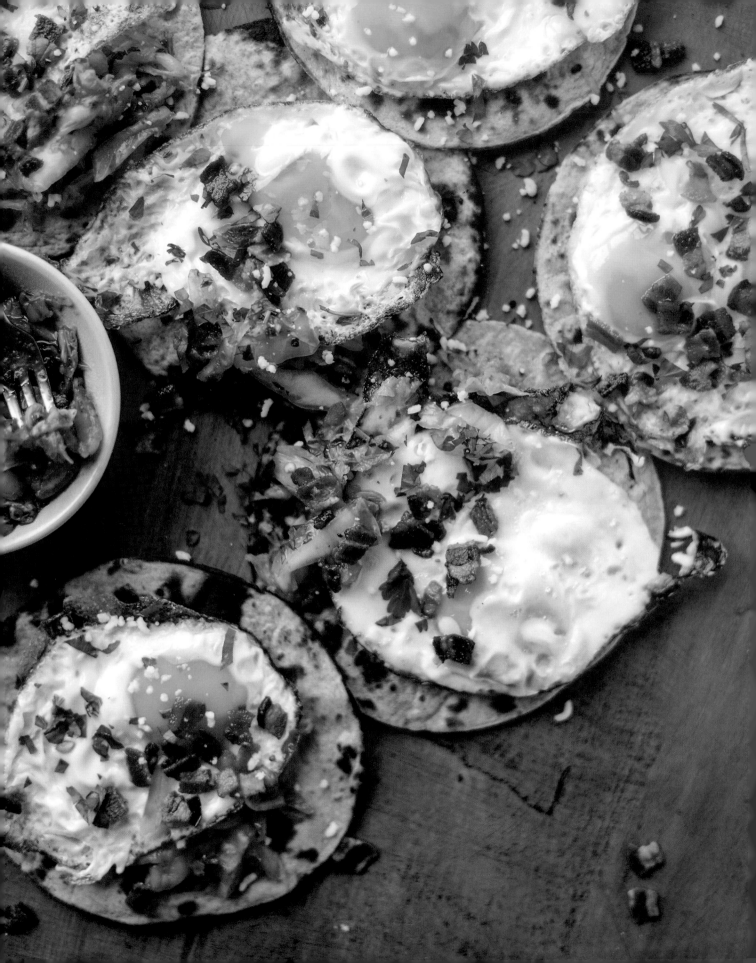

bacon, egg, and kimchi tacos

While I love a good breakfast taco, I actually eat them more in the morning with scrambled eggs, avocado, and occasionally, potatoes. It seems ridiculous, but if you're adding a fried egg to my taco? Oh heck, it's lunch! Or dinner.

The bacon and egg are a given here. Runny yolk, crunchy bacon. The star of the show, obviously, is the kimchi. It's unexpected and crunchy.

People either love or hate kimchi. For me, it's an easy love. With my infatuation for all things briny, vinegary, and pickled, it would be weird if I didn't enjoy it. I've tried my hand at making it myself, but I just cannot replicate that authentic flavor, probably since it's not in my blood. I don't have the magic touch! I find my kimchi from a local vendor here in Pittsburgh, and the flavor is unbeatable.

And finally, while it may be a little frowned upon, I still love some queso fresco on top of my kimchi tacos! It pulls the ingredients together and adds that little bit of creaminess to offset the crunchy tang. Deeeeelish.   MAKES 2 SERVINGS

2   tablespoons unsalted butter, divided

4   large eggs

1   avocado, thinly sliced

4   corn or flour tortillas (4" diameter), heated or at room temperature

½   cup kimchi

4   slices bacon, cooked

1   scallion, thinly sliced

¼   cup chopped fresh cilantro

¼   cup salsa, for topping

¼   cup crumbled queso fresco cheese

In a large nonstick skillet, melt 1 tablespoon of the butter over medium-low heat. In a bowl, lightly beat the eggs until just combined. Pour the eggs in the skillet and cook, stirring and tossing. Right before they firm up, stir in the remaining 1 tablespoon butter and toss until it's incorporated into the scrambled eggs.

To assemble the tacos, divide the avocado among the tortillas. Top with the eggs, kimchi, bacon, scallion, cilantro, salsa, and queso fresco.

jalapeño butternut squash tacos

One more taco, then I'll leave you alone! I think. I hope. But probably not.

I don't need meat in my tacos. One of the best tacos I've ever had was full of wild mushrooms and sweet corn, topped with avocado and a chipotle crema. It was fantastic. Then the taco joint went out of business, and I cried a long, hard tear.

While squash doesn't necessarily impart a meaty texture like mushrooms can, I find that roasted squash cubes (in this case, spicy ones!) can work perfectly in tacos as long as there is some other texture to work against the soft squash. Black beans and crunchy cabbage do that for us here in these tacos, along with fresh jalapeños. Heat and sweet! The combination is lovely. MAKES 2 TO 4 SERVINGS

LIME CREMA

- 3 tablespoons full-fat or 2% plain Greek yogurt
- ¾ cup half-and-half
- 1 tablespoon adobo sauce (from a can of chipotles in adobo)
- Grated zest and juice of ½ lime
- ⅛ teaspoon salt

TACOS

- 3 tablespoons coconut oil, melted
- 3 tablespoons brown sugar
- 1 teaspoon chili garlic paste
- 2 cups cubed butternut squash
- ¼ teaspoon salt
- ¼ teaspoon ground black pepper
- Corn tortillas (4" diameter), warmed or at room temperature

TOPPINGS

Sliced red cabbage

Black beans

Sliced avocado

Sliced jalapeño chile peppers

Crumbled queso fresco

TO MAKE THE LIME CREMA

In a bowl, whisk together the yogurt, half-and-half, adobo sauce, lime zest and juice, and salt until combined. Set aside.

TO MAKE THE TACOS

Preheat the oven to 400°F. In a small bowl, whisk together the coconut oil, sugar, and chili garlic paste.

Place the squash on a baking sheet and pour the mixture over top. Season with the salt and pepper and toss well to coat. Roast for 40 minutes, tossing a bit halfway through.

Assemble the tacos by filling the tortillas with the squash. Top with the cabbage, black beans, avocado, jalapeños, and queso fresco. Top with the lime crema!

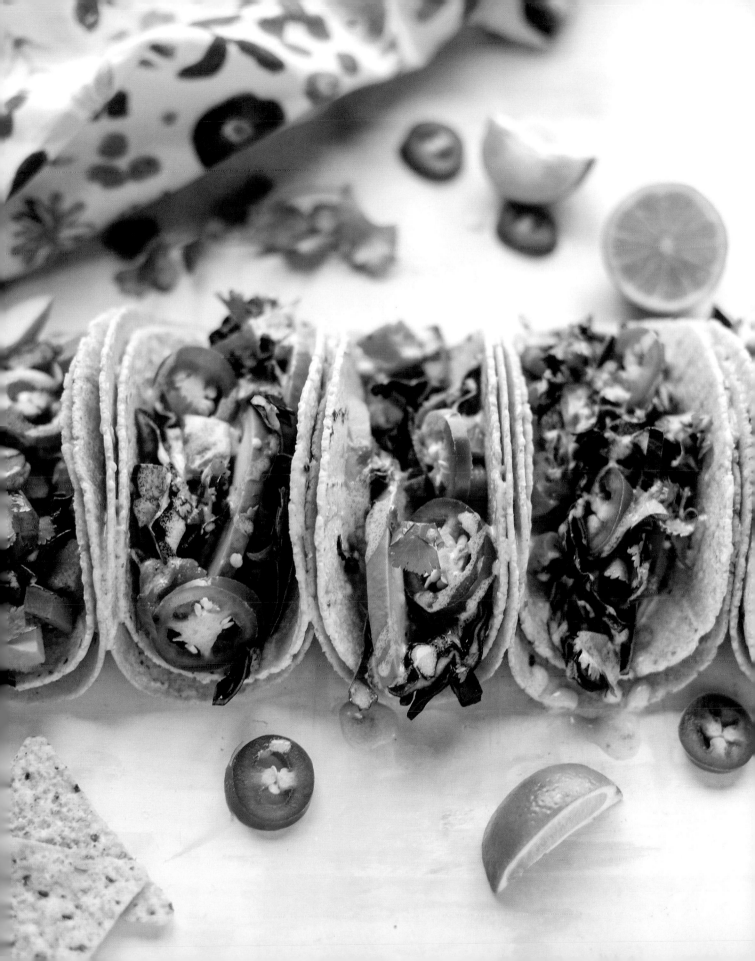

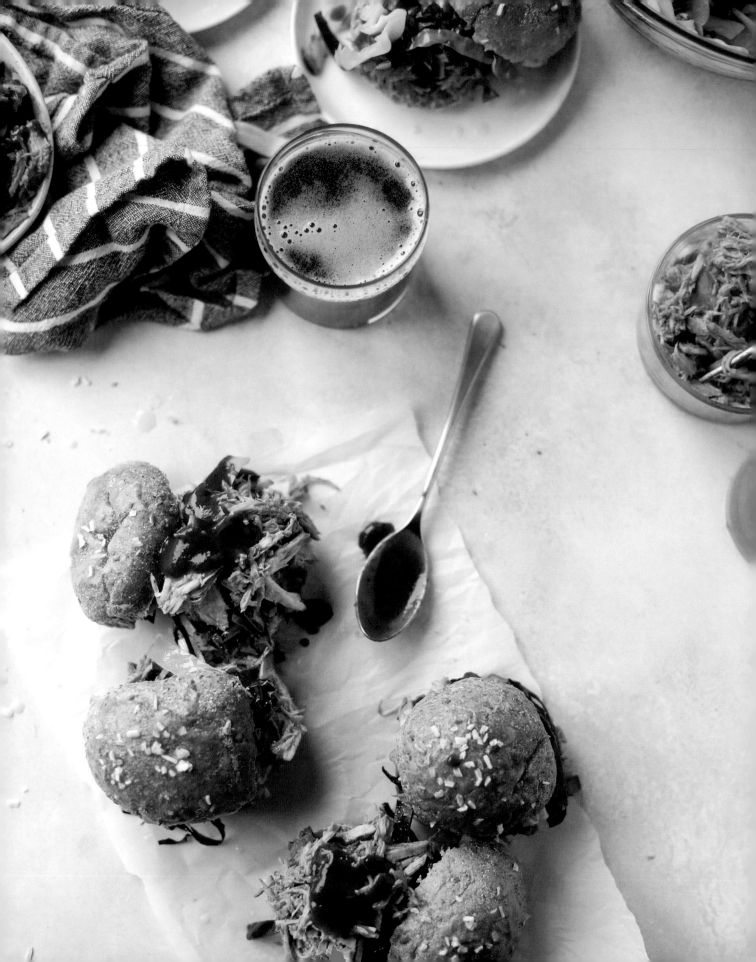

apple cider pulled pork sliders

This slow cooker pulled pork breaks our 60-minute meal rule, but the prep won't take that long, and I promise it will be worth it. After eight hours of downtime cooking, you will be thrilled to have this delicious, slightly apple-spiced pork in your house.

This pork can be used any way you like. It is perfect for game day to serve to a crowd, sandwiched in between kaiser rolls or buns. I'm partial to sliders, as you see here. It's also great when piled high on mashed sweet potatoes or mashed squash, for one of those stick-to-your-bones meals. And my favorite part? The slaw topping. Cold, crunchy slaw on top of hot pulled pork just works together. There is nothing I love more for a garnish. It's a lovely, refreshing crisp take on an otherwise heavy dish. MAKES 6 TO 8 SERVINGS

PORK

1 pork shoulder roast (4 pounds)
2 teaspoons coarse salt
½ teaspoon ground black pepper
2 tablespoons grapeseed or canola oil
1 tablespoon liquid smoke
4 cloves garlic, minced
½ cup apple cider

SLAW

1 cup shredded red cabbage
1 cup shredded Napa cabbage
⅓ cup shredded carrots
¼ cup chopped fresh cilantro
1 tablespoon extra-virgin olive oil
1 teaspoon apple cider vinegar
Juice of 1 lime
Pinch of salt and ground black pepper

APPLE CIDER BARBECUE SAUCE

⅔ cup ketchup
⅔ cup apple cider
½ cup honey
3 cloves garlic, minced
5 tablespoons apple cider vinegar
2 tablespoons Dijon mustard
1 teaspoon Worcestershire sauce
½ teaspoon onion powder
½ teaspoon smoked paprika
¼ teaspoon ground black pepper

FOR SERVING

Slider buns or dinner rolls
8 slices Havarti cheese

TO MAKE THE PORK

Season the pork with the salt and pepper. In a large skillet or pot, heat the oil over medium-high heat. (If you have a slow cooker that sears meat for you, do it in the slow cooker!) Add the pork and sear on all sides until deeply golden brown.

Place the pork shoulder in the slow cooker and cover it with the liquid smoke, turning a few times to coat. Add the garlic and apple cider. Cover and cook on low for 8 to 10 hours. After 8 to 10 hours, the pork will easily shred with a fork.

TO MAKE THE SLAW

In a bowl, combine the cabbages, carrots, and cilantro and toss. Drizzle the olive oil and vinegar over the top. Add the lime juice. Toss well. Season with the salt and pepper and toss again.

TO MAKE THE APPLE CIDER BARBECUE SAUCE

In a saucepan, whisk together the ketchup, apple cider, honey, garlic, vinegar, mustard, Worcestershire, onion powder, paprika, and pepper until combined. Bring to a boil over medium heat, then reduce the heat to low and cook, stirring occasionally, for 30 to 60 minutes, or until thickened. Let sit at room temperature until it cools and thickens even more.

Store leftovers in a jar or sealed container in the fridge.

To assemble the sliders, top the bottom of the buns with the shredded pork. Add a slice of cheese, barbecue sauce, and slaw!

lobster burrata pasta

I feel like this dish needs no explanation.
    Butter- and garlic-soaked lobster tails.
    Creamy burrata cheese.
    Warm, fresh pasta.
    Bright herbs on top.
    This is a special meal that needs no introductions or justifications. It's indulgent, it's soul warming, it tastes like heaven. MAKES 4 SERVINGS

1   pound pasta

2   large lobster tails

¼   teaspoon salt

¼   teaspoon ground black pepper

¼   cup unsalted butter

1   tablespoon olive oil

4   cloves garlic, minced

½   cup dry white wine

2   balls (8 ounces each) burrata cheese

¼   cup finely grated Parmesan cheese

Handful fresh herbs (such as oregano, basil, and parsley)

Bring a large pot of salted water to a boil and prepare the pasta according to the package directions. While the water is heating up, start the lobster.

Season the lobster with the salt and pepper. In a large skillet, heat the butter and olive oil over medium heat. Let it melt; it's even okay if it starts to brown slightly, but don't let it come close to browning all the way!

Add the lobster tails and cook for 6 to 8 minutes, turning a few times, or until they are opaque. Add the garlic. Add in the wine and let it simmer until it's reduced by about half. Turn off the heat.

Add the cooked pasta to the skillet (if your skillet is too small, you can throw everything in a large bowl!) and toss well. Add the burrata, pulling the balls of cheese apart, and toss well to distribute the cheese. Top with the Parmesan and herbs. Slice the lobster tails in half. Serve immediately.

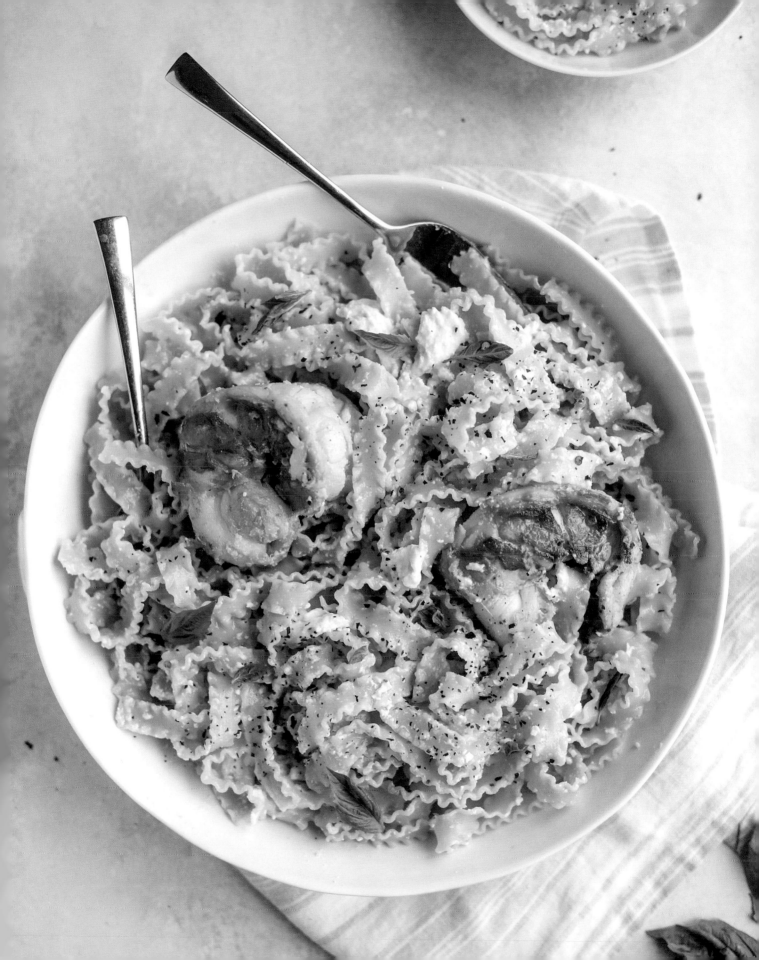

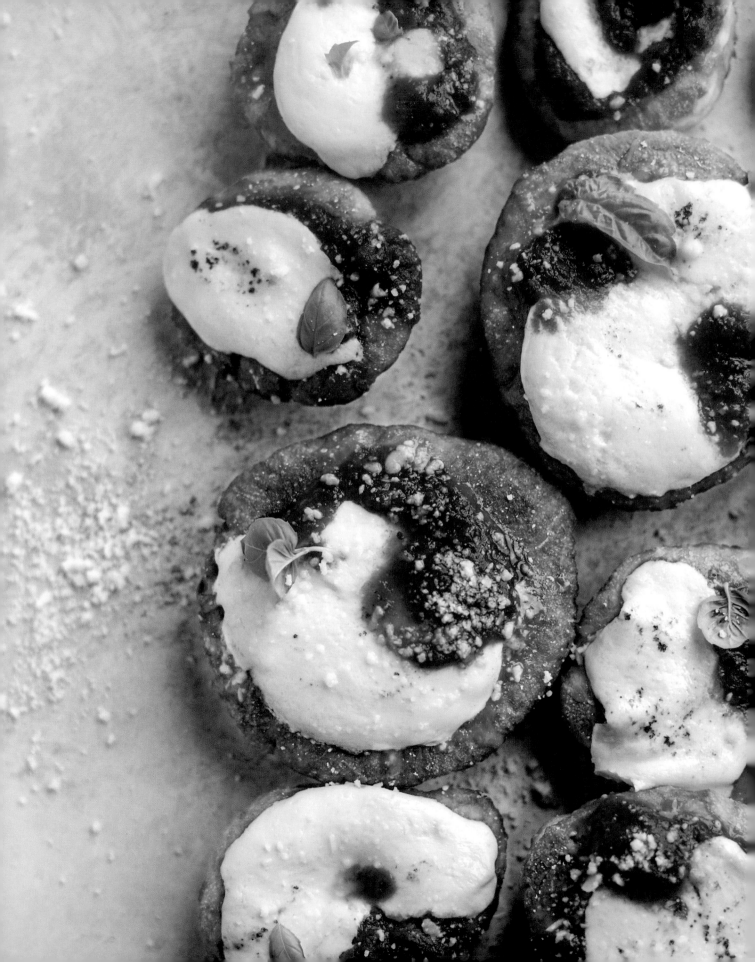

fried margherita pizzas

I almost want to tell you that these are pizza doughnuts. They aren't . . . but they sort of look like it, right?

What they are, are tiny pieces of pizza dough, fried until golden and puffy and topped with fresh mozzarella, tomato sauce, and a basil leaf for good measure. Essentially, margherita pizza doughnuts.

I know. Let's make them a thing!

These are wonderfully doughy and cheesy. A pizza lover's dream. A neat little change of pace for pizza fiends and a snack that kids go absolutely crazy over.

I have to credit my friend Giuliana for this recipe, as she has made her own perfect version of pizza fritta that I so often try to copy at home. They are an indulgent treat, but oddly enough, the dough remains light. Like a pizza funnel cake!

Now isn't that what we all want to consume. Pizza funnel cake. Oh, my goodness. MAKES 4 TO 6 SERVINGS

1⅛ cups warm water

1 tablespoon active dry yeast

1 tablespoon honey

1 tablespoon olive oil

3 cups all-purpose flour, divided

1 teaspoon salt

2 cups canola or vegetable oil, for frying

FOR TOPPING

2 cups tomato sauce

2 balls (8 ounces each) fresh mozzarella cheese, sliced

Fresh basil, for topping

In a large bowl, combine the water, yeast, honey, and olive oil. Mix with a spoon, then let sit until foamy, about 10 minutes. Add in 2½ cups of the flour and the salt, stirring with a spoon until the dough comes together but is still sticky. Using your hands, form the dough into a ball and work in the remaining ½ cup flour, kneading it on a floured surface for a few minutes. Rub the same bowl with olive oil and then place the dough inside, turning to coat. Cover with a towel and place in a warm place to rise for about 1 to 1½ hours, or until it has doubled in size.

After the dough has risen, punch it down and place it back on the floured surface. Using a rolling pin or your hands, form it into 6 mini personal pan pizza crusts.

In a pot or heavy skillet, heat the canola or vegetable oil over medium heat until it reaches 350°F. Add the pizza dough in batches and fry until golden brown on 1 side, then turn and fry for 2 to 3 minutes, or until golden on the other side. Repeat with the remaining dough. Immediately cover the fried crusts with the tomato sauce, cheese, and the basil.

summer garden pizza

Crunchy kale, sweet corn, and burst tomatoes are what should be on all of our pizzas this summer. It's a garden on our pizza, and I'm going to enjoy every bite.

Ricotta lightens up the cheese situation here, along with a touch of mozzarella for meltiness. Garlic and herbs finish it off (garlic butter crust might be my favorite thing, forever), and each bite is full of flavor. Just how it should be. MAKES 4 SERVINGS

CRUST

1⅛ cups warm water

1 tablespoon active dry yeast

1 tablespoon honey

1 tablespoon olive oil

3 cups all-purpose flour, divided

1 teaspoon salt

PIZZA

1 head kale, stems removed

¼ cup grated Parmesan cheese

2 tablespoons olive oil, divided

⅔ cup full-fat ricotta cheese

8 ounces mozzarella cheese, freshly grated

1 cup grape tomatoes, halved

2 ears sweet corn, cut from the cob

Fresh herbs, such as oregano, basil, or cilantro, for topping

GARLIC BUTTER

2 tablespoons unsalted butter

1 minced clove garlic

TO MAKE THE CRUST

In a large bowl, combine the water, yeast, honey, and olive oil. Mix with a spoon, then let sit until foamy, about 10 minutes. Add in 2½ cups of the flour and the salt, stirring with a spoon until the dough comes together but is still sticky. Using your hands, form the dough into a ball and work in the remaining ½ cup flour, kneading it on a floured surface for a few minutes. Rub the same bowl with olive oil and then place the dough inside, turning to coat. Cover with a towel and place in a warm place to rise for about 1 to 1½ hours, or until it has doubled in size.

After the dough has risen, punch it down and place it back on the floured surface. Using a rolling pin or your hands, form it into your desired shape and place on a baking sheet or pizza peel that's covered with a little bit of cornmeal. Place the towel back over the dough and let it sit in the warm place for 10 minutes.

Preheat the oven to 350°F.

TO MAKE THE PIZZA

Cut the kale into slices and place in a bowl. Add the Parmesan and 1 tablespoon of the olive oil and toss well to coat. Place on a baking sheet and roast for 20 minutes, tossing halfway through the cooking time.

Increase the oven temperature to 450°F.

Brush the pizza dough with the remaining 1 tablespoon olive oil. Top with the ricotta and half of the mozzarella. Add the tomatoes, crispy kale, and corn. Add the remaining mozzarella. Bake for 20 to 25 minutes, or until the pizza crust is golden and the cheese is bubbly.

TO MAKE THE GARLIC BUTTER

In a small bowl, stir together the butter and garlic.

When the pizza is finished baking, brush the crust with the garlic butter. Sprinkle with the herbs, slice, and serve!

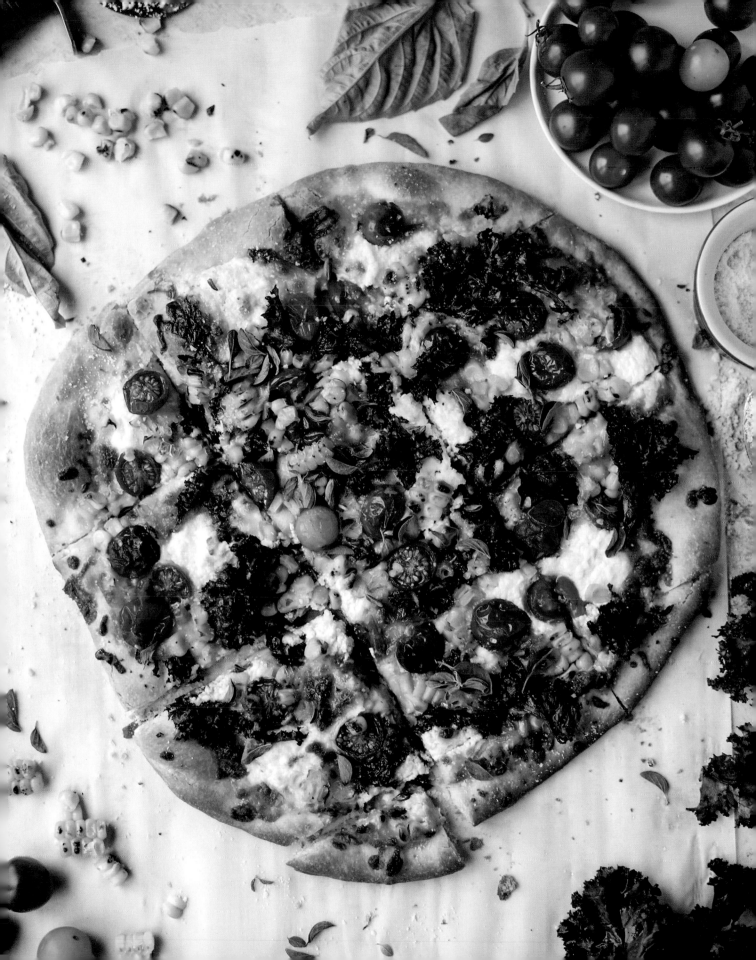

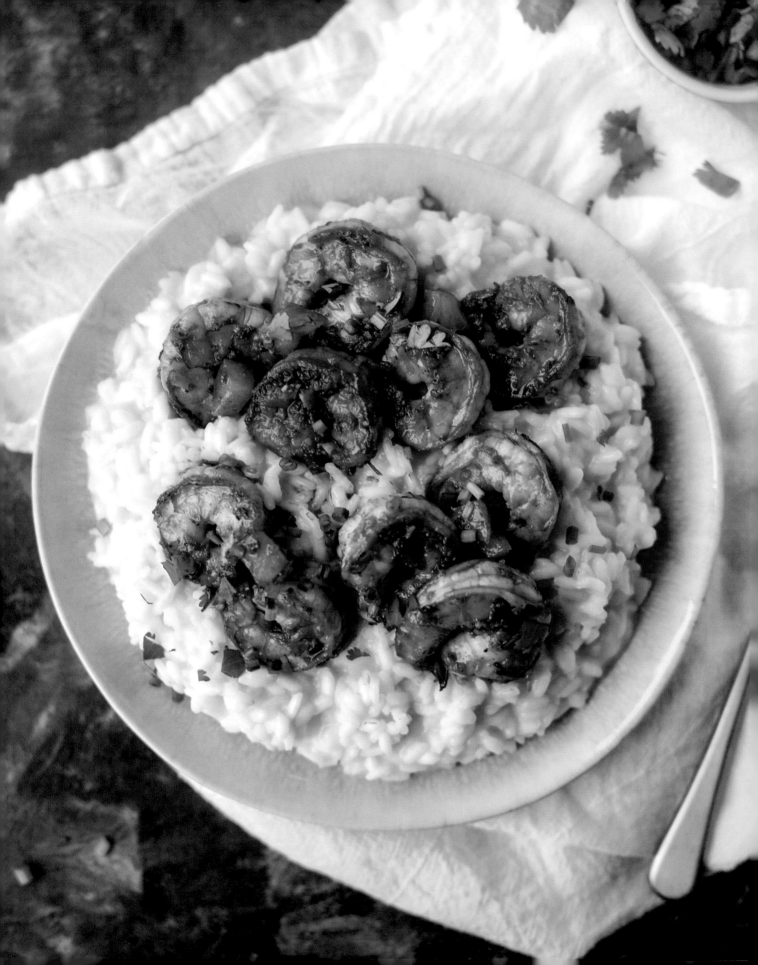

coconut risotto

WITH PINEAPPLE CHILI SHRIMP

A change of pace on comfort food, this risotto is made with coconut milk and is super creamy. It almost reminds me of rice pudding, but it's still a bit too savory for that, especially when topped with the spicy pineapple shrimp!

Chili garlic paste is one condiment that is always in our fridge. It's so flavorful and full of heat, and I love to blend it with fresh pineapple for a quick shrimp marinade. You should be able to find it in the Asian section of your grocery store. The pineapple juice caramelizes a bit on the shrimp when cooked, and the whole bowl is a mess of creamy, spicy, and sweet flavors. MAKES 2 TO 4 SERVINGS

1   cup cubed fresh pineapple

1   teaspoon chili garlic paste

1   pound raw peeled and deveined medium shrimp

3   tablespoons coconut oil, divided

1½ cups Arborio rice

3   cloves garlic, minced

½   teaspoon grated fresh ginger

1   cup dry white wine

4   cups (1 quart) low-sodium vegetable stock, warmed, divided

1   can full-fat coconut milk

Chopped fresh cilantro, for topping

In a food processor, combine the pineapple and chili garlic paste. Blend until smooth. Place the shrimp in a shallow dish and pour the pineapple mixture over it. Marinate in the refrigerator for 15 to 20 minutes—no longer.

Meanwhile, in a large saucepan, heat 2 tablespoons of the coconut oil over medium-low heat. Add the rice and toast, stirring often, for 5 minutes, or until it's somewhat translucent. Stir in the garlic and ginger and cook for another minute. Add the wine and stir constantly until it's absorbed. Add in 1½ cups of the stock and stir very frequently until the rice absorbs all of it. Repeat this 2 or 3 more times, until all of the stock has been added and the rice is al dente. You want it to appear "hydrated" and also want there to be some liquid left when serving. This process should take about 15 to 20 minutes. Finish by adding the coconut milk and stirring until most of it is absorbed.

In a large skillet, heat the remaining 1 tablespoon coconut oil over medium heat. Remove the shrimp from the marinade and cook for 2 to 3 minutes, turning once, or until opaque. Top with the cilantro.

To serve, scoop the risotto into a bowl and add the shrimp on top. Delicious!

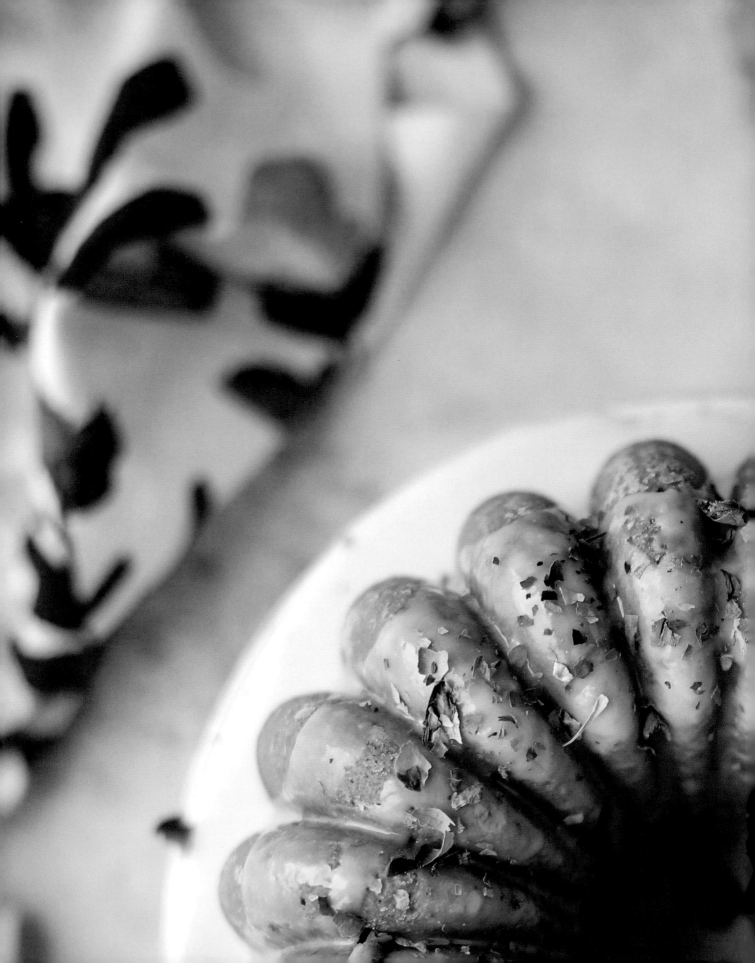

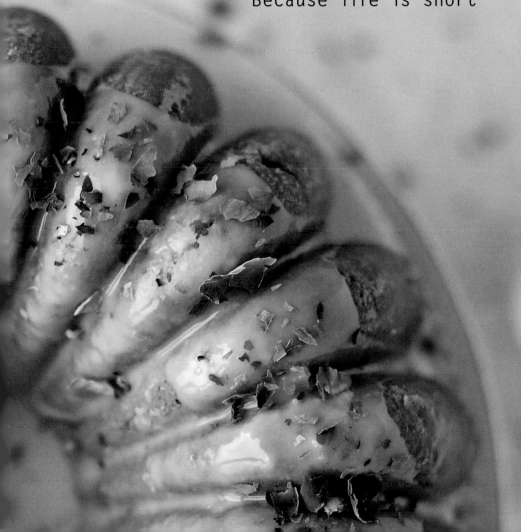

chapter 4

eat dessert first

Because life is short

WHILE I LOVE TO EAT AND INDULGE IN desserts, they aren't my favorite type of recipes to whip up in the kitchen. I much prefer to cook savory ingredients where a recipe is lightly followed or, let's be honest, not followed at all. I have rebellion syndrome, where the moment I am told that I *have* to do something, I automatically do not want to do it. It doesn't mean that I *won't* do it; I'm not that much of a brat. But it means that it may not be as enjoyable for me as it would have been if I could improvise mid-project.

And when I say mid-project, I mean during the process of recipe development. Recipes that require lots and lots of instruction just aren't my jam. You feel me?

There are some recipes that I have to make an exception for because they are just so fantastic every time. I also love to have dessert at my home when we have guests. I totally want to be that house that always has fresh-baked cookies in a cookie jar when people stop over, but I don't think I could ever be that house because Eddie and I would know that the cookies are there. And we would probably eat them all. Ourselves! In a matter of days . . . or hours.

Still, I'm always on the search for that signature dessert—an easy baked good that year after year, people will know me by. This doesn't bode well for my millennial brain, which always wants to try new things, every single day.

But I'm not giving up! In this chapter you will find my favorite celebration desserts, as well as some delicious staples (hello, Autumn Monster Cookies!).

lemon cupcakes
WITH MOJITO FROSTING

It took me a while to get into lemon desserts, but once I did, I was sold. This is how I view the light and citrusy treats:

I'm either in a chocolate mood or I'm in a lemon mood. And that's that. If I don't want something super rich and decadent? Something indulgent and fudgy? Then I want something lemon. It just feels lighter and is bright and happy. I mean, who doesn't want to eat something bright and happy?

These fluffy lemon cupcakes are piled high with mojito frosting, meaning fresh lime and—better yet—rum! Mojito buttercream might not be a cocktail, but it's pretty darn close. **MAKES 12**

1½ cups cake flour

1   teaspoon baking powder

¼   teaspoon salt

½   cup unsalted butter, at room temperature

1   cup sugar

1   large egg + 1 large egg white

2   tablespoons vegetable oil

1   tablespoon freshly grated lemon zest

1   teaspoon vanilla extract

½   teaspoon pure lemon extract

½   cup whole milk

MOJITO FROSTING

½   cup unsalted butter, at room temperature

½   cup cream cheese, at room temperature

2½ cups powdered sugar

1   teaspoon vanilla extract

1   teaspoon freshly grated lime zest

2   teaspoons rum

Fresh mint leaves, for garnish

Preheat the oven to 350°F. Place paper liners in a 12-cup muffin pan.

In a small bowl, whisk together the flour, baking powder, and salt.

In the bowl of an electric stand mixer, beat the butter until creamy. Add the sugar and beat for 3 to 4 minutes, or until light and fluffy. Add the egg and egg white, beating on medium speed until combined. Add the oil, lemon zest, vanilla, and lemon extract and beat for 1 to 2 minutes, or until combined. With the mixer on low speed, add half of the dry ingredients. Pour in the milk with the mixer on and mix to combine. Pour in the rest of the dry ingredients and mix on medium speed until the batter is combined.

Fill the cupcake liners three-quarters of the way full. Place the pan on a baking sheet and bake for 16 to 18 minutes, or until golden on top and set in the center. Let cool completely before frosting.

TO MAKE THE MOJITO FROSTING

In the bowl of an electric stand mixer fitted with the paddle attachment, combine the butter and cream cheese and beat until creamy. With the mixer on low speed, gradually add the powdered sugar. Increase the speed of the mixer and beat the frosting, scraping down the sides of the bowl as needed, until fluffy and combined. Beat in the vanilla, lime zest, and rum.

Frost the cupcakes and garnish with the fresh mint.

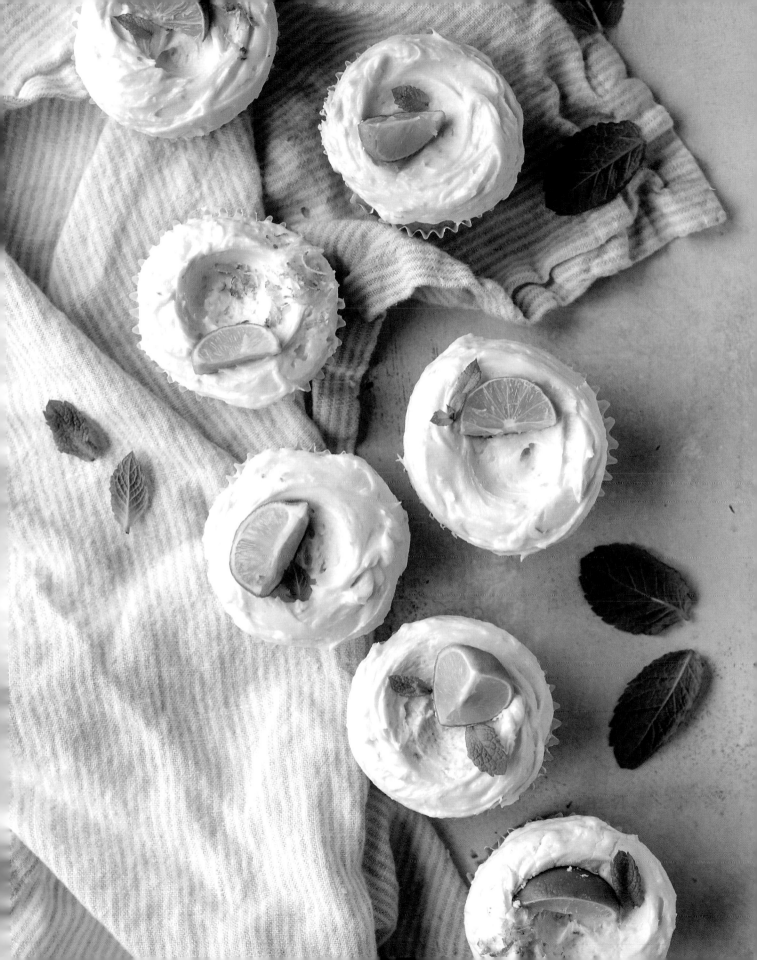

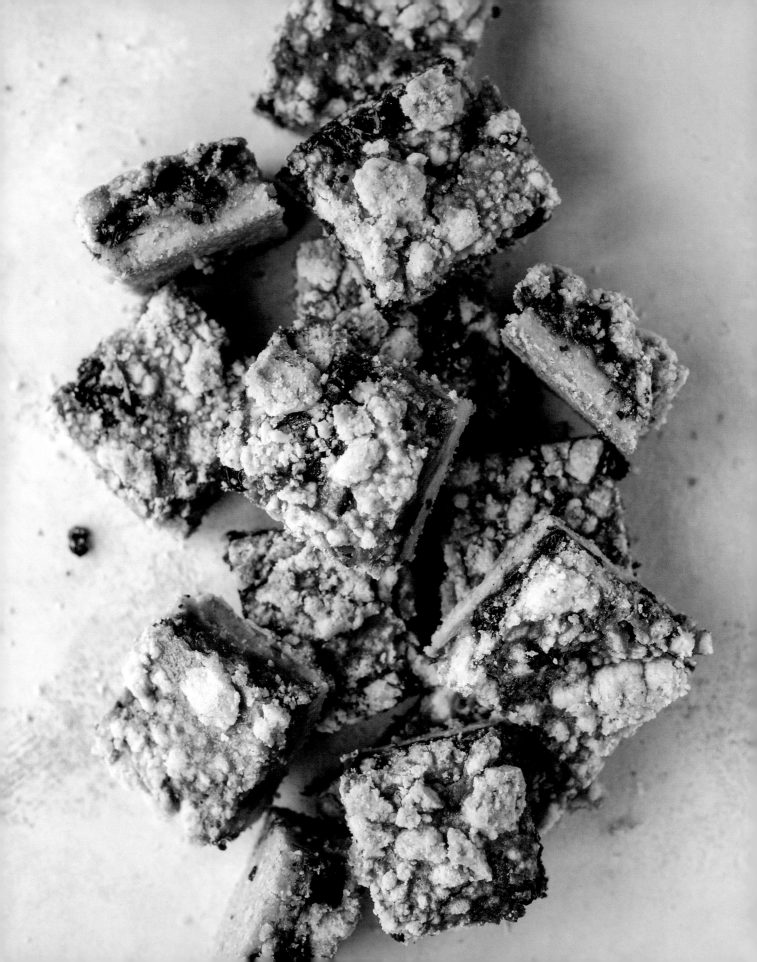

blueberry peach cobbler bars

My mom made peach cobbler only a handful of times when I was a kid, and even though the recipe came from a box (I know! Blasphemy!), I still remember just how much I enjoyed it. It was so fabulous right out of the oven, piled high with ice cream. It's one dessert I will never forget her making . . . ever.

Since I write a food blog and am always looking for the next best thing, I have tested a lot of cobbler recipes with many different fruits. I adore the combination of peaches and blueberries (which also happens to be one of my favorite pies!) and wanted to make a bite-size bar that was an easy grab-and-go treat. It also makes for a great summer dessert that you can bake the night before and take to a party. Huge hit all around. MAKES 16

CRUST AND TOPPING

3   cups all-purpose flour

1   cup granulated sugar

½   teaspoon salt

¾   cup unsalted butter, melted

FILLING

3   large eggs

⅓   cup half-and-half

1   cup firmly packed brown sugar

1   tablespoon cornstarch

1   teaspoon vanilla extract

¼   teaspoon ground cinnamon

Pinch of salt

2   cups fresh blueberries

1   cup chopped fresh peaches

Preheat the oven to 350°F. Spray a 13" x 9" baking dish with cooking spray.

TO MAKE THE CRUST AND TOPPING
In a large bowl, stir together the flour, granulated sugar, and salt. Add the butter and stir until a shortbread-like dough comes together. Press half of the dough into the bottom of the baking dish.

TO MAKE THE FILLING
In another bowl, whisk together the eggs, half-and-half, brown sugar, cornstarch, vanilla, cinnamon, and salt. Gently fold in the blueberries and peaches.

Pour the mixture over the crust and spread evenly. Crumble the rest of the dough over the blueberry mixture. Bake for 40 to 45 minutes, or until the bars are set and no longer jiggly. Cool completely before slicing into squares!

chai latte cheesecake

I'm not so much a fan of actual chai lattes. It's the truth. But chai-flavored treats? Count me way in.

It's also of note to mention that my all-time favorite dessert, like last-meal style, is cheesecake. It's so rich and creamy. I will pick it over a brownie or cookie any day, and homemade always wins the game.

That's why I have been dying to tell you about this chai latte cheesecake. There is a touch of espresso powder in here for just the teeeeeniest hint of coffee flavor, but the main flavor is chai spice. Cinnamon and ginger and cardamom combined with that lovely creamy texture and a cookie crust.

There really is no reason not to make it! **MAKES 8 SERVINGS**

CRUST

- 2 cups crushed gingersnaps
- 6 tablespoons unsalted butter, melted

FILLING

- 4 packages (8 ounces each) cream cheese, softened
- 1 cup sugar
- 1½ teaspoons ground ginger
- 1 teaspoon ground cinnamon
- 1 teaspoon instant espresso powder + additional, for sprinkling
- ½ teaspoon ground cardamom
- ½ teaspoon ground allspice
- 2 teaspoons vanilla extract
- 3 large eggs

Preheat the oven to 350°F.

TO MAKE THE CRUST

In a bowl, stir together the gingersnap crumbs and butter. Press the mixture into a 9" springform pan. Bake for 5 to 6 minutes, or until just slightly set. Let cool completely.

TO MAKE THE FILLING

In the bowl of an electric stand mixer, beat the cream cheese until smooth and creamy. Add the sugar, ginger, cinnamon, espresso powder, cardamom, and allspice. Beat on medium speed, scraping down the sides of the bowl as needed, for 1 to 2 minutes, or until combined and fluffy. Beat in the vanilla, then beat in the eggs 1 at a time until just combined. Pour the mixture into the crust, smoothing out the top. Place the pan on a baking sheet.

Bake for 50 to 55 minutes, or until the center is almost set. Let cool completely. Refrigerate overnight. When ready to serve, remove from the springform pan and sprinkle with additional espresso powder.

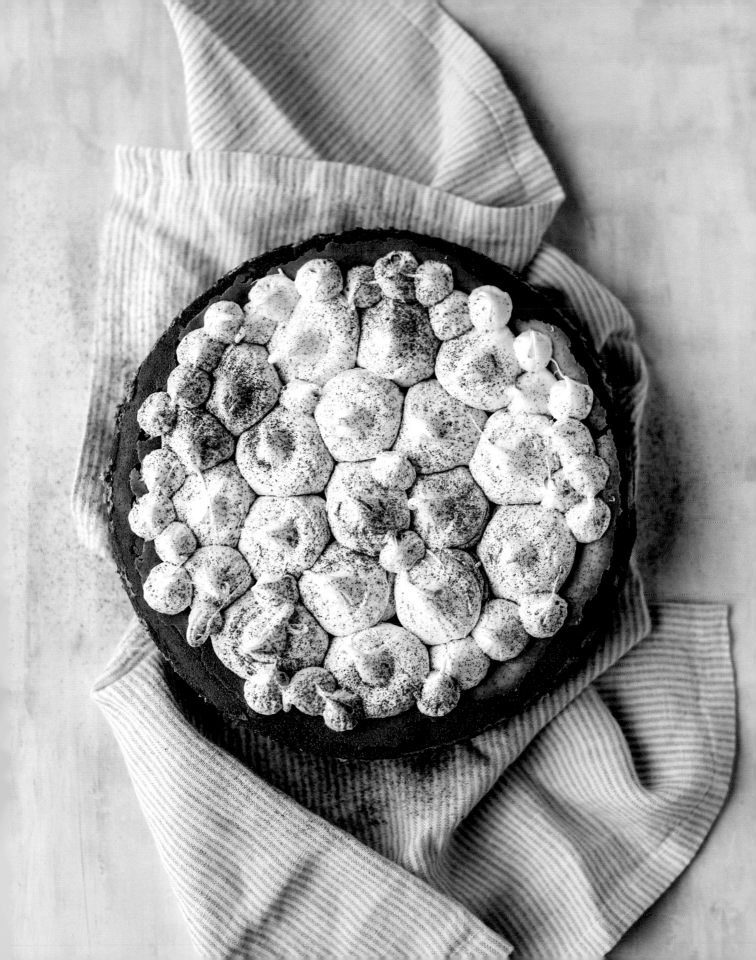

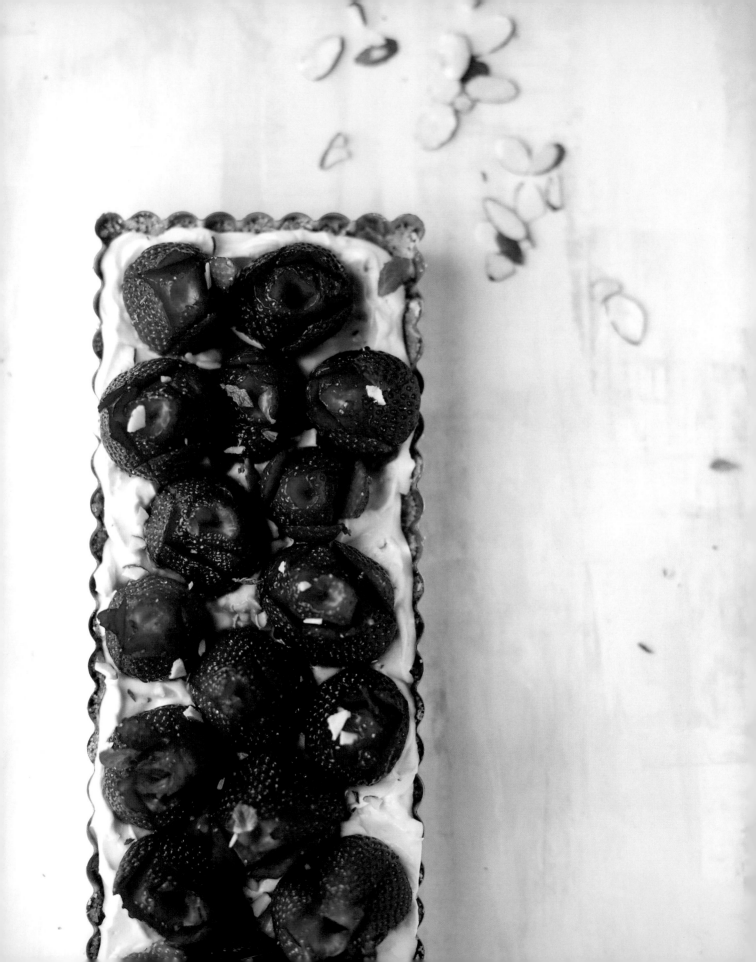

strawberry almond mascarpone tart

I promise that slicing your strawberries into little roses is not that difficult. And they look super cute! I had to share this take on one of the most popular recipes on my website—the strawberry rose tart. It looks super fancy but is pretty easy. It doesn't require a ton of ingredients. And it tastes fantastic.

Let's talk about why I love it so much. The crust is graham crackers and almonds, which is my favorite kind of crust. It's crunchy and sweet, and it adds a wonderful texture to the filling.

The filling is almond-flavored mascarpone and oh-so creamy. A bit like cheesecake, but creamier and not as rich. Plus, it comes together in minutes.

The strawberries are drizzled with honey and toasted sliced almonds.

This tart is ideal as a spring or summer dessert and looks way more impressive than it actually is. Plus, it's super fun to eat! MAKES 4 SERVINGS

CRUST
- ¾ cup graham cracker crumbs
- ¾ cup almond meal
- 5 tablespoons unsalted butter, melted
- 5 tablespoons almond butter, melted

FILLING
- 12 ounces mascarpone cheese, at room temperature
- ¼ cup powdered sugar
- 1 teaspoon almond extract
- 2 pints strawberries, cut into roses if you're feeling fancy
- 1 tablespoon honey
- 3 tablespoons sliced almonds, toasted
- 1 handful fresh mint leaves

TO MAKE THE CRUST
In a bowl, stir together the graham cracker crumbs, almond meal, butter, and almond butter until combined and all the crumbs are moistened. Press the crust into a 14" x 4" tart pan, pressing it up along the sides until packed. This will also work in an 8" round tart pan.

TO MAKE THE FILLING
In a bowl, stir together the mascarpone, sugar, and almond extract until creamy and combined. Spread evenly over the graham crust. Refrigerate for at least 1 hour.

While the tart is in the fridge, cut the strawberries. To slice them into "roses," slice off the tops so the strawberries can sit upright. Use a paring knife to make small slits in the berry, going around the tip and down to the thicker part. Press the knife barely ⅛" into the berry and push back gently, repeating all around the berry. You can also just slice the berries like a regular person!

Place the strawberries on the mascarpone tart. Drizzle with the honey. Top with the sliced almonds and mint. You can serve immediately, or keep in the fridge until ready to serve.

grapefruit rose pound cake

My favorite thing about Bundt cakes is that they can totally pass for breakfast. I mean, they are basically coffee cake. Almost. Maybe this one doesn't have the streusel . . . or the cinnamon. But it looks like some coffee cakes I've made before, and therefore seems perfectly acceptable to have for breakfast and brunch.

As a longtime lover of all things grapefruit, I have to admit that my favorite way to consume it is in desserts. Because when grapefruit is mixed with sugar? Oooh, is it delicious.

This lovely Bundt cake is another citrus treat that's covered in a grapefruit glaze and dried culinary rose petals. They are super adorable but also edible, which is always fun.

It also makes an awesome somewhat-light dessert after dinner. It's not necessarily light in calories, but that whole citrus thing gets me every time! It just seems light and wonderful, and before you know it, you're onto your 2nd piece. It's totally deserving, by the way. MAKES 8 SERVINGS

3 cups all-purpose flour

2 teaspoons baking powder

½ teaspoon salt

1 cup unsalted butter, softened

¾ cup granulated sugar

4 large eggs

1 teaspoon vanilla extract

1 cup whole milk

3 tablespoons freshly grated grapefruit zest

GRAPEFRUIT GLAZE

Zest and juice of ½ grapefruit

2 cups powdered sugar

Crushed dried culinary rose petals, for topping (see note)

Preheat the oven to 350°F. Butter and flour a 10-cup Bundt pan. (With Bundt pans, I find it imperative to use butter *and* flour and not a cooking spray!)

In a bowl, whisk together the flour, baking powder, and salt.

In the bowl of an electric stand mixer, beat together the butter and granulated sugar for 5 minutes, or until fluffy. Beat in the eggs 1 at a time, scraping down the sides of the bowl as needed. Beat in the vanilla.

With the mixer on low speed, beat in a third of the dry ingredients, then beat in half of the milk. Add another third of the dry ingredients and the rest of the milk. Finish with the rest of the dry ingredients. Beat in the grapefruit zest.

Scoop the batter into the Bundt pan and place the pan on a baking sheet. Bake for 65 to 75 minutes, or until a toothpick inserted in the center comes out clean. Let cool before glazing.

TO MAKE THE GRAPEFRUIT GLAZE

In a medium bowl, whisk together the grapefruit zest, juice, and powdered sugar until combined. If the glaze is too runny, add a bit more powdered sugar ¼ cup at a time. If it is too thick, add in more juice 1 teaspoon at a time.

Drizzle the glaze over the cooled cake. Sprinkle the crushed rose petals over top. Serve!

NOTE: I find my culinary rose petals on Amazon!

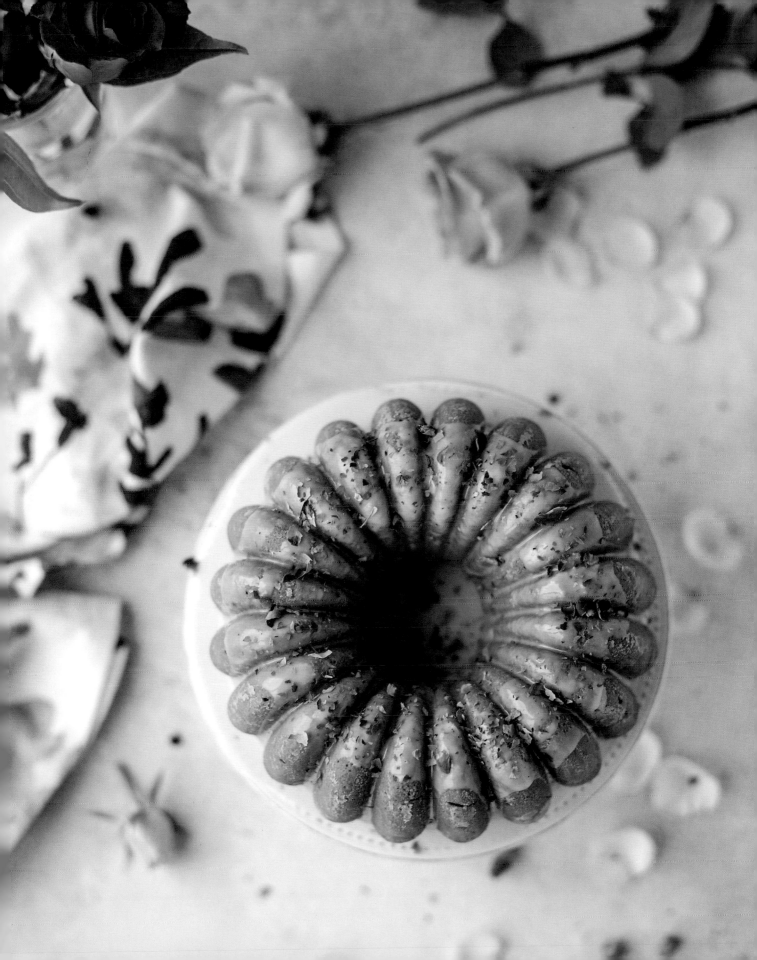

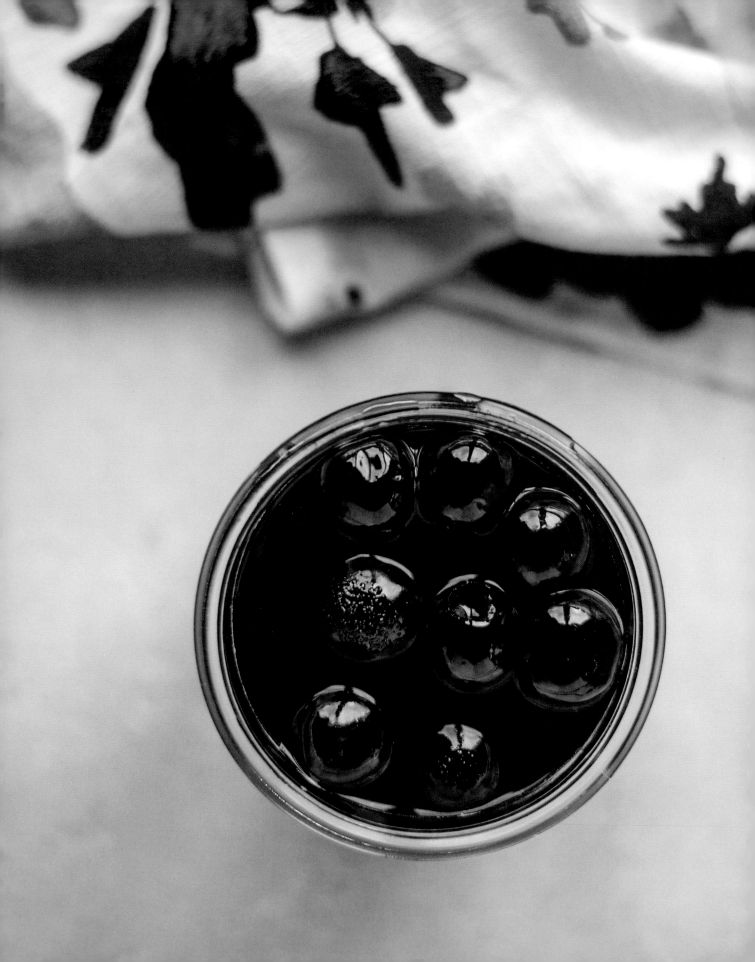

boozy soaked bing cherries

Boozy soaked cherries to use any way you please! I'm partial to tossing mine into cocktails (yes, I guess that technically means more booze), but spooning them over angel food cake instead of straw-berries or on ice cream or cheesecake is another great way to go.

Amaretto is my favorite liqueur to use for these, but bourbon works, too. The key is whatever you like to drink? That's what you should soak your cherries in. MAKES 2 CUPS

2   cups amaretto liqueur

½   cup sugar

2   cups pitted Bing cherries, stems removed

In a saucepan, combine the amaretto and sugar and heat over low heat. Whisk constantly until the sugar dissolves. Turn off the heat and let the mixture cool completely.

Place the cherries in a large jar. Cover them with the amaretto mixture. Stick in the fridge and let soak for at least 2 days. These will stay good in the fridge for about a month. They are excellent in cocktails, on pancakes, and over ice cream!

chocolate cupcakes

WITH BOURBON FROSTING

I have never been a huge frosting person. While my mom, aunt, and generally anyone on their side of the family can eat frosting on a spoon alone, I've never been that excited over it. I want a bite of the cake and the frosting—together. The perfect taste, if you will.

That is . . . until I made my frosting with bourbon. Trust me, I'm still really into eating the cake with the frosting (I can have my cake and frosting, too, right?), but this buttercream is just irresistible. It's so lightly flavored with bourbon that it makes you think, "What is that?" And combined with the butter and sugar, the bourbon almost takes on a butterscotch-like, almost brown butter flavor. Without the brown butter!

But hey. If you wanted to brown the butter? I'm not going to stop you.   MAKES 12

1½ cups all-purpose flour

½ cup unsweetened cocoa powder

1 teaspoon baking powder

½ teaspoon baking soda

¼ teaspoon salt

1 cup granulated sugar

1 large egg

⅓ cup vegetable oil

2 tablespoons butter, melted

2 teaspoons vanilla extract

1 cup milk

½ cup mini chocolate chips

BOURBON FROSTING

½ cup unsalted butter, softened

1 package (8 ounces) cream cheese, softened

3½ cups powdered sugar

2 tablespoons bourbon

1 teaspoon vanilla extract

Preheat the oven to 350°F. Place paper liners in a 12-cup muffin pan.

In a bowl, stir together the flour, cocoa, baking powder, baking soda, and salt.

In the bowl of an electric stand mixer, beat the granulated sugar and egg until slightly fluffy and combined. Add the oil and butter, beating until combined. Add in the vanilla and beat on medium speed, scraping down the sides of the bowl if needed. Add in half of the dry ingredients while beating on low speed. Add in the milk, continuing to beat on low speed. Add in the dry ingredients. Beat until a smooth, silky batter forms. Stir in the chocolate chips with a spatula.

Use a ¼-cup measure to evenly fill the liners three-quarters of the way full. Bake for 18 to 20 minutes, or until the tops are set. Let the cupcakes cool completely before frosting.

TO MAKE THE BOURBON FROSTING
In the bowl of an electric stand mixer, combine the butter and cream cheese. Beat on medium speed until creamy and blended. With the mixer on low speed, gradually add the powdered sugar. Add in the bourbon and vanilla, then beat the frosting on medium to high speed until creamy, scraping down the sides of the bowl when needed.

Frost the cooled cupcakes with the bourbon frosting.

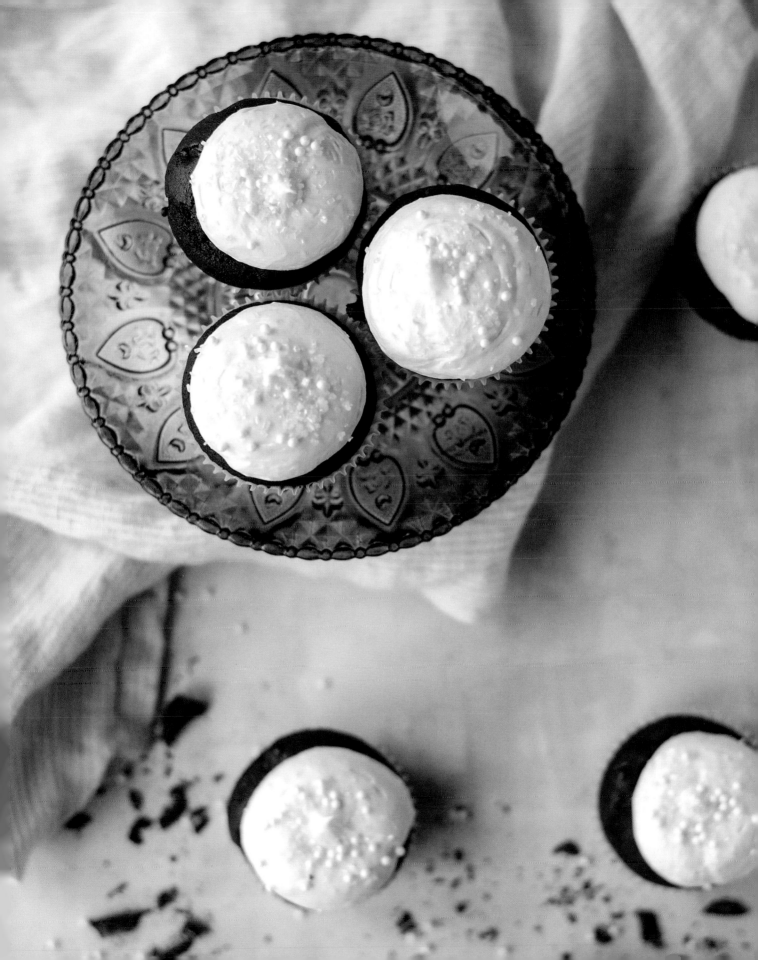

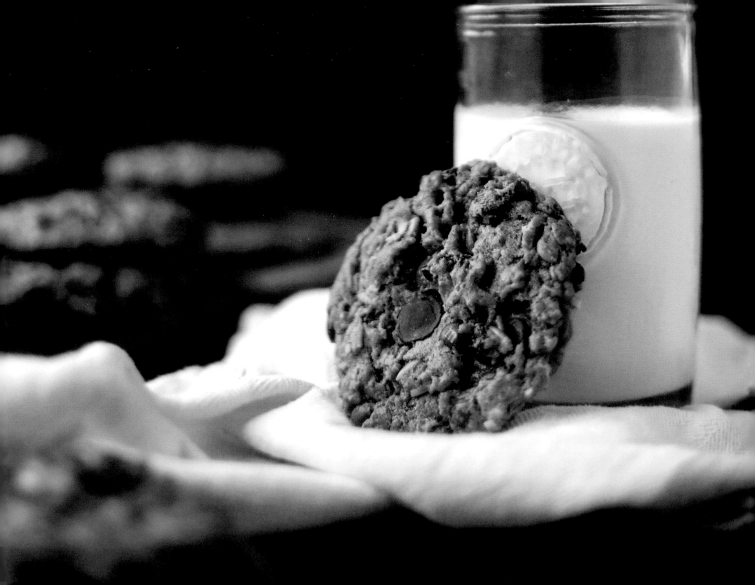

autumn monster cookies

Traditional monster cookies kind of include everything but the kitchen sink. Autumn monster cookies? Think of all the fall flavor that we can pack into these babies.

We have almond butter, roasted and creamy. Oh, so good!

Chocolate chips, of course. M&M's, a bit of pumpkin spice, some pepitas for crunch, and shredded coconut.

Oh. And the very best part. Dried cranberries soaked in bourbon, so they get all plump and juicy.

This cookie is certainly a monster in the best way possible. Pass the (almond) milk! MAKES 24

½ cup dried cranberries

⅓ cup bourbon

2 cups all-purpose flour

1 teaspoon ground cinnamon

1 teaspoon baking soda

1 teaspoon salt

1 cup sweetened shredded coconut

1 cup unsalted butter, at room temperature

½ cup almond butter

1 cup firmly packed light brown sugar

¼ cup pure maple syrup

2 tablespoons molasses

1 large egg

2 teaspoons vanilla extract

3 cups old-fashioned rolled oats

½ cup mini M&M's chocolate candies

1 cup milk chocolate chips

½ cup roasted, salted pepitas

Preheat the oven to 325°F. Line a baking sheet with parchment paper.

Place the cranberries in a microwaveable bowl and cover them with the bourbon. Microwave for 1 minute. Let them sit and soak for at least 10 minutes—or even longer.

In a bowl, stir together the flour, cinnamon, baking soda, and salt. Add the coconut and stir to combine.

In the bowl of an electric stand mixer fitted with the paddle attachment, beat the butter, almond butter, and sugar for 5 minutes, or until fluffy. Add the maple syrup and molasses and mix to combine.

Add the egg and vanilla and beat until well combined, scraping down the sides of the bowl as needed. With the mixer on low speed, add the flour mixture in 2 batches; mix until just combined. Add the oats, cranberries (along with the remaining bourbon, if you wish), M&M's, chocolate chips, and pepitas and mix on low speed until combined.

Using a 2" ice cream scoop or a spoon, scoop 3 tablespoons and drop the dough 2" apart onto the baking sheet. Bake for 15 to 17 minutes, or until the edges begin to turn golden brown. Do not overbake even if the center looks a bit soft; they will set while cooling. Let the cookies cool on the baking sheet for about 2 minutes, or until firm enough to remove to wire racks.

The cookies can be kept in an airtight container for about 2 weeks. They also freeze well in an airtight bag for up to 3 months.

tiramisu bread pudding

Would you believe that until last year, I could count the number of times I've had bread pudding on one hand?

Well, that all changed with this recipe.

Brioche bread is the key. Its buttery, general sponginess allows it to soak in so many delicious flavors, from coffee liqueur to legit espresso to the mascarpone drizzle.

This dessert is soft and fluffy and tastes exactly like tiramisu, in bread pudding form. The mascarpone glaze is simply divine—a rich drizzle over espresso-soaked bread cubes that are baked until lightly crunchy. The top is crispy, and the inside melts in your mouth, like the best French toast you'll ever taste. Espresso syrup is also one of the biggest delights of this recipe, and I'm convinced we all need to store some in our fridge for emergencies. **MAKES 8 SERVINGS**

2   tablespoons butter, melted

8   cups brioche bread cubes

4   cups (1 quart) whole milk

5   large eggs

¾   cup granulated sugar

¼   cup coffee liqueur

2   shots freshly brewed espresso

2   teaspoons unsweetened cocoa powder + additional for garnish

½   teaspoon espresso powder

½   teaspoon salt

ESPRESSO SYRUP

4   ounces freshly brewed espresso

½   cup granulated sugar

MASCARPONE GLAZE

8   ounces mascarpone cheese, at room temperature

1½   cups powdered sugar

2   teaspoons vanilla extract

4– 5 tablespoons milk

Preheat the oven to 350°F. Brush a 13" x 9" baking dish with the melted butter. Line a baking sheet with parchment paper and place the bread cubes on the sheet. Bake for 20 minutes, tossing once while baking, or until the cubes are just toasted. Place them in the baking dish.

In a large bowl, whisk together the milk, eggs, granulated sugar, coffee liqueur, espresso, cocoa, espresso powder, and salt. Pour it over the bread cubes, just until it's about three-quarters of the way up the cubes, so the top of the bread is poking out. Cover the dish and refrigerate for at least an hour, or overnight.

When ready to bake, preheat the oven to 350°F. Bake the bread for 45 minutes, or until golden and slightly crunchy on top.

TO MAKE THE ESPRESSO SYRUP
In a saucepan, heat the espresso and granulated sugar over medium heat, whisking just until the sugar dissolves. Let the mixture simmer for 1 to 2 minutes, then remove it from the heat and let it sit at room temperature. It will thicken slightly as it cools.

TO MAKE THE MASCARPONE GLAZE
Add the mascarpone to a large bowl and whisk until creamy. Whisk in the powdered sugar and vanilla, then stream in the milk and stir until a glaze forms. You will have to stir for a minute or 2 to remove any lumps and bring the glaze together. If the mixture still seems too thick, add more milk 1 tablespoon at a time, whisking well until smooth.

To serve, drizzle the bread pudding with the espresso syrup and mascarpone glaze. Garnish with a sprinkle of cocoa.

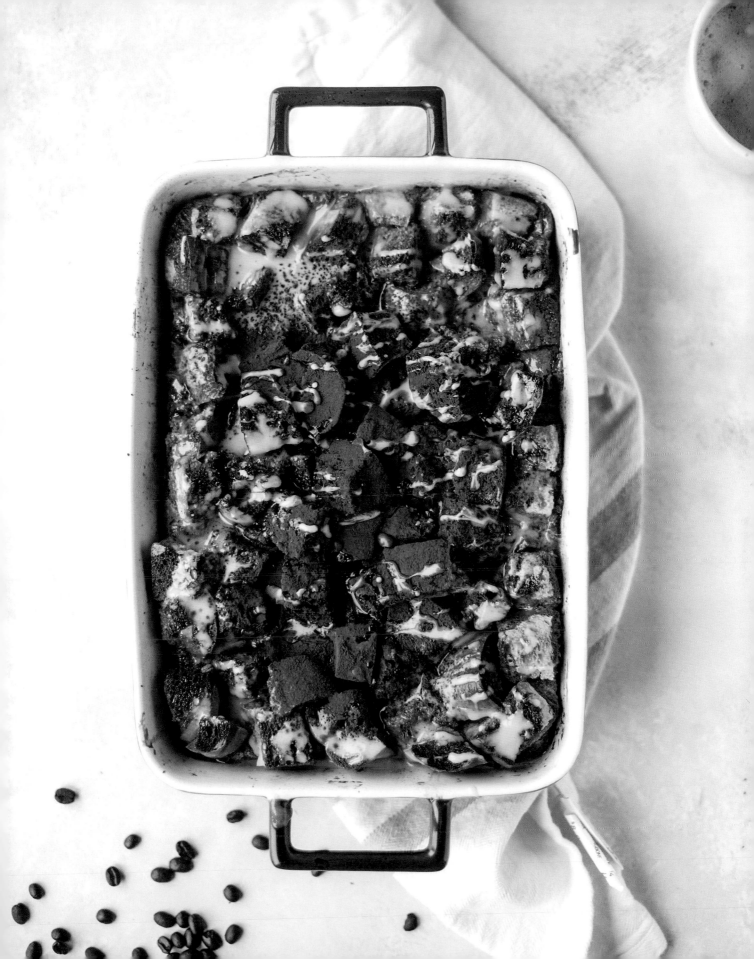

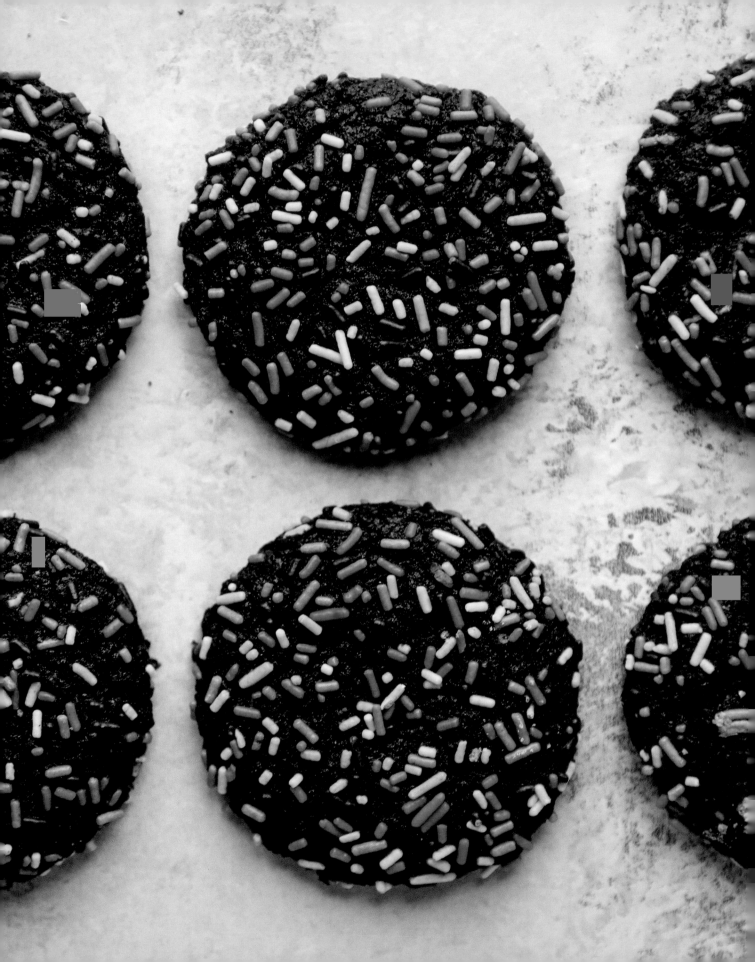

chocolate crinkle sprinkle cookies

These cookies! Oh, how they are so fudgy and chewy, you cannot stop at just one.

You know that traditional chocolate crinkle cookie recipe? The ones you dip in powdered sugar at Christmastime? This is my take on my grandmother's recipe for crinkle cookies.

These spread a bit more in the oven and taste like a chewy brownie, coated in rainbow sprinkles. They are plain fun to eat, but they also taste so good. They are rich and gooey, and it's almost necessary to make a double batch because they won't ever last long in your house. MAKES 24

1   cup all-purpose flour

1   teaspoon baking powder

½   teaspoon salt

½   cup unsweetened cocoa powder

¾   cup sugar

⅓   cup vegetable oil

2   eggs

1   teaspoon vanilla extract

⅓   cup assorted rainbow sprinkles

In a small bowl, stir together the flour, baking powder, and salt.

In the bowl of an electric stand mixer, stir together the cocoa, sugar, and vegetable oil. Beat the eggs in 1 at a time and add the vanilla.

Beat in the dry ingredients until combined. The mixture will be super sticky! Transfer it to a bowl and refrigerate for at least 4 hours or even overnight.

Preheat the oven to 350°F. Line a baking sheet with parchment paper. Place the sprinkles in a bowl.

Roll the dough (it will still be sticky) into 1" balls. Roll the balls in the sprinkles, pressing gently to adhere. Place the balls 2" apart on the baking sheet.

Bake for 10 to 12 minutes, or until the cookies have spread a bit and look set. They will remain soft and chewy! Let the cookies cool completely before removing them from the sheet.

chocolate pumpkin crumble snack cake

I go through phases with pumpkin-flavored things. I like pumpkin desserts that are mostly pumpkin, but I do not love baked goods with tons of pumpkin spice, which is a bit too heavy for me. A little touch of it? I can handle that.

What I have recently started to love, though, is pumpkin and chocolate together. It all started when I was pregnant with Max and would swirl Nutella into pumpkin yogurt. And then put Nutella on pumpkin pancakes. It just went downhill from there.

But this is very . . . uphill. Fudgy chocolate cake with a little hint of pumpkin.

Dreamy! MAKES 12 SERVINGS

1   cup all-purpose flour

⅓   cup unsweetened cocoa powder

1¼ teaspoons baking powder

1   teaspoon pumpkin pie spice

¼   teaspoon salt

¼   cup unsalted butter, melted

½   cup loosely packed brown sugar

1   large egg, lightly beaten

½   cup pumpkin puree

¼   cup milk

2   teaspoons vanilla extract

½   cup dark chocolate chunks or chips

CRUMB TOPPING

⅔   cup firmly packed brown sugar

3   tablespoons unsweetened cocoa powder

¼   teaspoon ground cinnamon

¼   teaspoon salt

½   cup unsalted butter, melted

1½ cups all-purpose flour

Preheat the oven to 350°F. Spray an 8" x 8" baking dish with cooking spray.

In a small bowl, whisk together the flour, cocoa, baking powder, pumpkin pie spice, and salt. Set it aside.

In a large bowl, whisk together the butter and sugar. Once smooth, whisk in the egg, pumpkin, milk, and vanilla until smooth. Gradually add in the dry ingredients and stir with a spoon until just combined. Stir in the chocolate chunks or chips. Spread the batter in the baking dish.

TO MAKE THE CRUMB TOPPING

In a medium bowl, whisk together the sugar, cocoa, cinnamon, salt, and butter until combined. Whisk for a good minute or 2 until the sugar begins to dissolve, then use a wooden spoon to stir in the flour. The mixture will be crumblike and dry, almost like a sludge or paste. This is what you want! Sprinkle the crumbs on top of the cake batter.

Bake for 30 to 35 minutes, or until a toothpick inserted in the center comes out clean. Let cool in the pan for 20 minutes.

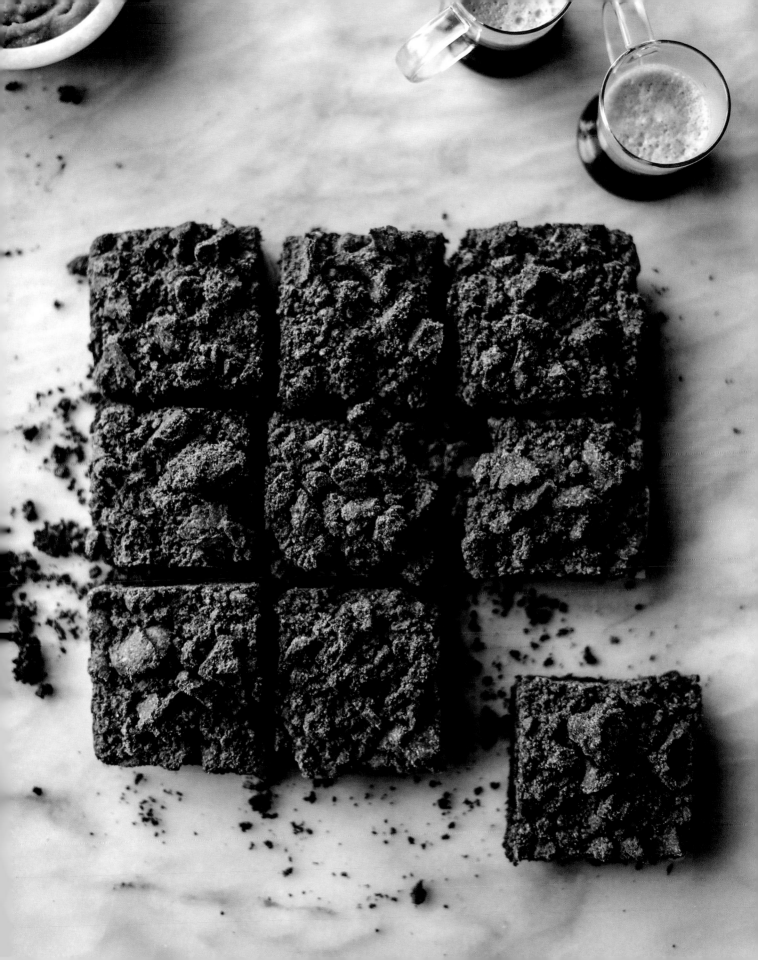

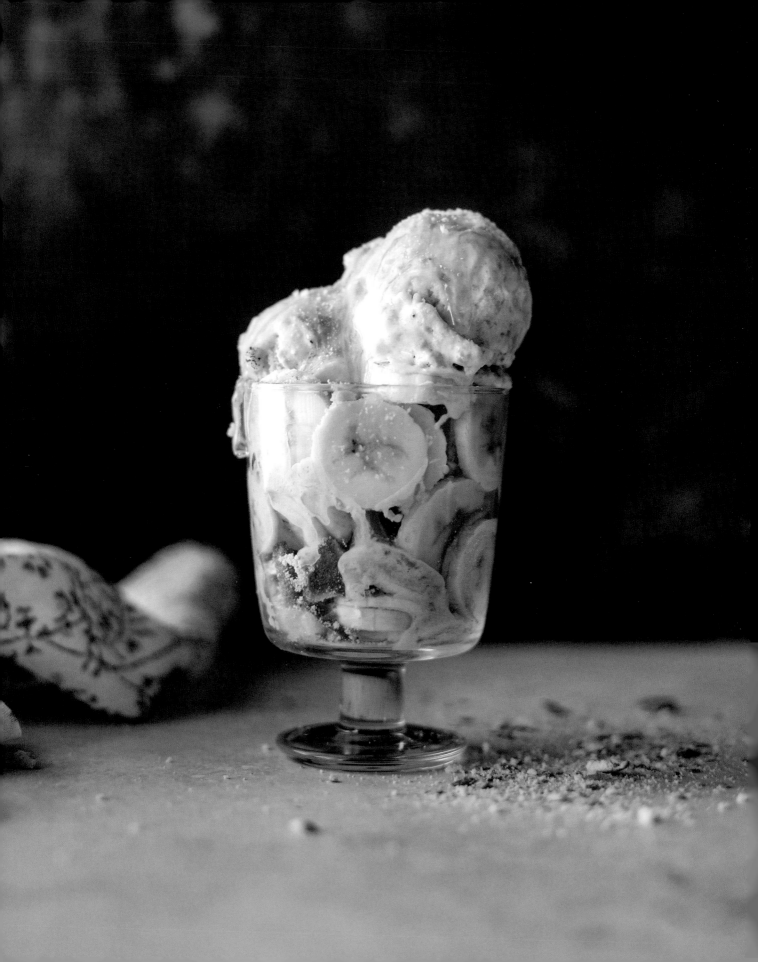

banana cream pie ice cream

One of my first jobs was at an ice cream shop. I burnt the heck out of my fingertips making home-made waffle cones (they smelled so wonderful, though!) and practically developed tendonitis from scooping ice cream daily. It was such a fun job as a teenager, even if we were pretty sure that two people met in the parking lot daily to carry on an affair in the front seat of their car.

My favorite ice cream there was a banana pudding ice cream that I've never been able to find anywhere else. It was banana ice cream swirled with marshmallow, graham cracker crumbs, and vanilla wafer cookies, and it was so good. I remember stealing bites and wanting to take a container home every night!

Banana ice cream these days on the Internet usually consists of frozen bananas blended in a food processor or blender, called banana froyo. I won't lie: I make that and I love it, because I love bananas. It's even better with peanut butter and chocolate chips on top.

But it's certainly not ice cream, and it's definitely not the banana pudding ice cream of my youth. This version is more pie-like (with graham cracker crumbs, of course!) than pudding-like, but I have come so close to hitting the nail on the head with this recipe. It's a traditional ice cream base with lots of bananas, marshmallow fluff, and the aforementioned vanilla wafers. It's even better with a drizzle of honey on top! MAKES ABOUT 1 QUART

2½ cups heavy cream

1½ cups whole milk

½ cup granulated sugar

¼ teaspoon salt

6 medium bananas, mashed

1 tablespoon vanilla extract

1½ cups marshmallow fluff

1½ cups vanilla wafer cookies, crushed

Honey, for drizzling

In a saucepan, combine the cream, milk, sugar, and salt and heat over medium heat. Stir constantly until the sugar dissolves. Continue to heat until the mixture becomes warm and begins to bubble around the edges. Remove from the heat. Add the bananas and vanilla. Pour the mixture into a bowl and refrigerate for at least 30 to 60 minutes, or until cold.

Add the mixture to an ice cream maker and churn according to the manufacturer's directions. A few minutes before it's finished churning, add in 1 cup of the marshmallow fluff in a few increments and 1 cup of the vanilla wafer cookie crumbs. Once it's finished churning, scoop the ice cream into a freezer-safe container. Stir in the remaining ½ cup marshmallow fluff and the remaining ½ cup vanilla wafer cookie crumbs, then freeze for at least 4 to 6 hours.

Let sit for a few minutes before serving so the ice cream can soften. Serve with a drizzle of honey, if desired.

peanut butter mousse

If you are a peanut butter lover, this one is for you.

It's exactly as it sounds: rich and fluffy peanut butter cream, topped with the fluffiest, slightly charred homemade marshmallow. It's rich and very sweet, so a little goes a long way. A small jar of this is the most decadent after-dinner dessert. And the true cherry on top? Sea salt! It is perfection.

MAKES 4 SERVINGS

1   cup cold heavy cream

1   package (8 ounces) cream cheese, softened

¾   cup creamy peanut butter

1   cup powdered sugar

1   teaspoon vanilla extract

Coarse sea salt, for topping

TOASTED MARSHMALLOW

3   large egg whites

¾   cup granulated sugar

½   cup cream of tartar

1   teaspoon vanilla extract

Pour the cream into the bowl of an electric stand mixer. Beat on medium-high speed until peaks form. Transfer the whipped cream to another bowl and set the bowl in the fridge.

Wash and dry the stand mixer bowl. Add the cream cheese and peanut butter to it and beat until creamy and combined. Gently stir in the powdered sugar and vanilla, beating until combined.

Remove the whipped cream from the fridge and fold it into the peanut butter mixture. Spoon the mousse into 4 glasses or jars. Refrigerate for 4 hours before serving.

TO MAKE THE TOASTED MARSHMALLOW

Bring some water to a simmer in the bottom of a double boiler. In a heatproof bowl, preferably the bowl of your electric stand mixer, combine the egg whites, granulated sugar, and cream of tartar. Place over top of the double boiler and whisk constantly for 3 to 4 minutes, or until the sugar has dissolved and the egg whites are slightly warm. Immediately remove the bowl and place it on your stand mixer fitted with the whisk attachment. Beat slowly at first and then gradually increase the speed to high. Beat for 6 to 7 minutes, or until glossy and thick. Beat in the vanilla for another minute, or until combined.

Right before serving, scoop the marshmallow on top of the mousse and use a culinary torch to toast it, if desired. Sprinkle with sea salt!

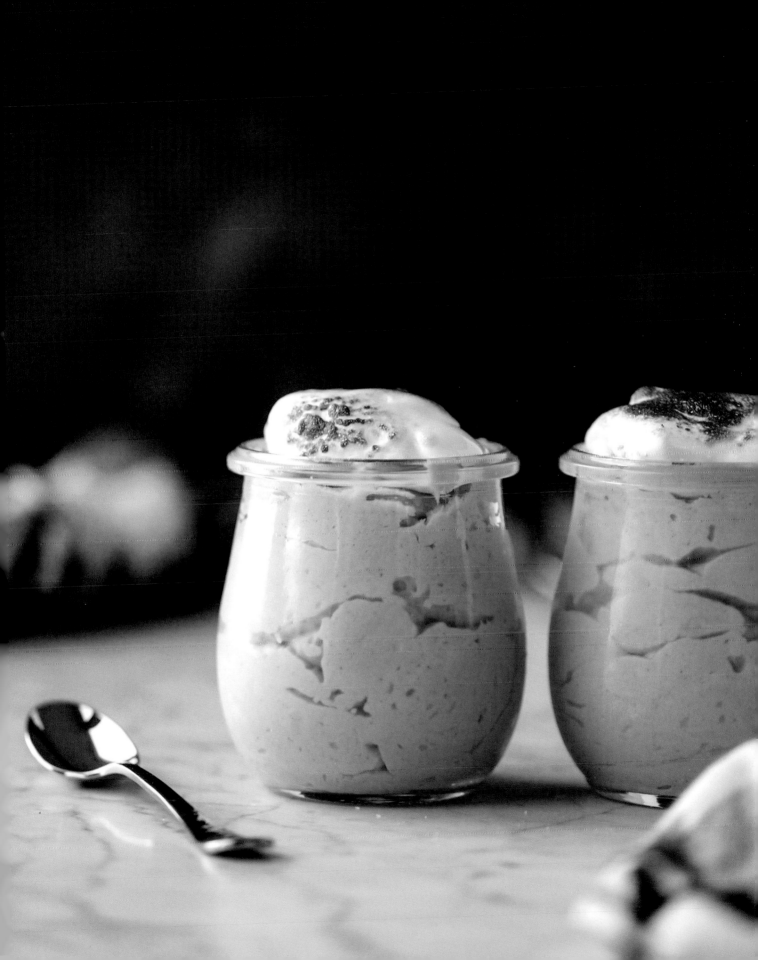

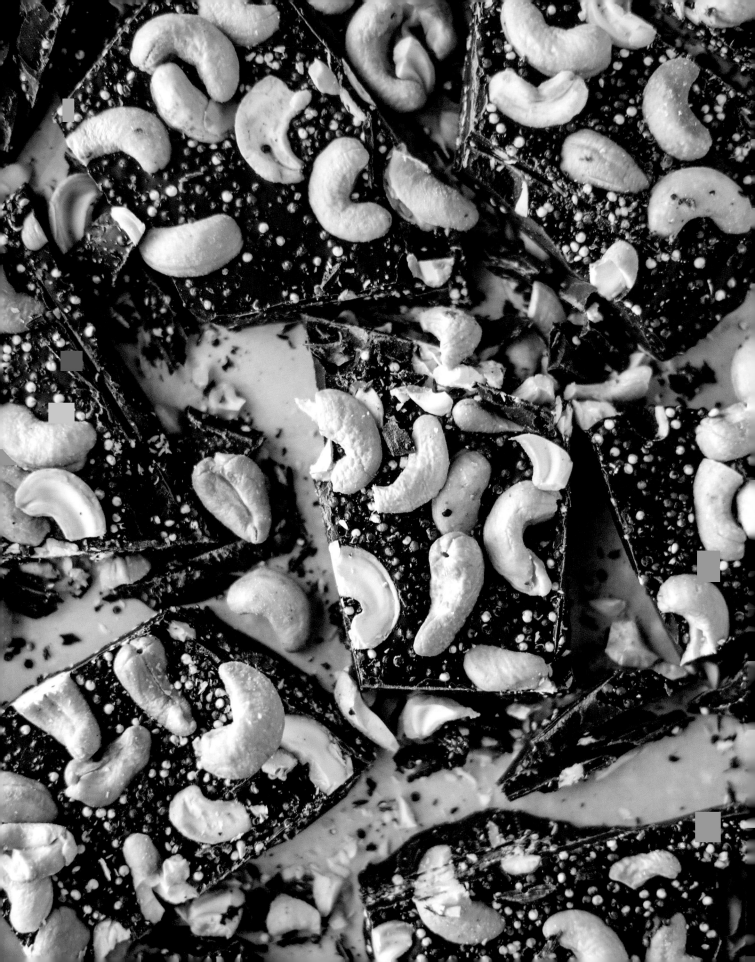

toasted quinoa cashew chocolate bark

If quinoa is a super food and packed with protein, and we combine it with dark chocolate that is loaded with antioxidants, and cashews that have a dose of healthy fat, are we technically eating a super super food?

That is the question. MAKES 8 SERVINGS

1   cup dry quinoa

1   pound high-quality dark chocolate, chopped

1   cup cashews, chopped

4   ounces white chocolate, chopped

Line a baking sheet with parchment paper.

Add the quinoa to a skillet and place over medium heat. Cook, stirring and tossing often, for 5 to 6 minutes, or until the quinoa becomes fragrant and pops—and also turns golden if you're using white quinoa. Set aside.

Place the dark chocolate in a heatproof bowl. You can melt it over top of a double boiler that contains simmering water or microwave it at 50 percent power. If microwaving, I heat it in 30-second increments, stirring well after each until the chocolate is melted.

Spread the chocolate on the parchment paper in a big rectangle (or any shape you'd like!) and immediately sprinkle it all over with the toasted quinoa. Sprinkle the cashews over top, too. Let it sit until firm, about 1 hour. If you're impatient like me, you can stick it in the fridge!

Melt the white chocolate using the double-boiler or microwave method. Remove the bark from the fridge and drizzle it with the melted white chocolate. Let sit until firm, then break it into pieces.

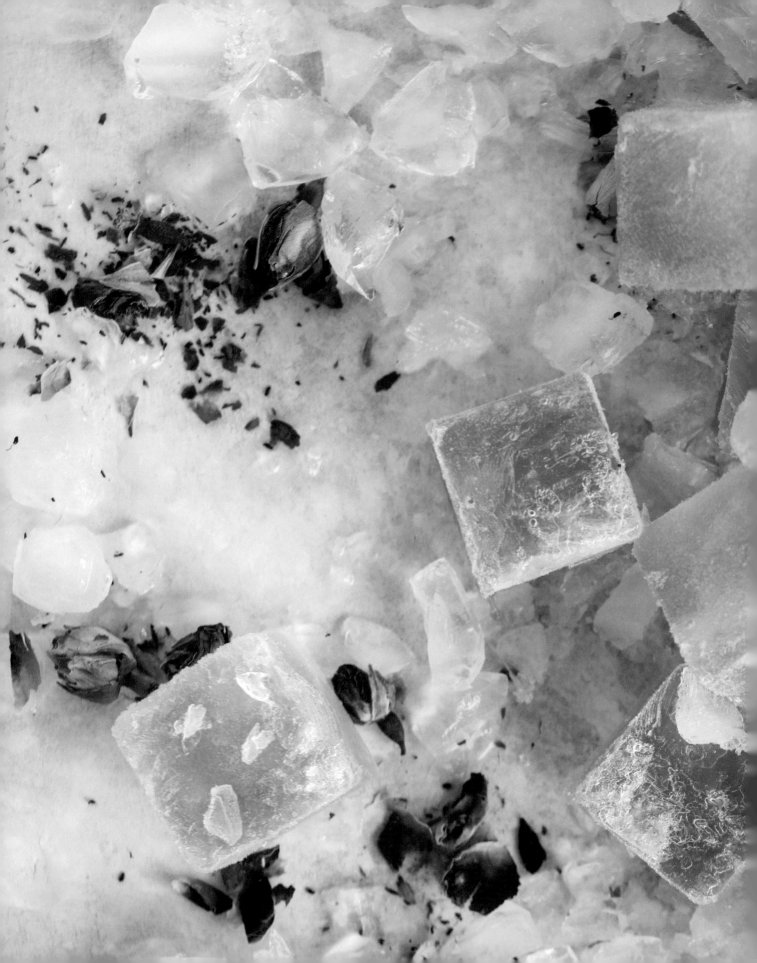

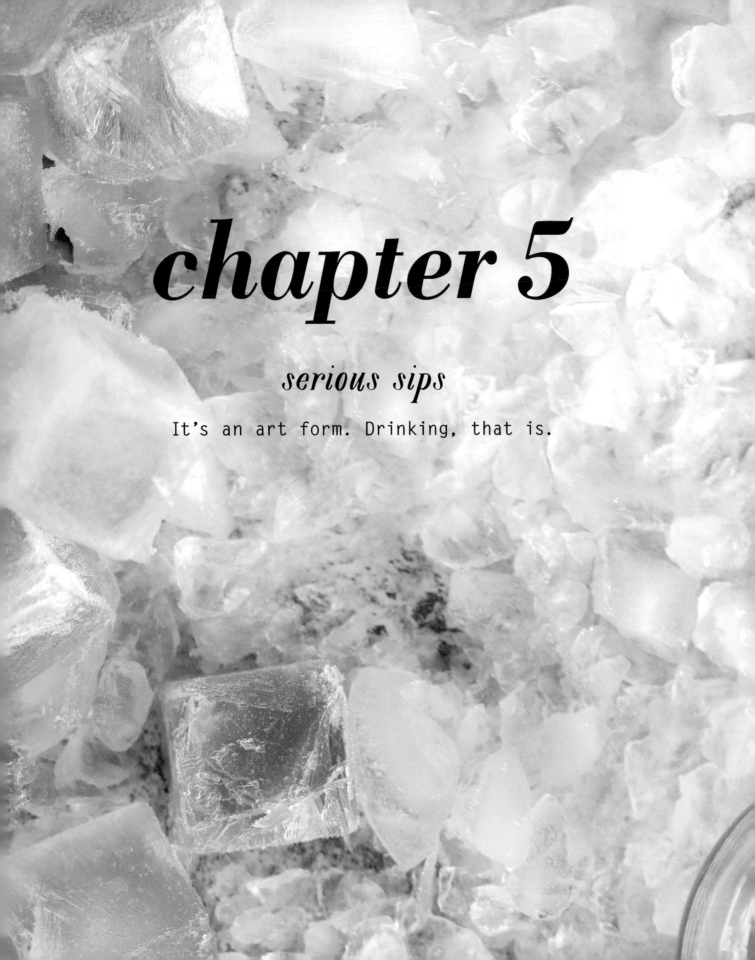

chapter 5

serious sips

It's an art form. Drinking, that is.

A FEW YEARS AGO, I STARTED A THIRSTY Thursday series on my blog, sharing mostly cocktails, but also drinks in general. I wanted a way to bring some creativity into my life when it came to party drinks, and I figured that sharing 1 cocktail a week would definitely be a challenge that I was up for.

Since then, I have discovered so many combinations that I adore, but it remains true that my favorite cocktail will forever be a margarita. On the rocks. Lots of salt.

However! The Thirsty Thursday series has also been all about mocktails and milkshakes—basically anything I can sip through a straw. It has been so much fun to take beverages and turn them into something wild and delicious.

This chapter is chock-full of some of my favorite creative cocktails—a few classics and a few wild ones. There are some mocktail options, too!

cider beergaritas

When I first heard of beergaritas a few years ago, I was completely turned off. Most recipes combined cheap beer and sours mix, and nothing sounded worse to me. And that's saying something, since I shamefully love one of those super cold, canned beer margaritas at the beach in the summer.

It wasn't until I started making my own margarita mix and adding beer that I fully committed.

This beergarita uses hard cider and apple cider (pumpkin cider is also a good bet!) along with tequila, lime, and orange. Plus a salty sugar rim, because everything is better with that.

The key to making these super delicious is to use frosty glasses! So a few hours (or the night) before, stick your glasses in the freezer. I suggest making a single serving first and tasting it so you can add more or less tequila or syrup to your liking. Everyone is different and prefers their drinks a different way, so feel free to add more or less tequila, simple syrup, lime juice, etc. **MAKES 1 SERVING, AND IS EASILY MULTIPLIED**

SIMPLE SYRUP

1 cup sugar

1 cup water

1 tablespoon coarse salt + 1 tablespoon sugar + 1 teaspoon ground cinnamon, for the rim

2 ounces fresh lime juice

2 ounces hard cider

1½ ounces silver tequila

½ ounce Grand Marnier liqueur

1 ounce apple cider

1 ounce simple syrup

Fresh apple and orange slices, for garnish

TO MAKE THE SIMPLE SYRUP

In a saucepan, combine the sugar and water and heat over medium-low heat. Whisk until the sugar dissolves, let the mixture simmer for a minute, then turn off the heat and let it cool to room temperature. (Leftover simple syrup can be stored in the refrigerator for 2 to 3 weeks.)

On a plate, stir together the salt, sugar, and cinnamon.

Rim the edge of a glass with an orange slice and then dip it in the salt mixture to coat. Fill the glass with just a few ice cubes or even with crushed ice—my ice preference of late.

In a cocktail shaker, combine the lime juice, hard cider, tequila, Grand Marnier, apple cider, and simple syrup. Shake well for 30 seconds, then pour it over the ice. Garnish with the apple and orange slices.

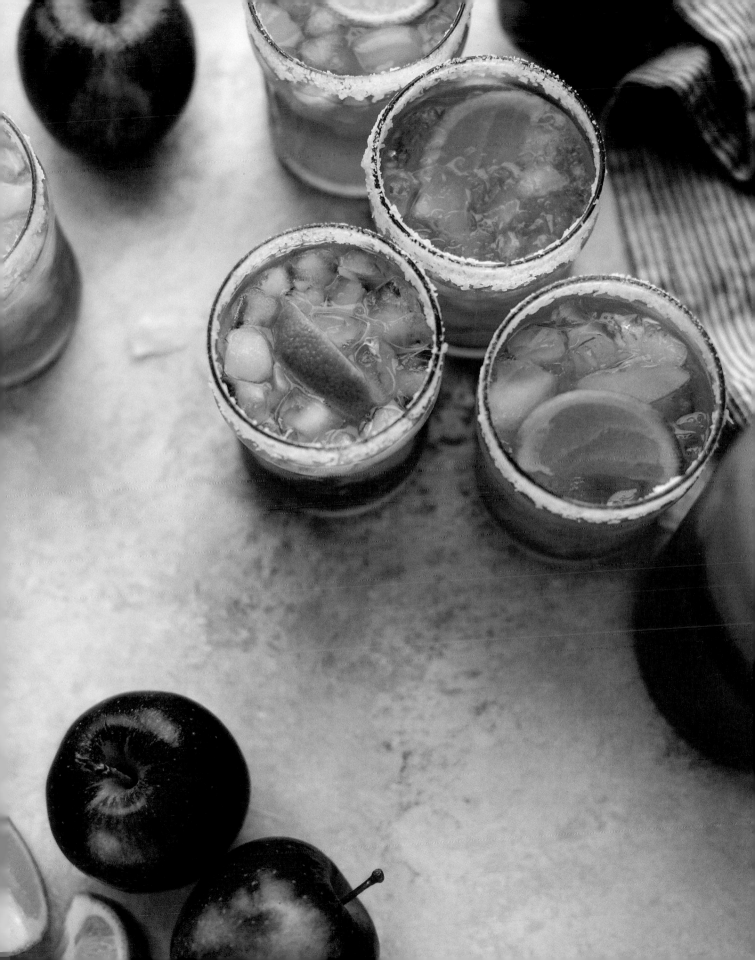

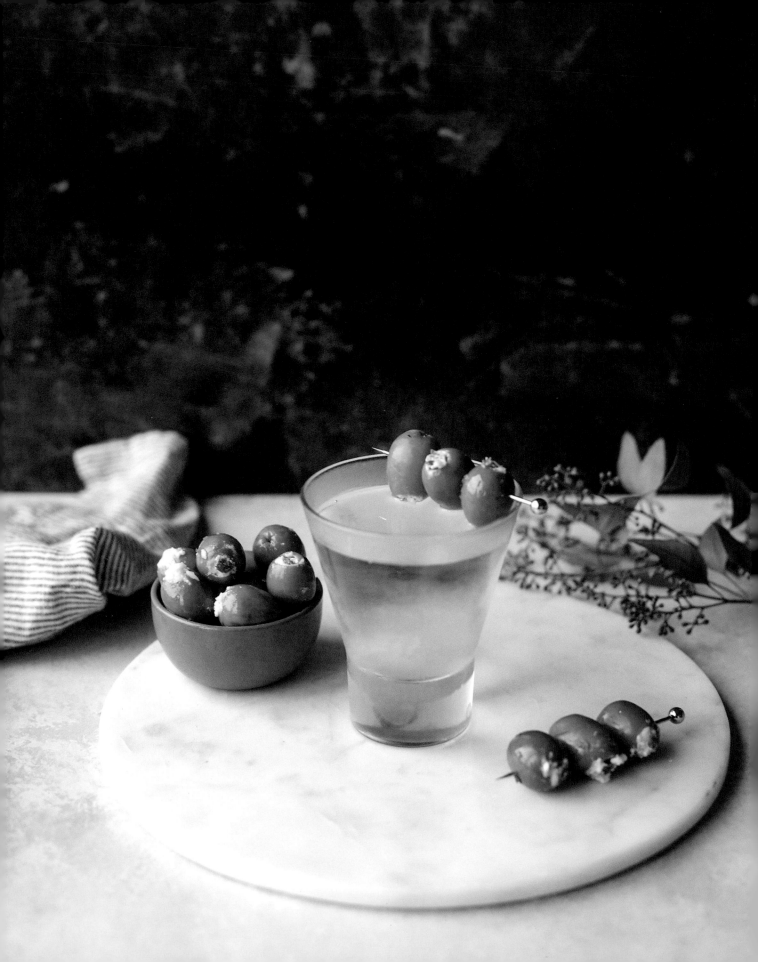

pimiento cheese olive dirty martini

I believe that I've been an olive lover since birth. We are talking a serious olive lover. As in, I used to pop them like candy when I was a toddler, and I basically have not stopped since.

For years, one of my go-to orders has been an extra dirty martini with blue cheese–stuffed olives. The creaminess of the cheese, the briny olive juice . . . oh my gosh, just the thought of one makes my mouth water.

I switched it up just a touch here, using the pimiento cheese–stuffed olives from Chapter 2 as garnish. If you're a pimiento cheese fan, this is such a welcome, interesting change. It's also the perfect cocktail for crunchy pretzels and cashew snacking. MAKES 1 SERVING, IS EASILY MULTIPLIED

4　ounces vodka

2　ounces juice from a jar of olives

½　ounce dry vermouth

Pimiento Cheese–Stuffed Olives
　　(page 54)

In a cocktail shaker, combine the vodka, olive juice, and vermouth. Shake for 20 seconds. Pour into a frosty, chilled glass. Garnish with a few pimiento cheese–stuffed olives.

pickle margaritas
WITH POTATO CHIP SALT

Yep. You heard me right.

I may have taken my pickle love a bit too far here, huh? We shall see.

If you are a pickle fan, you will totally get this. If you are my husband, there is absolutely no chance that you will.

I may sound like a freak, but I love pickle juice. I add a touch of it to my egg salad, and I dip my chips in it if I have residual pickle juice left over on a barbecue plate. Some of us have the pickle tastebuds and some of us . . . don't.

These aren't overly pickle-y, but they definitely have that pickle juice hint. They are rimmed with crushed potato chips, which don't stay as firm as coarse salt, so it's imperative that you enjoy immediately and drink this baby up. MAKES 1 SERVING, IS EASILY MULTIPLIED

Crushed kettle-cooked potato chips, for rimming the glass

1½ ounces tequila

2 ounces fresh lime juice

1 ounce pickle juice from a jar of pickles

1 ounce simple syrup (page 218)

Lime slices and/or pickles, for garnish

The key to rimming the glass with potato chips is to do only a small section of the glass since they can become soggy quickly. Rim a glass with a wedge of lime and dip in the crushed potato chips. Fill a glass with ice.

In a cocktail shaker, combine the tequila, lime juice, pickle juice, and simple syrup. Shake well for 30 seconds. Pour over the ice. Garnish with lime slices and/or pickles.

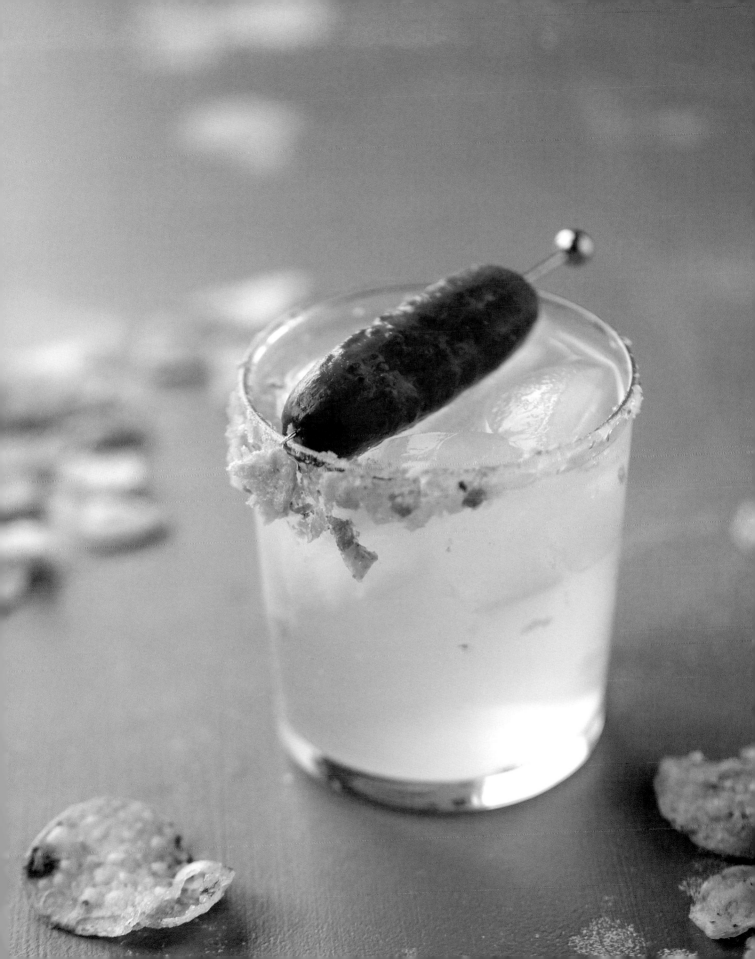

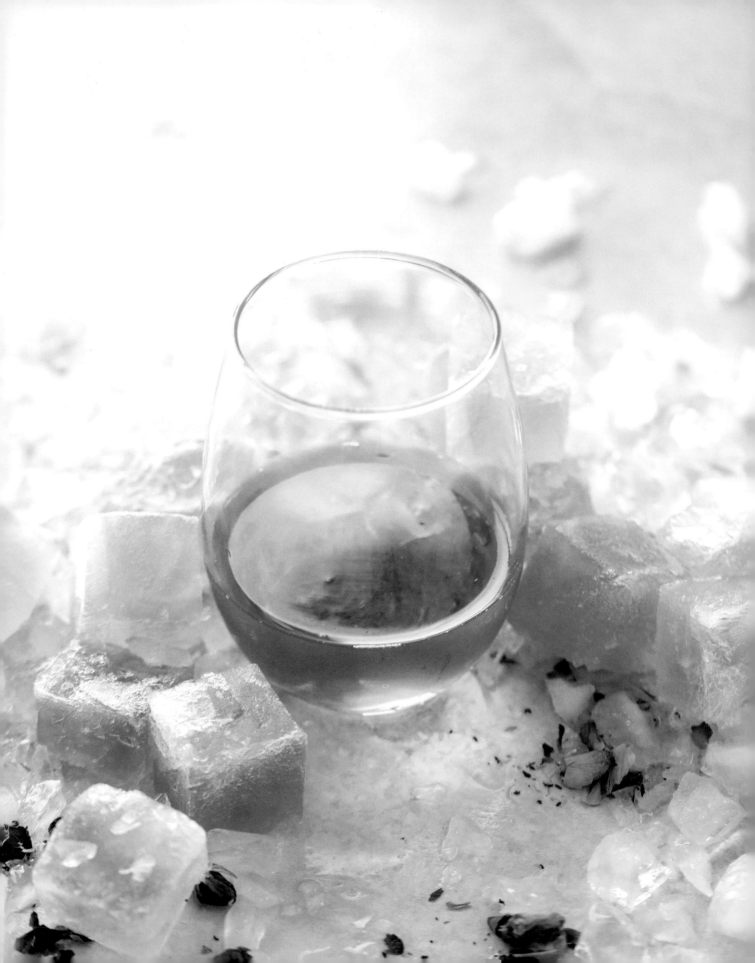

rosé ice cubes

I discovered rosé ice cubes on Instagram. If that isn't the most cliché millennial statement ever, I don't know what is. But it's true!

This is such a simple idea, but it's fantastic if you're a summer rosé lover. All embarrassing traits aside, I occasionally will throw an ice cube in my wine (I know) to chill it even more. I love my white wine and rosé ice-cold, so this is necessary in the hot summer heat.

Not only can you toss these in your wine glass without watering down your drink, you can use them in punches or sangrias, too. Even in a glass of club soda so it melts into a spritzer! MAKES 2 TRAYS

1   bottle (750 milliliters) rosé wine
2   ice cube trays

Fill the ice cube trays with the rosé and freeze overnight. Use the cubes in your wine, sangria, or punch!

mint iced tea

WITH PINEAPPLE ICE CUBES

Another super simple ice cube idea, but this time, I'm telling you exactly where I love them: minty summer iced tea! I love using these pineapple ice cubes to sweeten the tea naturally. It is refreshing and bright and adds an unexpected punch of flavor.

Of course, these pineapple ice cubes can work wonders in other places, too. Think punches, sangrias, lemonades, and soda water alike. They will turn into your new favorite thing. **MAKES 1 QUART**

2 cups pineapple juice

4 cups (1 quart) water

4 tea bags (your favorite variety)

2 handfuls fresh mint leaves, plus extra for garnish

¼ cup sugar

Pour the pineapple juice in an ice cube tray (or 2, depending on the size of your tray) and freeze overnight.

In a saucepan, bring the water to a boil. Turn off the heat. Place the tea bags and mint in the water and let it steep for 30 minutes. Remove the tea bags and the mint. Stir in the sugar. Pour the mixture into a pitcher and refrigerate for 2 hours.

To serve, pour the tea over the pineapple ice cubes! Garnish with fresh mint, if you wish.

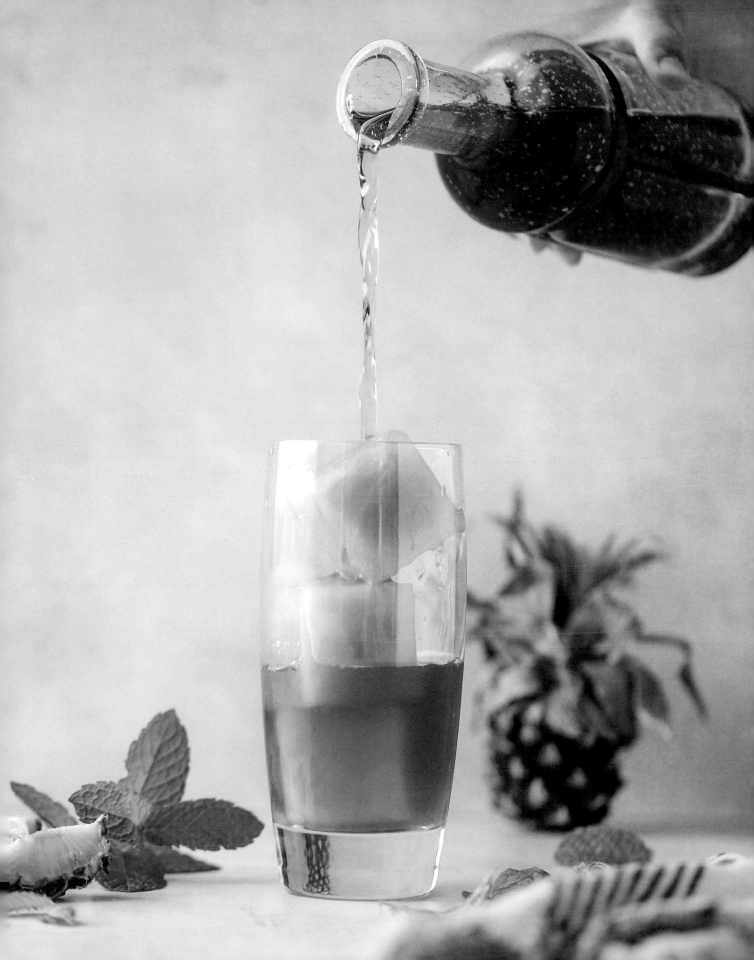

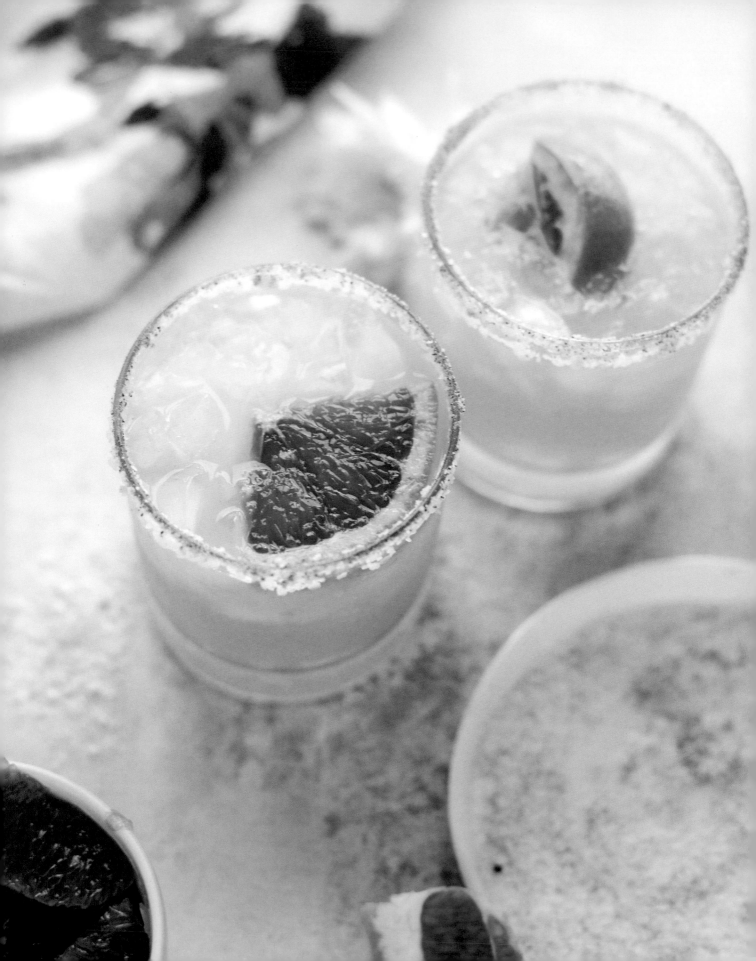

grapefruit salty dog

The salty dog is usually an acquired taste, with the grapefruit juice and all. But since I've been drinking grapefruit juice all my life, it was a taste I instantly loved.

The thing about my salty dogs, though, is that I want them to be super grapefruit-y. I want the grapefruit to overpower the vodka—almost. Because of this, I like using a grapefruit simple syrup to intensify the flavor and add just a touch of sweetness.

This drink is so refreshing. And it tastes even better with friends on a hot summer night. MAKES 1 SERVING, AND IS EASILY MULTIPLIED

GRAPEFRUIT SIMPLE SYRUP
½   cup fresh grapefruit juice
½   cup sugar

Coarse salt, for rimming the glass
Grapefruit wedge
4   ounces vodka
4   ounces fresh grapefruit juice
1   ounce grapefruit syrup

TO MAKE THE GRAPEFRUIT SIMPLE SYRUP
In a saucepan, combine the grapefruit juice and sugar and heat over medium heat. Whisk until the sugar dissolves. Simmer for 1 to 2 minutes, then turn off the heat. Let cool to room temperature.

Place the salt on a plate and rim a glass with the grapefruit wedge. Dip the glass in the salt and fill it with ice. Pour in the vodka, grapefruit juice, and grapefruit syrup. Stir and serve!

blood orange smash

This bourbon smash is one of the most popular winter recipes on my blog and one of my all-time favorites. I couldn't leave it out of my book because it's too good not to share with everyone. I mean, look at the color alone! It's stunning.

Garnished with a few pieces of fresh rosemary or even thyme, and sweet and citrusy with a hint of bourbon, it's a gorgeous and warming holiday cocktail or even a perfect one for early spring.

MAKES 1 SERVING, AND IS EASILY MULTIPLIED

SPICY VANILLA SUGAR

½ cup sugar

Pinch of cayenne pepper

1 vanilla bean, seeds scraped

1½ ounces simple syrup, or more if you want it sweeter! (page 218)

Few drops of bitters

1 or 2 blood orange slices, plus extra slices for garnish

6 ounces blood orange juice

1½ ounces bourbon

2 ounces club soda

Fresh herbs (such as rosemary or thyme), for garnish

TO MAKE THE SPICY VANILLA SUGAR

In a small bowl, combine the sugar, cayenne, and scraped vanilla bean seeds. Stir and mash together with a fork until the vanilla is distributed evenly. You can store this sugar in a jar if you make it ahead of time, and in that case, keep the vanilla bean in the jar! Make a double or triple batch . . . hint hint.

Use an orange slice to rim the glass and dip it in the sugar. Next, combine the simple syrup, bitters, and an orange slice or 2 in a chilled glass. Muddle together until the orange slices have broken down. Add crushed ice and pour the blood orange juice and bourbon over the top. Stir to mix. Top off with the club soda, and garnish with an orange slice and fresh herbs for color.

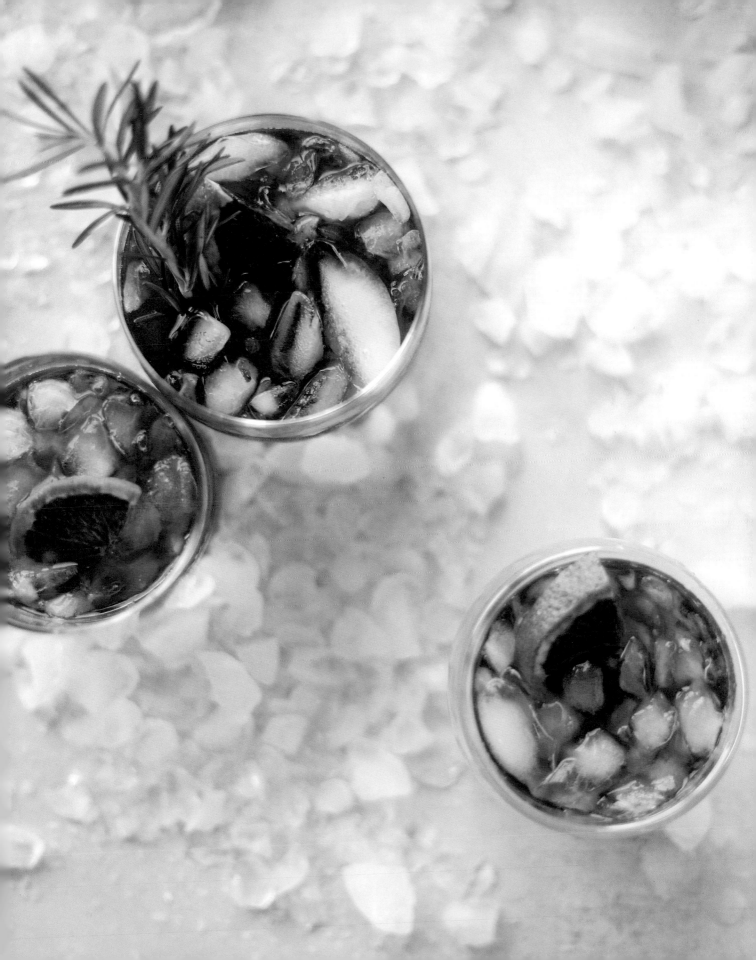

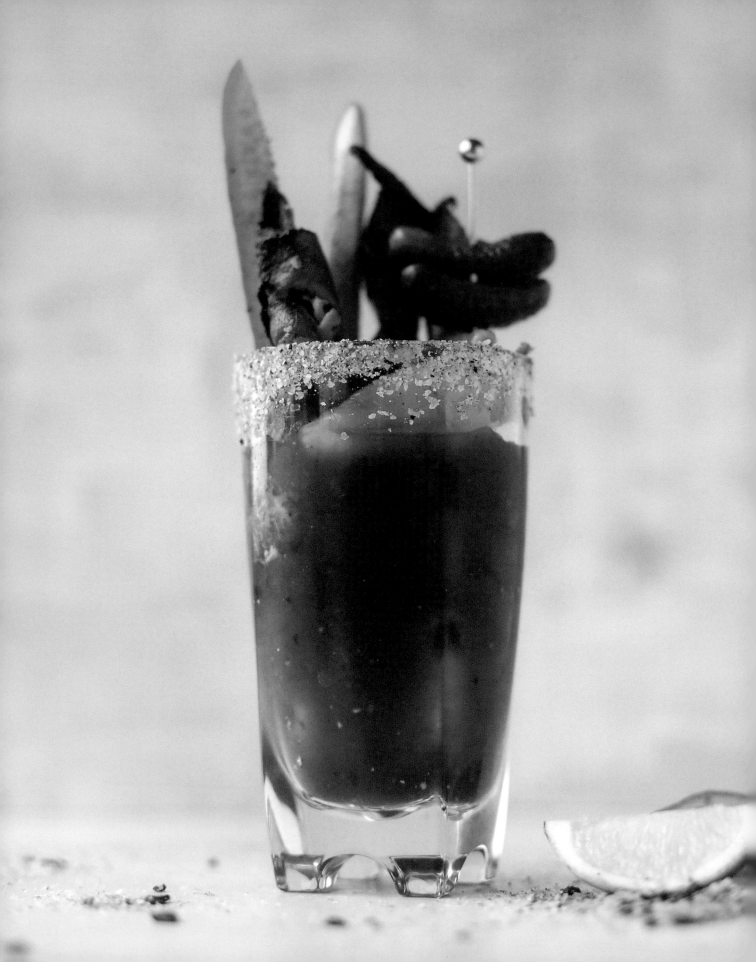

bacon bloody maria

Bloody Marys are a cocktail that I've always wanted to love, but just never could. With my distaste for tomato sauce–based things (most of the time!), the idea of mixing tomato juice with vodka and serving it with something else I don't love, celery, was my worst cocktail nightmare.

That is, until I tried it with lots of bacon and . . . tequila! And more pickle juice, of course.

A Bloody Mary made with tequila is called a Bloody Maria, and I personally like that name a whole lot better anyway. I like the taste of tequila so much better than vodka, so when it's mixed with the tomato juice and a little lime, I was completely hooked.

This Bloody Maria is practically brunch with all of its snacks attached, and that's just the way I like it.   MAKES 1 SERVING, AND IS EASILY MULTIPLIED

⅓ cup fresh tomato juice

3 ounces fresh lime juice

2 ounces pickle juice from a jar
   of pickles

1 teaspoon Worcestershire sauce

¼ teaspoon celery salt

¼ teaspoon garlic powder

Pinch of ground black pepper

Drop of hot-pepper sauce

1½ ounces tequila

GARNISH

3 fried bacon pieces

2 cornichons

1 pepperoncini pepper

1 pickle

In a cocktail shaker or blender, combine the tomato juice, lime juice, pickle juice, Worcestershire, celery salt, garlic powder, pepper, and hot-pepper sauce. Shake or blend until mixed. Pour over ice in a chilled glass and stir in the tequila. Garnish with the bacon, cornichons, pepperoncini, and pickle.

cucumber gin fizz

If you're into refreshing cocktails on hot summer days, this has your name all over it. Be sure to choose a gin that has lots of botanical undertones (like Hendrick's) and use cold, bubbly club soda. These go down like water! MAKES 1 SERVING, IS EASILY MULTIPLIED

CUCUMBER SYRUP

1   cucumber, peeled and cubed

¼   cup sugar

3   ounces gin

1   ounce cucumber syrup

½   ounce fresh lime juice

2   cucumber ribbons or slices

5   ounces club soda

TO MAKE THE CUCUMBER SYRUP

Place the cucumber in a blender and puree until smooth. Strain the mixture through a fine-mesh strainer until you have ¼ cup of cucumber "juice."

In a saucepan, combine the cucumber juice and sugar and heat over medium heat. Whisk until the sugar dissolves. Simmer for 1 to 2 minutes. Turn off the heat and let the mixture cool completely.

In a cocktail shaker, combine the gin, cucumber syrup, and lime juice. Shake until mixed. Fill a glass with ice and the cucumber ribbons or slices. Pour the mixture into the glass. Top it with the club soda and serve.

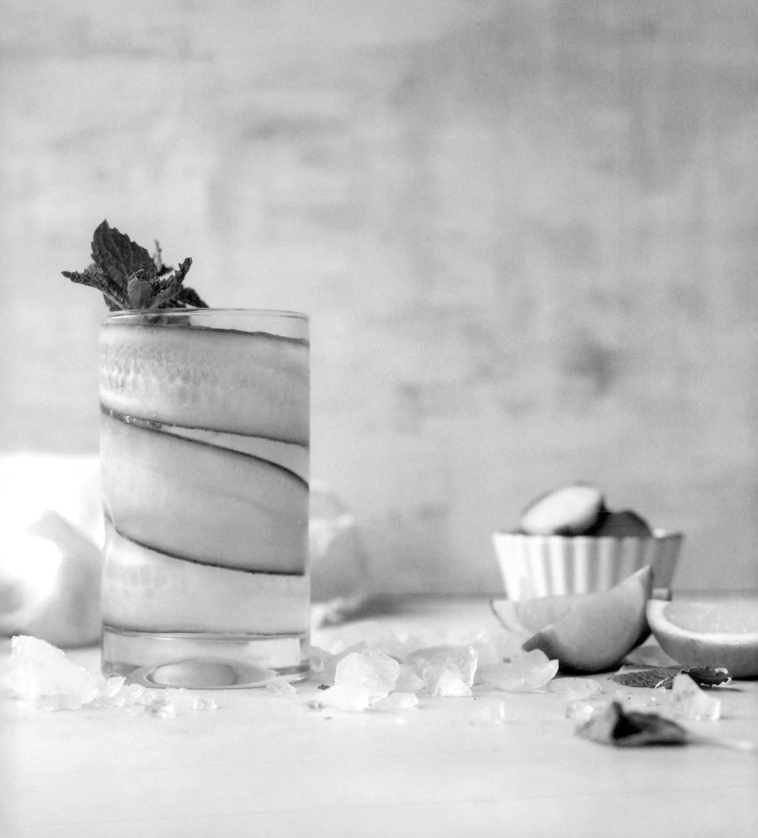

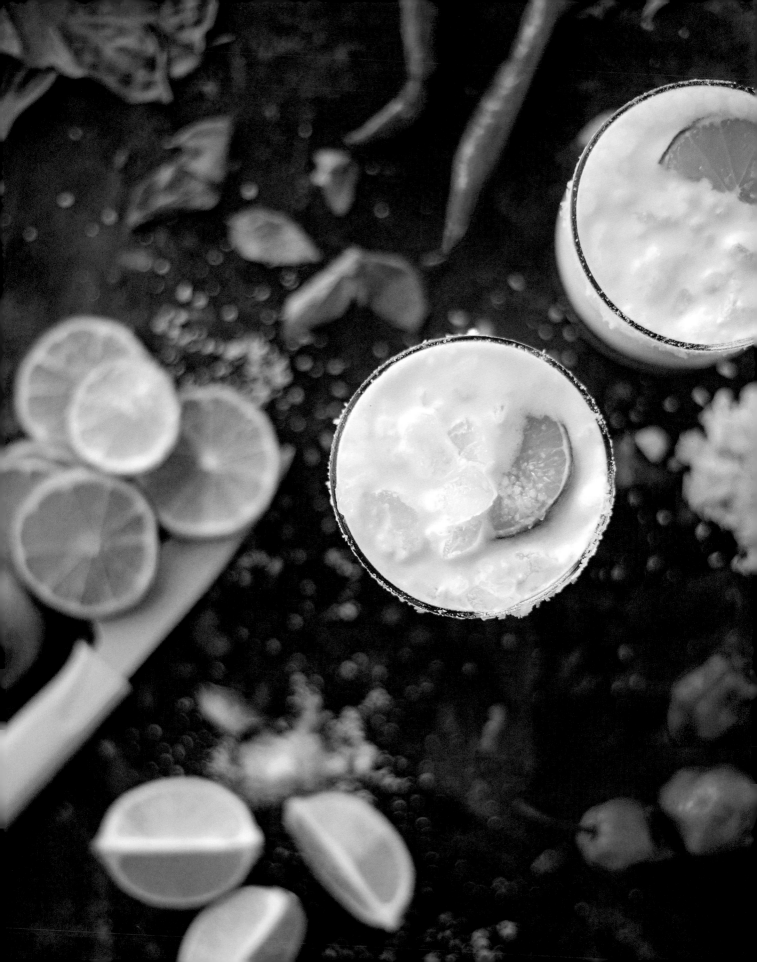

thai coconut margaritas

Just look at this creamy, dreamy concoction! In what is my favorite indulgent cocktail, this creamy coconut margarita on the rocks takes the cake. I love to garnish it with a spicy pepper, which you may or may not consume, depending on how brave you are. Thai basil makes it even better! MAKES 1 SERVING, AND IS EASILY MULTIPLIED

COCONUT SALTED RIM

2 tablespoons coarse salt

1 tablespoon sugar

1 tablespoon flaked unsweetened coconut

1 lime wedge

2 ounces silver tequila

1 ounce Grand Marnier

1 ounce fresh lime juice

1 ounce coconut water

1 ounce canned coconut milk

1 ounce coconut cream

1 ounce coconut rum

1 ounce simple syrup (page 218)

1 drop coconut extract (optional)

GARNISH

Thai basil

Serrano pepper

TO MAKE THE COCONUT SALTED RIM

Combine the salt, sugar, and coconut on a plate. Rim a glass with the lime wedge and dip in the salt coconut mixture. Fill the glass with ice.

In a cocktail shaker with ice, combine the tequila, Grand Marnier, lime juice, coconut water, coconut milk, coconut cream, rum, simple syrup, and coconut extract (if desired). Shake for 30 seconds and pour over the ice in the glass. Garnish with the basil and pepper and serve.

frozen avocado margaritas

Say what? Frozen? Avocado? Margaritas? Is this too much?

It might be, but if you love the cooling and refreshing creaminess of avocado, you'll adore it frozen with lots of lime. It's one big adult slushy. Salted rim and all.

If your friends are super freaked out by this idea, I suggest starting off by serving them in shooters.   MAKES 4 SERVINGS (ABOUT 8 TO 10 SHOOTERS)

4   cups (1 quart) ice

2   avocados, pitted and peeled

½   cup silver tequila

½   cup fresh lime juice

¼   cup Grand Marnier

¼   cup simple syrup (page 218)

Pinch of salt

Coarse salt, for rimming the glasses

Lime wedges, for garnish

In a high-powered blender, combine the ice, avocados, tequila, lime juice, Grand Marnier, simple syrup, and salt. Blend until mixed. Taste and, if desired, add a little more tequila or simple syrup—whatever you need.

Place the coarse salt on a plate. Rim the glasses with lime wedges and dip the rims in the coarse salt.

Spoon the frozen margarita into the glasses and serve with lime wedges.

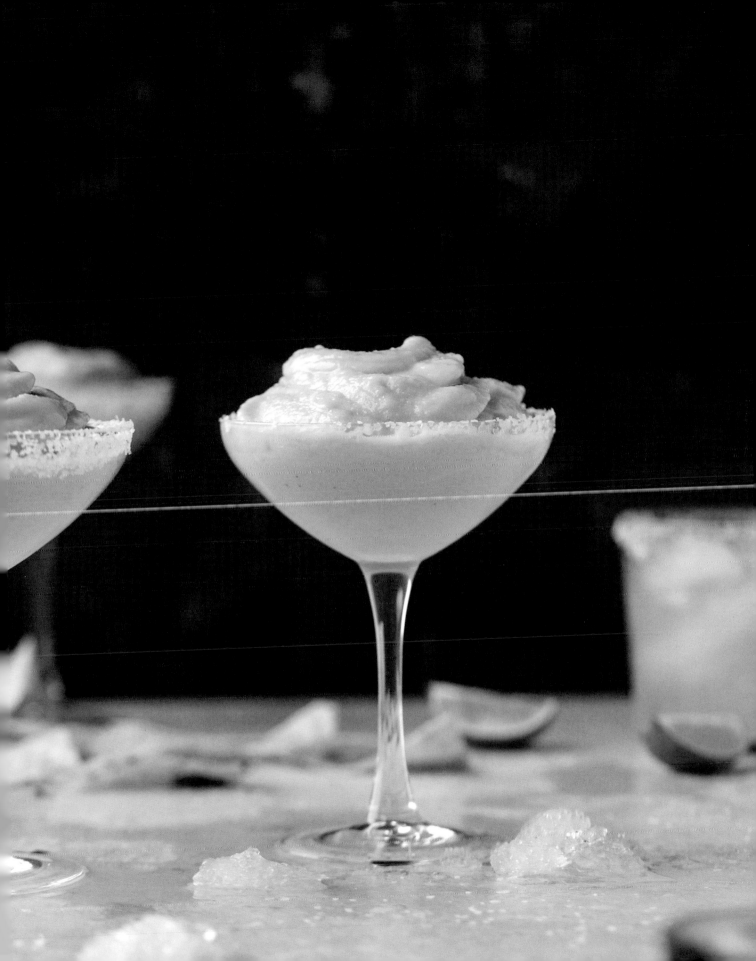

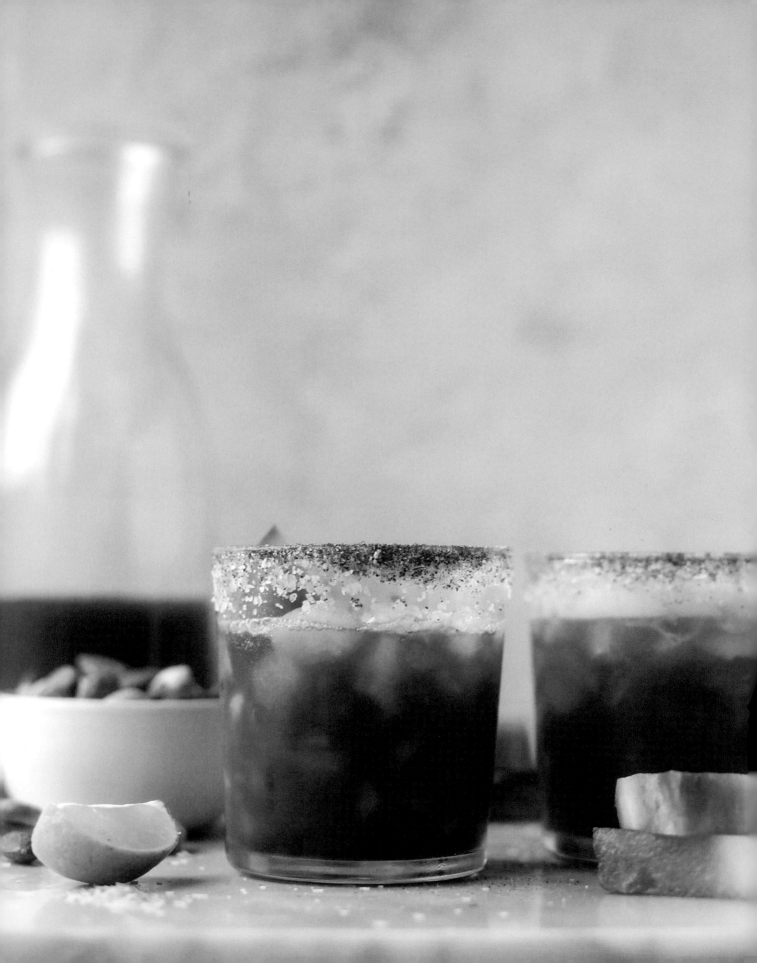

watermelon michelada

The first time I tried micheladas, I was instantly hooked. I loved the fizzy beer with the bit of tomato (or clamato!) juice, the lime and the soy sauce mixed together. It tasted particularly delicious on a late summer evening with a bowl of spicy mixed nuts, and I've dreamed of it ever since.

I've made a few micheladas at home before, but I knew that I wanted to make a version that incorporated a little fruit juice for summer sweetness. Enter beautiful, juicy watermelon. Oh my gosh, this cocktail is fantastic. **MAKES 2 SERVINGS, IS EASILY MULTIPLIED**

3   tablespoons coarse salt,
    for rimming the glasses

½   teaspoon chili powder,
    for rimming the glasses

Lime wedges

⅓   cup cold tomato juice

½   cup fresh watermelon juice

¼   cup fresh lime juice

½   teaspoon Worcestershire sauce

¾   cup cold Mexican beer (I love
    Tecate or Corona)

Drop of hot-pepper sauce

Drop of Maggi sauce

Watermelon wedges, for garnish

Mix the salt and chili powder together on a plate. Rim 2 glasses with the lime wedges, then dip in the salt mixture to cover the rims.

Fill the glasses with ice. Divide the tomato juice and watermelon juice evenly between the glasses. Add half of the lime juice and Worcestershire to each glass. Fill each glass with the beer. Add a drop of hot-pepper sauce and Maggi sauce, then stir. Garnish each with a watermelon wedge and serve immediately.

NOTE: To make the watermelon juice, I simply blend 2 cups of fresh watermelon cubes in a blender, then strain the mixture through a fine-mesh sieve.

blackberry lemonade sangria

I am the queen of homemade sangria. There is no fruit or wine that I won't pair together with some brandy and soda—all combinations are a go. And my most recent favorite is blackberries, brandy, lemonade, and champagne. The combination is just divine!

It's refreshing and light and perfect for brunch! **MAKES 4 SERVINGS**

2   pints fresh blackberries, divided

1   bottle (750 milliliters) sparkling white wine or champagne, chilled

2   cups lemonade, chilled

2   cups lemon-lime soda or sparkling water (depending on the sweetness you want), chilled

½   cup brandy

2   lemons, cut into rounds

Place 1 pint of the blackberries in a bowl and mash them with a fork.

In a large pitcher or punch bowl, combine the mashed blackberries and any juice, the wine or champagne, lemonade, soda or sparkling water, and brandy. Refrigerate for 30 minutes before serving. Serve over ice with the remaining 1 pint blackberries and the lemons.

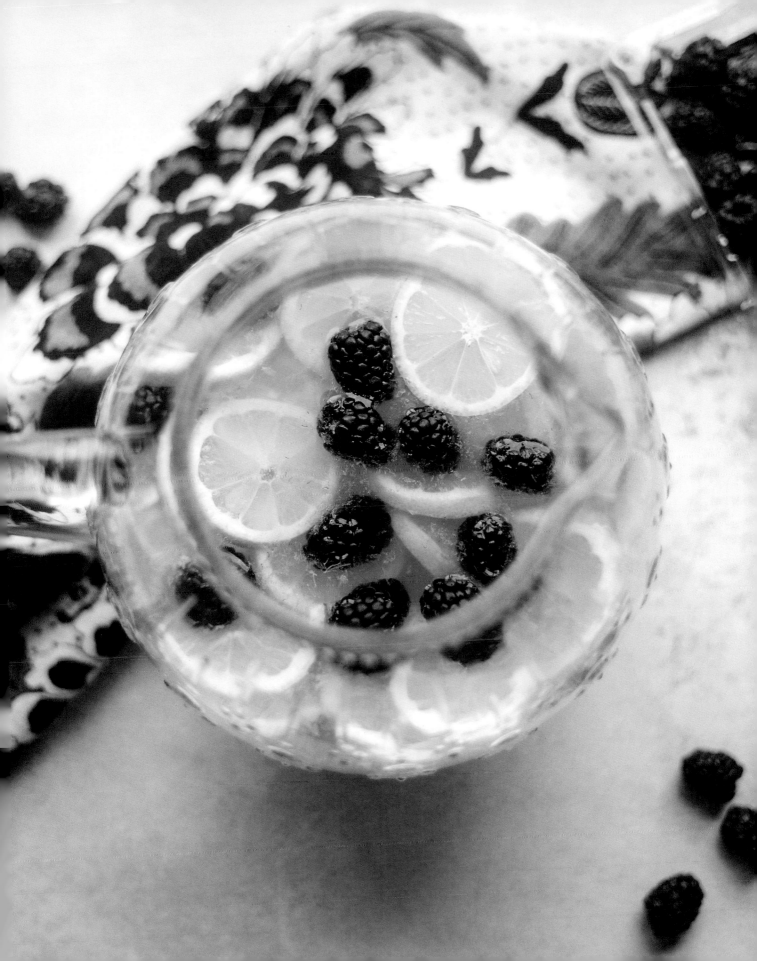

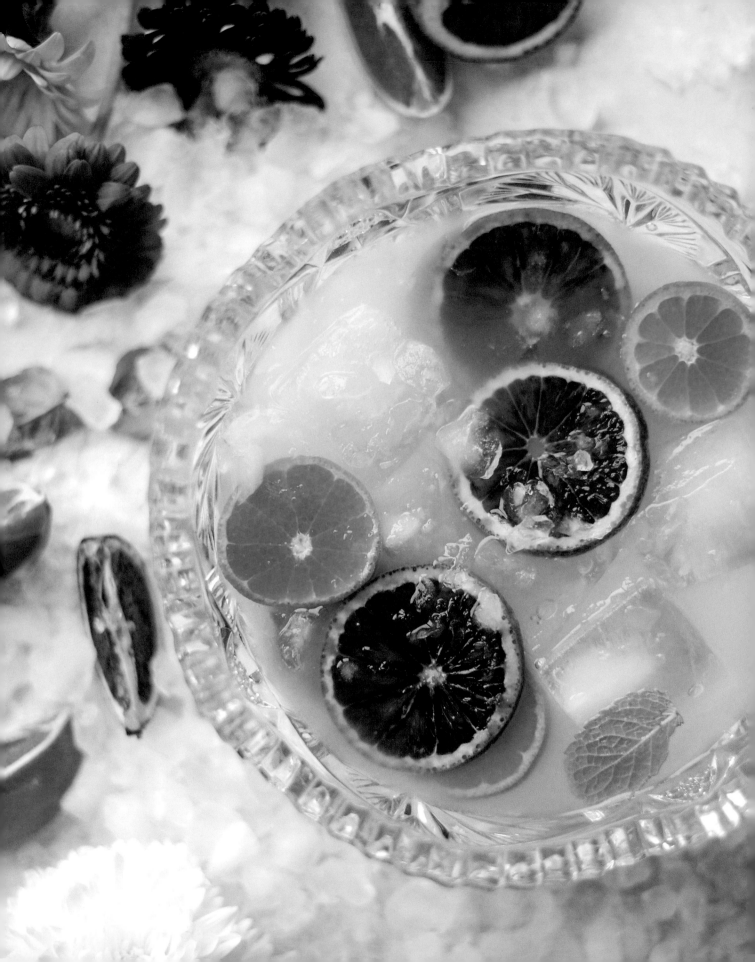

triple citrus mimosa punch

My love of blood oranges doesn't just exist in salads and with bourbon. One of the great things about blood orange soda is that you can find it year-round, with the Italian sodas in your grocery store. Perfectly sweet and tart and ready for your girls' brunch!

Extra champagne, please. MAKES 6 TO 8 SERVINGS

2   cups cold orange juice

2   bottles (750 milliliters each)
    champagne, chilled

1   bottle (16 ounces) blood orange
    Italian soda, chilled

½   cup vodka

2   navel oranges, sliced

2   Cara Cara oranges or tangerines,
    sliced

2   blood oranges, sliced

In a large pitcher or punch bowl, combine the orange juice, champagne, soda, and vodka. Add the orange slices and serve!

blueberry hibiscus mint juleps

Hello spring! That is exactly what a mint julep represents to me. The middle of spring when we're close to summer and the sun is shining bright and warm with the promise of so many sunny days to come!

In this version, we don't muddle the mint with sugar in the bottom of the glass, but instead use a blueberry mint puree and lots of fresh mint leaves. The hibiscus syrup is sweet without being too florally. It's refreshing and delicious. MAKES 1 SERVING, IS EASILY MULTIPLIED

MINT SIMPLE SYRUP

⅓ cup sugar

⅓ cup water

1 bunch fresh mint leaves

HIBISCUS SYRUP

1 cup dried culinary hibiscus flowers

1 cup hot water

⅔ cup sugar

BLUEBERRY MINT PUREE

⅔ cup fresh blueberries

2 tablespoons mint simple syrup

2½ ounces bourbon

2 ounces hibiscus syrup

1 ounce blueberry mint puree

Fresh mint leaves

Fresh hibiscus flower (optional)

TO MAKE THE MINT SIMPLE SYRUP
In a small saucepan, combine the sugar, water, and mint and heat over high heat until boiling, stirring constantly. Reduce the heat to low and cook for another minute or so, then set aside to cool completely. Remove the mint before using. You can do this ahead of time and store it in the fridge!

TO MAKE THE HIBISCUS SYRUP
Place the hibiscus flowers in a bowl and pour the water over top. Let sit and steep for 30 minutes. Strain to remove the flowers.

Pour the hibiscus water into a saucepan and heat over medium heat. Whisk in the sugar and bring the mixture to a simmer. Simmer for 2 minutes. Remove from the heat and let cool to room temperature. Store the syrup in a jar in the fridge for about a week. (You can also use this syrup in seltzer water for a sweet little hibiscus spritzer!)

TO MAKE THE BLUEBERRY MINT PUREE
In a mini food processor or blender, combine the blueberries and mint simple syrup. Blend until pureed.

In a cocktail shaker or glass, combine the bourbon, hibiscus syrup, and blueberry mint puree. Shake or stir well. Pour over crushed iced and serve with extra mint leaves and a fresh hibiscus flower, if desired.

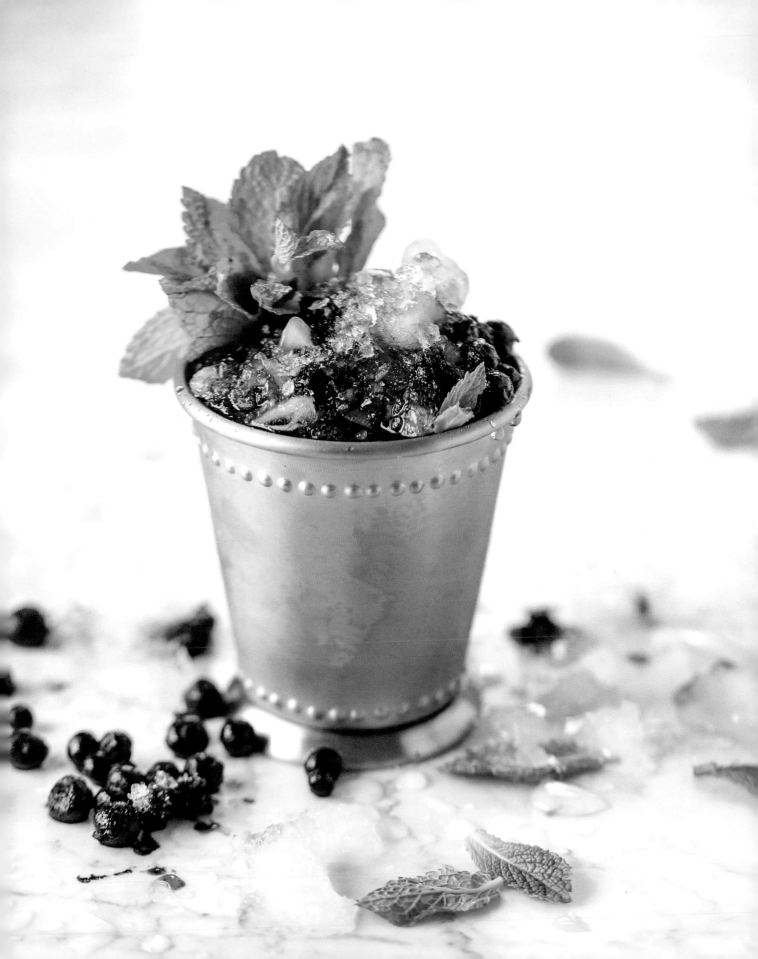

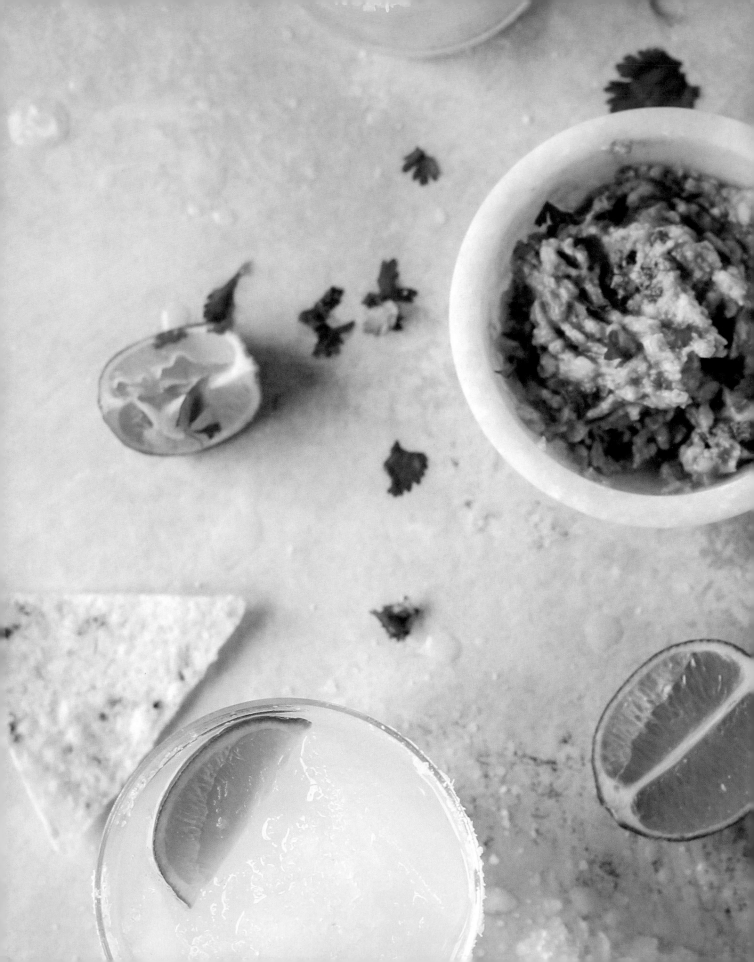

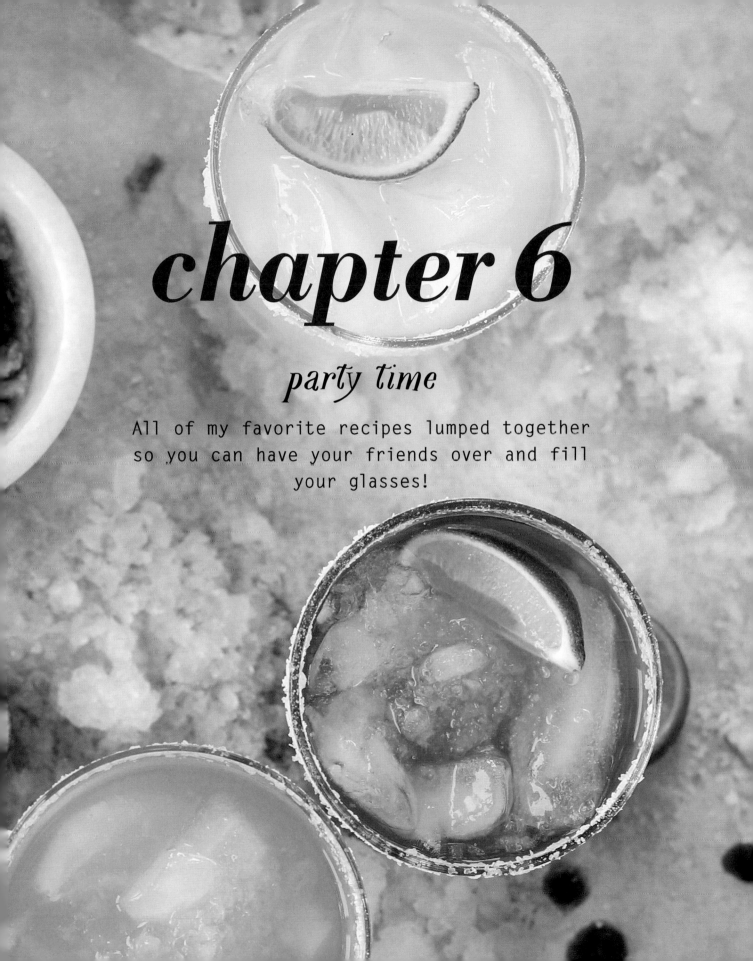

chapter 6

party time

All of my favorite recipes lumped together
so you can have your friends over and fill
your glasses!

AUTUMN HARVEST
BARBECUE PARTY

STARTER
Sweet and Spicy Pretzels
with Maple Beer Mustard
(page 62)

MAIN DISHES
Apple Cider Pulled Pork Sliders
(page 173)

Thai Peanut Acorn Squash
(page 119)

Apple Croissant Panzanella Salad
(page 77)

DRINK
Cider Beergaritas (page 218)

DESSERT
S'mores Stuffed Sweet Potatoes
(page 151)

Autumn Monster Cookies
(page 201)

FRIENDSGIVING PARTY

STARTER
Butternut Squash Queso
with Rustic Tortilla Chips
(page 53)

MAIN DISHES
Bread or biscuits
with Butternut Squash Sage
Compound Butter (page 124)

Any-Squash-You-Choose Shooters
with Buttered Popcorn
(page 135)

Winter Rice Bowls with
Crispy Shallots (page 104)

Fall-Spiced Pesto with pasta
or zucchini noodles (page 96)

DRINK
Cider Beergaritas (page 218)

DESSERTS
Chocolate Pumpkin Crumble
Snack Cake (page 206)

Autumn Monster Cookies
(page 201)

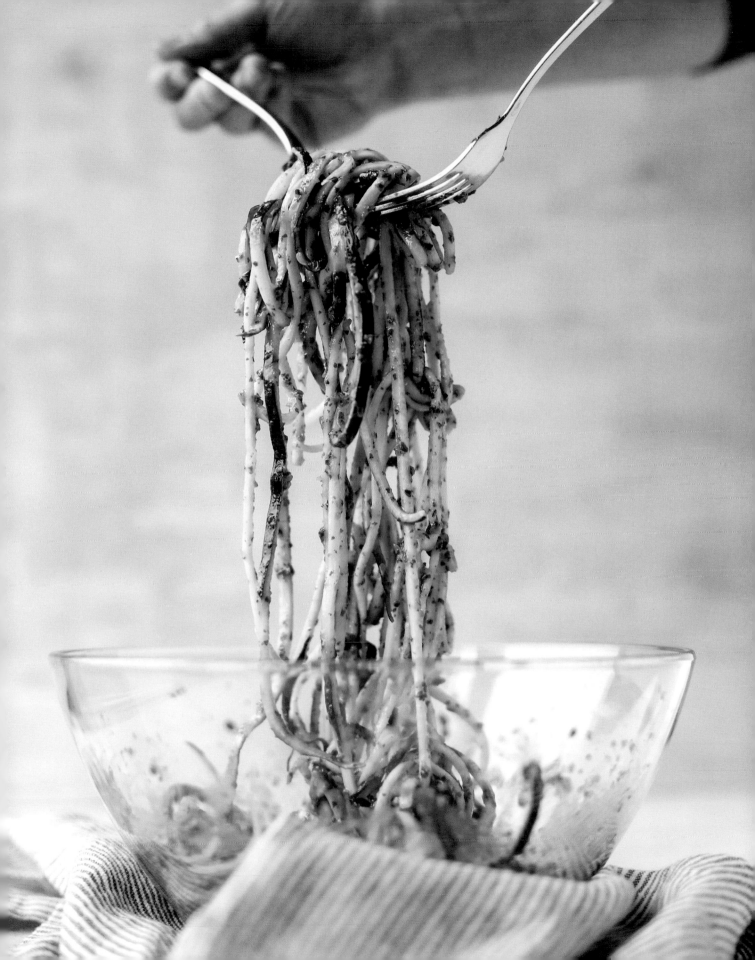

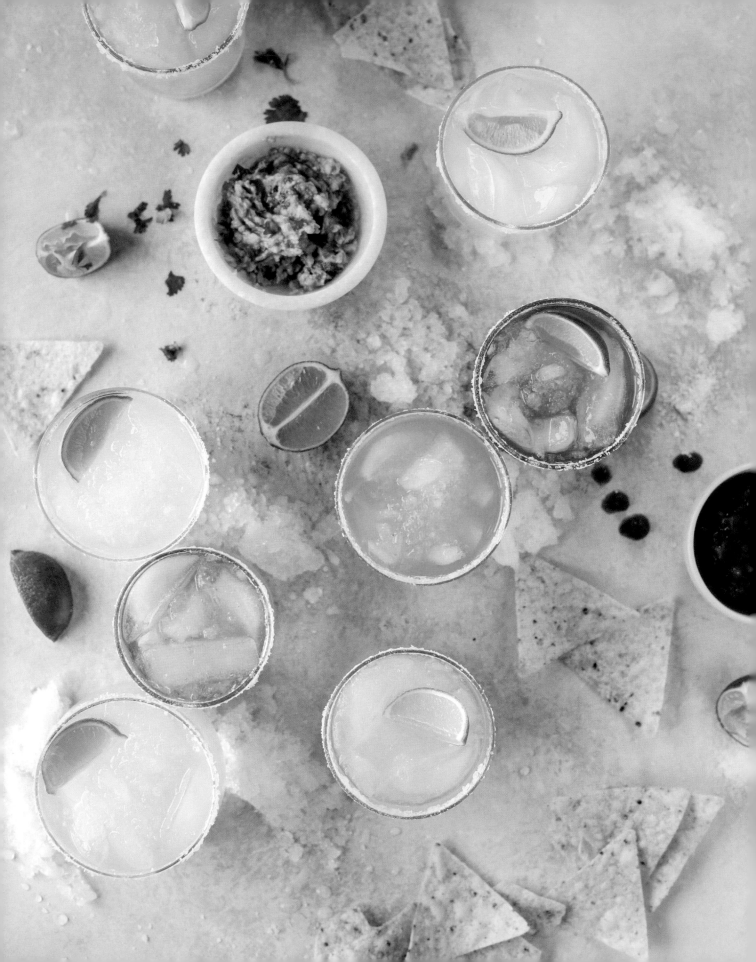

TACOS & TEQUILA PARTY

STARTERS

Watermelon Avocado Salsa
with tortilla chips
(page 61)

Spicy Corn and Peach Salsa
with tortilla chips
(page 58)

MAIN DISHES

Jalapeño Butternut Squash Tacos,
made into mini
bite-size tacos (page 170)

Carnitas Burrito Bowls (page 159)

DRINKS

Thai Coconut Margaritas
(page 237)

Bacon Bloody Marias
(page 233)

DESSERTS

Lemon Cupcakes with
Mojito Frosting (page 186)

Chocolate Crinkle Sprinkle
Cookies (page 205)

GIRLS' BRUNCH PARTY

STARTER

Vegetable and fruit
cheese board

MAIN DISHES

Charred Pineapple Salad
(page 84)

Hot Pink Hummus Avocado
Toast (page 87)

Asparagus with Shallots,
Bacon, and Parmesan
(page 116)

DRINKS

Iced Lavender Vanilla Lattes
(page 21)

Triple Citrus Mimosa Punch
(page 245)

DESSERT

Tiramisu Bread Pudding
(page 202)

DERBY DAY PARTY

STARTERS
Pimiento Cheese–Stuffed
Olives (page 54)

Extra Pimiento Cheese
with crackers

MAIN DISHES
Green Goddess Chicken Salad
Sandwiches (page 139)

Blood Orange, Avocado, and
Beet Salad (page 73)

Sweet Potato Corn Fritters (page 147)
with Homemade Bacon Mayo
(page 148)

DRINKS
Mint Iced Tea with Pineapple
Ice Cubes (page 226)

Blueberry Hibiscus Mint Juleps
(page 246)

DESSERTS
Strawberry Almond Mascarpone
Tart (page 193)

ONLY SUMMER CHEESE PLATE YOU'LL EVER NEED

CHEESE
White Cheddar
Smoky blue cheese
Humboldt Fog chèvre
Burrata

PRODUCE
Fresh and dried figs
Red and green grapes
Fresh strawberries
Grilled peaches
Melon balls

BREADS
Fresh baguette
Multigrain crackers
Hard breadsticks
Soft breadsticks

MEATS
Thinly sliced prosciutto
Thinly sliced soppressata

PICKLED
Olives
Cornichons
Pickled green beans or asparagus
Pickled onions (page 160)

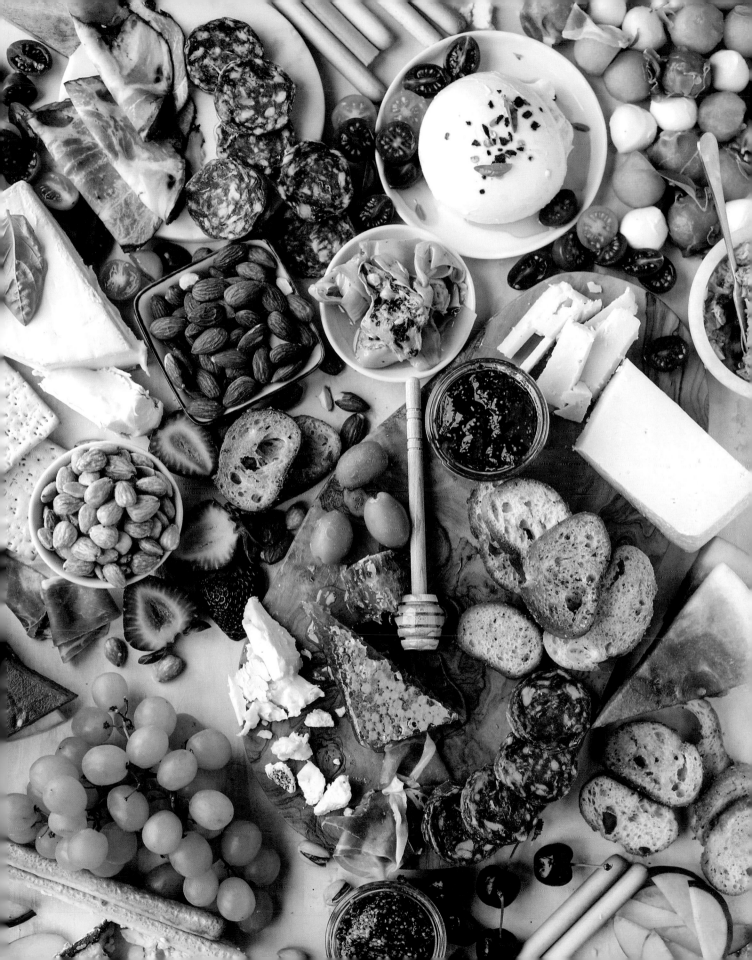

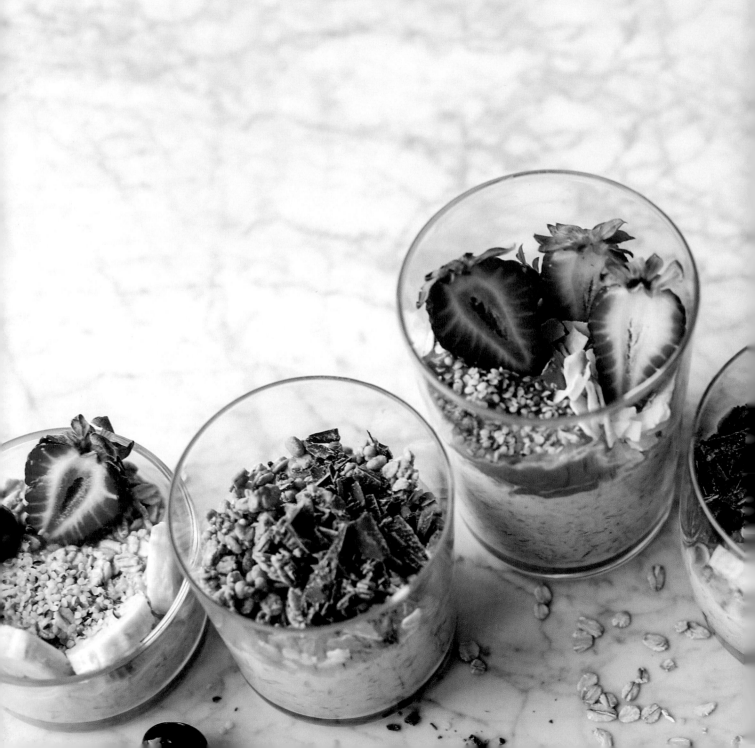

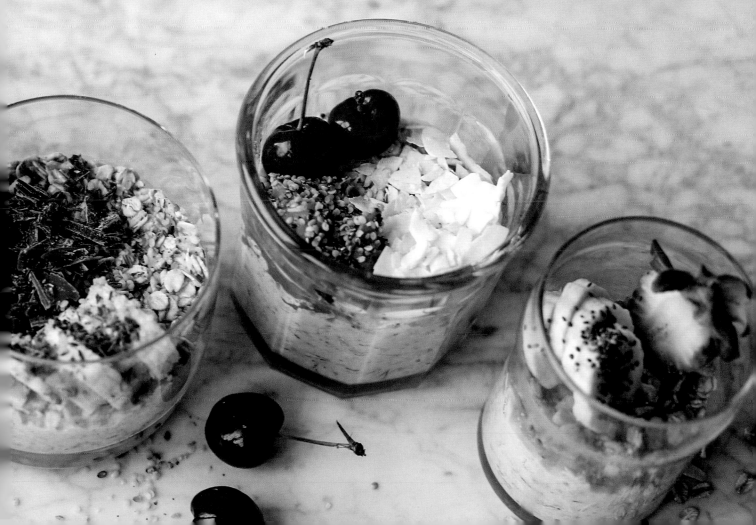

chapter 7

let's go to the bar

In fact, let's go to six of them!

OVERNIGHT OATS BAR

1. WHAT YOU NEED

Your basic overnight oats recipe! For each serving, you'll need: ½ cup rolled oats + ½ cup milk + 2 teaspoons sweetener of your choice

Toppings and add-ins, including but not limited to: nut butters, chia seeds, hemp seeds, chocolate chips, flaked and shredded coconut, granola, toasted nuts, fresh and frozen fruit, milks for drizzling (coconut, almond, cashew), honey, maple syrup, sprinkles for fun!

2. EQUIPMENT

Single-serve jars for the oats, as well as bowls for toppings and mix-ins, utensils.

3. HOW TO DO IT

Prepare the oats the night before, obviously! You can prepare a large batch in a bowl and portion them out into small bowls and jars for single-serving portions. Be sure to add a touch of sweetener into the oats, but not that much. It's also up to you on whether you add chia seeds to the oats at this point.

The morning of, prep your toppings and add-ins in an assembly line with utensils. Start with the basic add-ins (fruit, milk for drizzling) and then the additional toppings (chocolate chips, chopped nuts).

BUILD-YOUR-OWN PIZZA BAR

1. WHAT YOU NEED

A basic pizza dough recipe (see page 178). Plan on each dough recipe serving 3 to 4 people. Pizza sauce! + Traditional pizza cheeses, such as provolone and mozzarella.

Toppings including but not limited to: pepperoni, mushrooms, peppers (fresh, roasted, and/or pickled), shredded chicken, artichoke hearts, red onion, fresh spinach, olives, fresh arugula, goat cheese, crispy bacon, crumbled sausage, figs, fresh basil, fresh oregano, ranch dressing, barbecue sauce, hot-pepper sauce, truffle oil, eggs.

2. EQUIPMENT

pizza peels, rolling pins, parchment paper, bowls or plates for toppings, utensils.

3. HOW TO DO IT

Prepare your dough a day or 2 ahead of time and portion it into 2-ounce balls. Wrap it in plastic wrap or place it in a resealable plastic bag in the fridge. Remove it from the fridge 30 minutes prior to prepping the pizzas.

Have a designated workspace and pieces of parchment paper sprinkled with flour so people can roll or press out their dough.

Place the toppings in an assembly line that makes sense, starting with the sauce and the cheese, the most common toppings in the center, and more unique toppings toward the end.

Whether you're using your oven, a grill, or a wood fire, the doughs should be small enough that you can cook 2 at a time. Make sure the appliance is preheated and ready to go. Have extra pizza peels on hand, too!

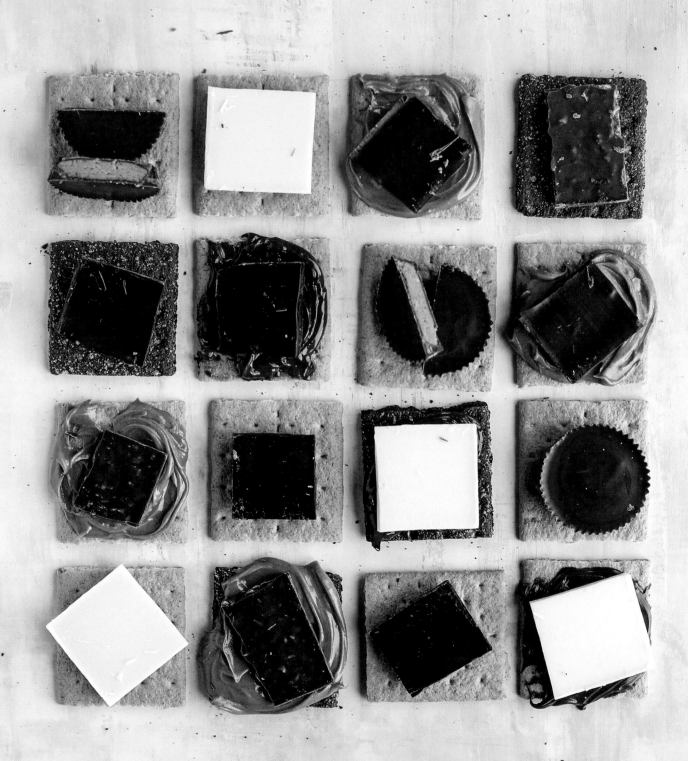

BUILD-YOUR-OWN S'MORES BAR

1. WHAT YOU NEED

A fire! + S'mores goodies, including but not limited to: graham crackers (honey, cinnamon, and chocolate), buttery Ritz crackers, sandwich cookies, peanut butter cookies, fudge stripe cookies, marshmallows (assorted flavors if desired!), peanut butter (as well as almond butter and other nut butters), Nutella, chocolate bars, white chocolate, cookies-and-cream bars, caramel-filled chocolate, mint-filled chocolate, peanut butter cups, strawberries, and bananas.

2. EQUIPMENT

skewers or wood sticks for roasting the marshmallows, plates for the finished s'mores, bowls and plates for toppings, utensils.

3. HOW TO DO IT

While I love homemade marshmallows more than anything, I find that they don't toast as wonderfully as the store-bought kind. For ease and convenience here, I suggest buying the store-bought ones and rolling with those!

Prep a bonfire or even a fire in a portable fire pit. Arrange the toppings in an assembly line for s'mores making, starting with the marshmallows. Having the marshmallows already skewered for the first go-round is the easiest option, but as long as the skewers are nearby, you're good to go!

The rest of the toppings should be arranged by crackers and cookies, any spreads (such as peanut butter), and finally the chocolate and fillings.

AFFOGATO BAR

1. WHAT YOU NEED

Your favorite ice cream flavors! I suggest going with about six to eight flavors. My favorites include chocolate, vanilla, peanut butter, pistachio, cookies and cream, blackberry, and coconut.

An espresso machine or an easy plan to brew a few ounces of strong coffee.

A variety of toppings, including but not limited to: flavored syrups (vanilla, caramel, mocha, hazelnut), cookies, chocolate chips, biscuits, and colorful sprinkles.

2. EQUIPMENT

bowls for the toppings; cute bowls, mugs, or jars for serving the affogato; utensils for serving.

3. HOW TO DO IT

The easiest way to serve ice cream to a crowd without it melting is to keep it in the containers, provide each container with its own scoop, and set the containers on a bed of ice. This can be in a cooler, in a large bowl, on a large platter with a lip (so the ice doesn't melt off!), or in a beverage bucket or tub.

Set up an assembly line starting with the mugs first and heading into the ice cream. Finish with a spot for the espresso to be poured over top (if you're not using an espresso machine, you can keep the strong coffee hot in a thermos) and toppings to be sprinkled on top.

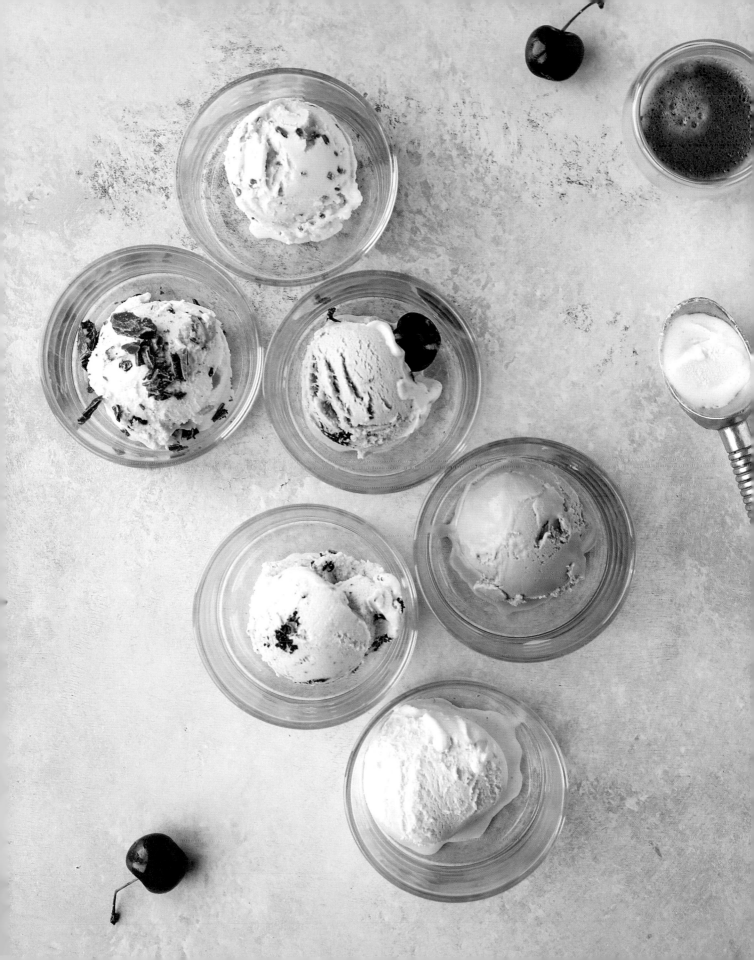

SAVORY SNACK TOAST BAR

1. WHAT YOU NEED

A variety of breads for toasting! Baguettes, sourdough, traditional wheat and white, marbled rye.

Spreads for the first layer of your snack toast. Including but not limited to: mashed or sliced avocado, ricotta cheese, hummus, fig jam (or another flavor you may love!), and softened goat cheese.

Toppings for the second layer of your toast, including but not limited to: crumbly cheese such as Gorgonzola or crumbled goat cheese, sliced almonds or toasted pistachios, sliced cherry tomatoes, crumbled bacon, pickled or roasted peppers and artichokes, fresh fruits and vegetables, pesto for drizzling, grilled corn, fresh herbs, smoked sea salt, and fresh pepper for grinding.

2. EQUIPMENT

bowls for spreads and toppings, plates, and utensils

3. HOW TO DO IT

Shortly before setting up the bar, toast the bread slices if possible. You don't want them to get soggy, but this also removes an extra step for your guests!

Set up an assembly line of different toasts, bowls with spreads, and then bowls of toppings. Be sure to check on spreads or toppings that don't keep for long (such as avocado) so you can do easy refills.

TIME FOR A CHILI BAR

1. WHAT YOU NEED

One or two chili recipes. I like to do a spicier one for those who like some heat! See pages 131 and 136 for chili recipes.

Tortilla chips and hot dogs on buns for those who prefer more than a bowl of chili.

A big bowl of butternut squash queso dip for drizzling! See page 53 for the recipe.

An assortment of toppings, including but not limited to: freshly grated cheese, queso fresco cheese, jalapeño peppers (fresh and pickled), banana peppers, diced red onion, sliced scallions, chives, corn chips (like Fritos!), chopped fresh tomato, salsa or pico de gallo, and fresh cilantro.

2. EQUIPMENT

one or two slow cookers, bowls for toppings, bowls and plates for serving.

3. HOW TO DO IT

Make your chili a day or two beforehand and keep it prepped in the fridge. The day of, transfer your chili to one or two slow cookers and heat them on low for a few hours before your guests arrive.

Set up an assembly line of toppings and chili "accessories," starting with the chili, then the cheeses, and moving on to the veggies, other toppings, and queso. I like to keep the tortilla chips and hot dogs nearby in case someone wants nachos or a hot dog first!

Be sure to periodically check the chili, hot dogs, and queso dip to make sure they're still warm.

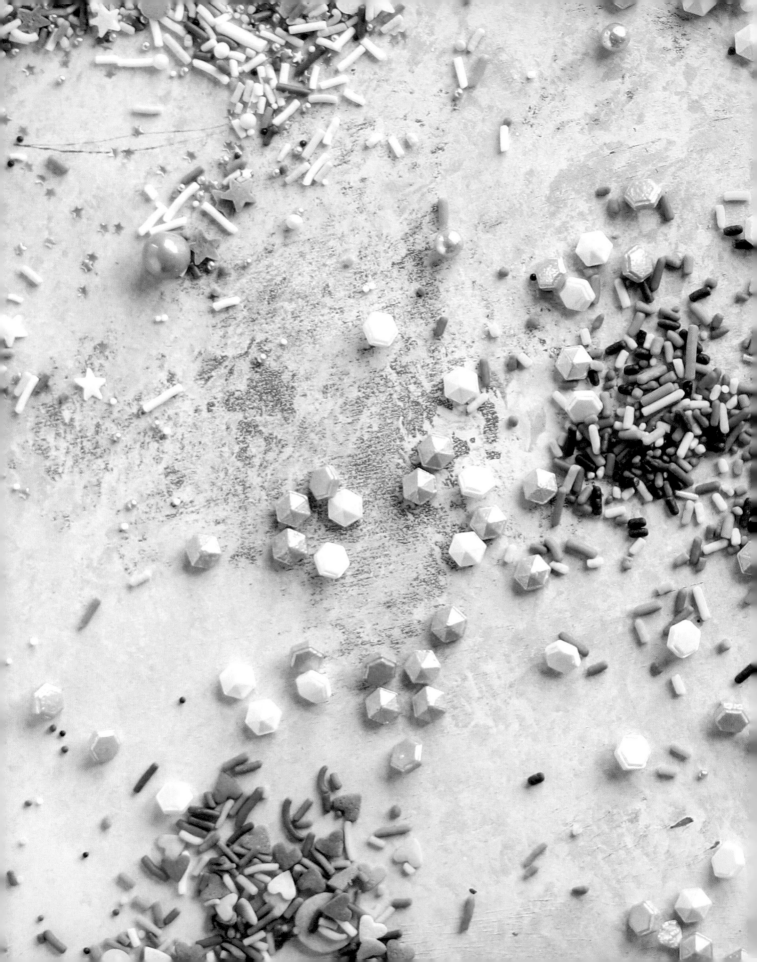

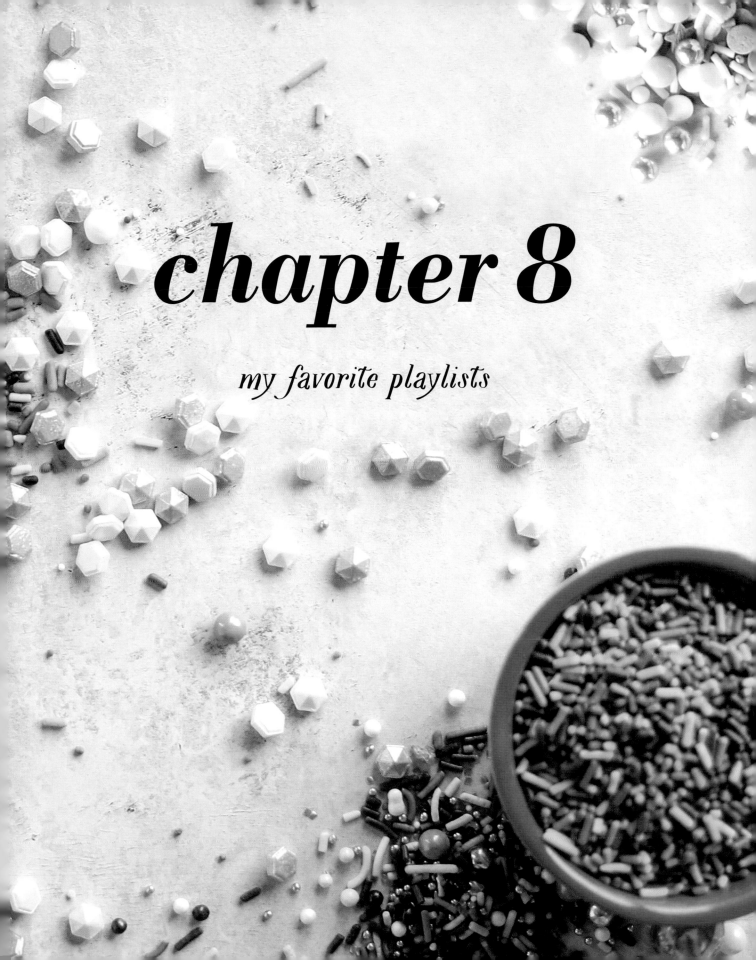

chapter 8

my favorite playlists

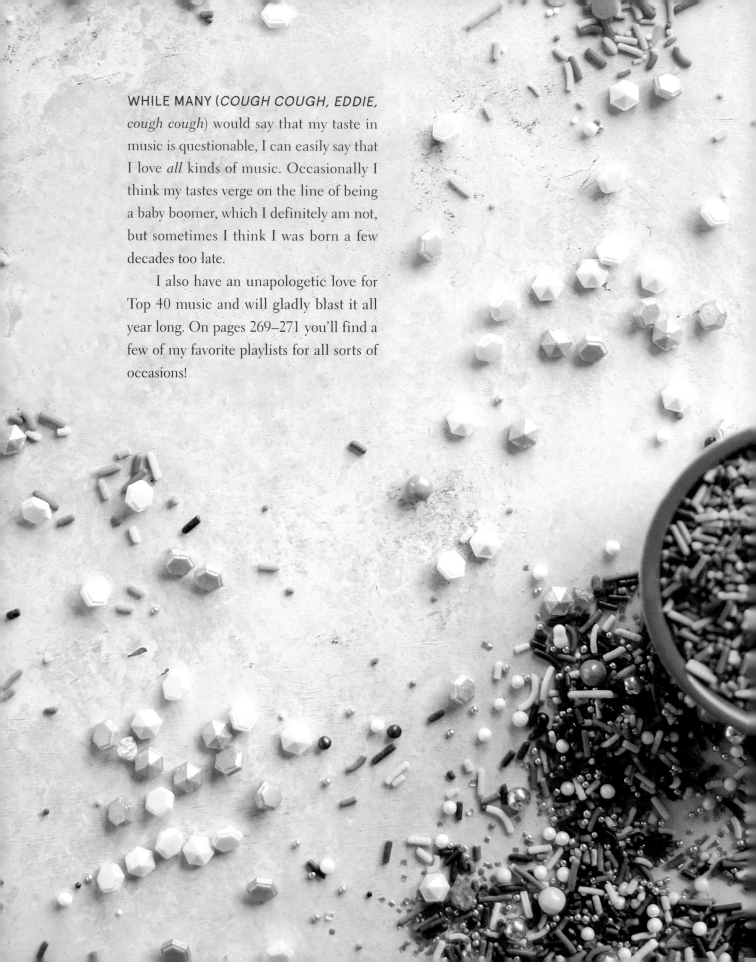

WHILE MANY (*COUGH COUGH, EDDIE, cough cough*) would say that my taste in music is questionable, I can easily say that I love *all* kinds of music. Occasionally I think my tastes verge on the line of being a baby boomer, which I definitely am not, but sometimes I think I was born a few decades too late.

I also have an unapologetic love for Top 40 music and will gladly blast it all year long. On pages 269–271 you'll find a few of my favorite playlists for all sorts of occasions!

A SUPER CHILL DINNER PARTY

"It Had to Be You"
by Steve Tyrell

"Let There Be Love"
by Nat King Cole

"The Way You Look Tonight"
by Maroon 5

"Ain't That a Kick in the Head"
by Dean Martin

"Beyond the Sea"
by Bobby Caldwell

"Love on Top"
by Beyoncé

"All I Do Is Dream of You"
by Michael Bublé

"I Could Write a Book"
by Harry Connick Jr.

"Sway"
by Dean Martin

"Stay with You"
by John Legend

"Wonderful World" by Sam Cooke

"Lovesong"
by Adele

"Thinking Out Loud"
by Ed Sheeran

A MORE UPBEAT DINNER PARTY

"You Beat Me to the Punch"
by Mary Wells

"September"
by Earth, Wind & Fire

"Sugar"
by Maroon 5

"Come Fly with Me"
by Frank Sinatra

"Feeling Good"
by Michael Bublé

"Moondance"
by Van Morrison

"The Sound"
by The 1975

"No One Else Like You"
by Adam Levine

"83" by John Mayer

"Don't Rush"
by Kelly Clarkson and Vince Gill

"Lady (You Bring Me Up)"
by Lionel Richie

"Don't Stop 'Til You Get Enough"
by Michael Jackson

"I Second That Emotion"
by Smokey Robinson

MORNING BRUNCH PLAYLIST

"A Sunday Kind of Love"
by Etta James

"Treasure" by Bruno Mars

"Coming Home"
by Leon Bridges

"Magic" by Coldplay

"Wedding Bell Blues"
by The 5th Dimension

"You Send Me"
by Aretha Franklin

"Everything"
by Michael Bublé

"Water under the Bridge"
by Adele

"I Feel It Coming"
by The Weeknd

"Closer"
by The Chainsmokers

"You Are the Best Thing"
by Ray LaMontagne

"Don't" by Ed Sheeran

"You've Got the Love"
by Florence + the Machine

SUMMER FUN PLAYLIST

"Return of the Mack"
by Mark Morrison

"Hey Ya!" by OutKast

"Summer Wind"
by Frank Sinatra

"Feels Like the First Time"
by Foreigner

"Vacation"
by Thomas Rhett

"How Will I Know"
by Whitney Houston

"One Love"
by Bob Marley

"Try Me" by Jason Derulo

"Carolina in My Mind"
by James Taylor

"Too Good"
by Drake and Rihanna

"Wouldn't It Be Nice"
by the Beach Boys

"Pontoon"
by Little Big Town

"Catch My Breath"
by Kelly Clarkson

ENERGIZING PLAYLIST

"Neon Lights" by Demi Lovato

"Work"
by Rihanna and Drake

"One Dance" by Drake

"Uptown Funk"
by Mark Ronson and
Bruno Mars

"Promiscuous"
by Nelly Furtado

"Emotions"
by Mariah Carey

"Get Me Bodied"
by Beyoncé

"Lose Control"
by Missy Elliott

"Birthday" by Katy Perry

"We Found Love"
by Rihanna and Calvin Harris

"Crazy in Love"
by Beyoncé and Jay-Z

"Bailando"
by Enrique Iglesias

"Forever" by Chris Brown

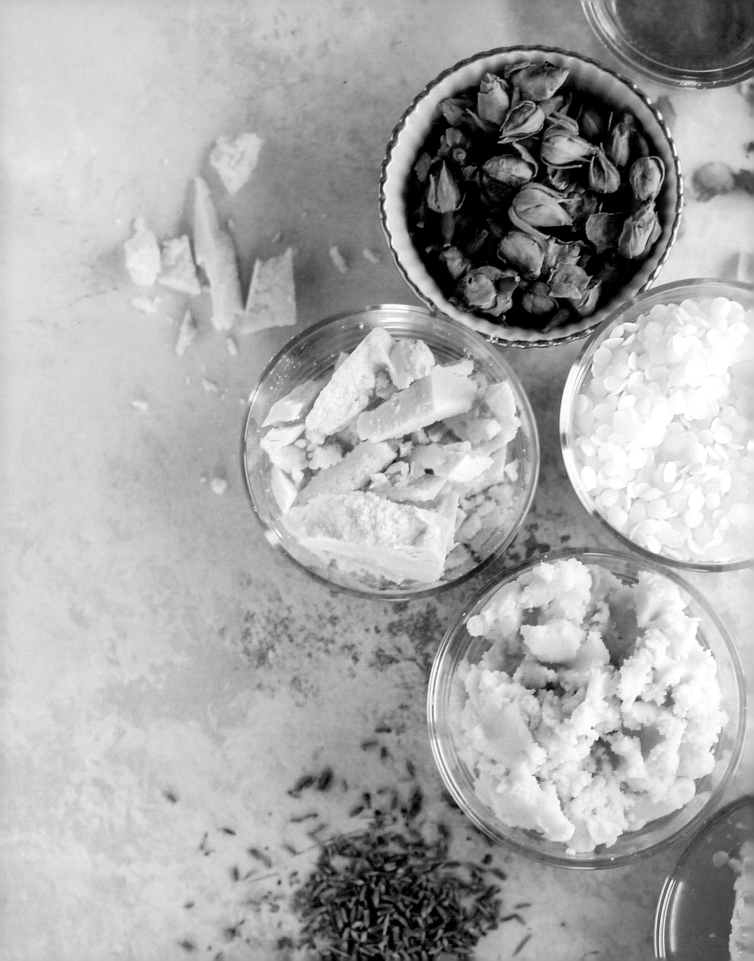

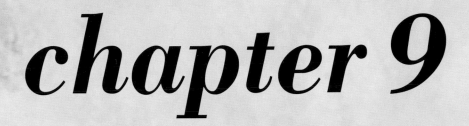

chapter 9

beauty DIYs

IT'S TIME FOR FOOD THAT YOU CAN PUT ON
your face! And your body.

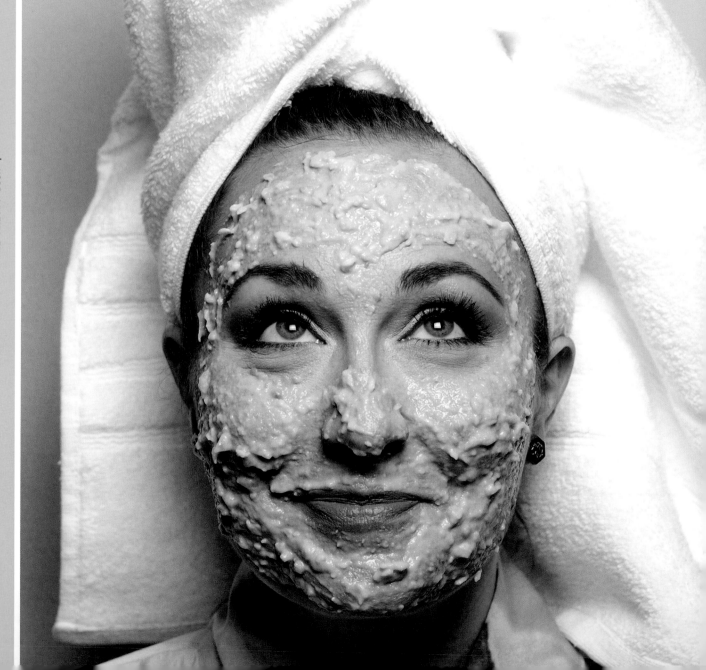

IT'S TIME FOR FOOD . . . THAT YOU CAN put on your face! And your body.

I've been experimenting with homemade beauty products since I was a tween. The first time I saw an article about putting smashed bananas in my hair or yogurt on my face, I was sold. My best friend and I used to test out our own "products" in her bathroom and even create pretend magazine articles and videos about them on a massive camcorder from the '90s.

To say I've upgraded that situation a little would be an understatement, but the ingredients remain mostly the same! Here you will find a bunch of fun homemade treats that you can make and share with your girlfriends.

homemade sugar scrubs

Exfoliating has been a part of my beauty routine for as long as I can remember, mostly because I've been "blessed" with the dry skin that my dad's side of the family has. Exfoliating once or twice a week, from the time I've been in high school, always felt like an extra little spa experience—even though I didn't even get to a spa for the first time until I was in my late twenties.

I'm very particular about my scrubs, however. I have been to spas where the scrub has felt like a million tiny bees stinging my legs. I like a balance of moisturizing oils and larger exfoliating granules. I want it to feel like it's working, but leave my skin moisturized. I am also a much bigger proponent of sugar scrubs, rather than ones made with salt, on the skin and face. Way too often I'd have a tiny paper cut or a brush burn that I missed and using a salt scrub on that? Oh boy. Pain city.

After going through countless pounds of sugar, I've discovered the formula that I love, one that closely resembles my favorite store-bought sugar scrub. These are moisturizing and exfoliating at the same time. They make for the cutest gifts because they look beautiful sitting near your tub or shower.

Most of my scrubs include a few drops of essential oils to heighten the scent experience. You can always leave these oils out and receive the same benefits of exfoliation. I find that these scrubs stay fresh for two to three months.

(continued)

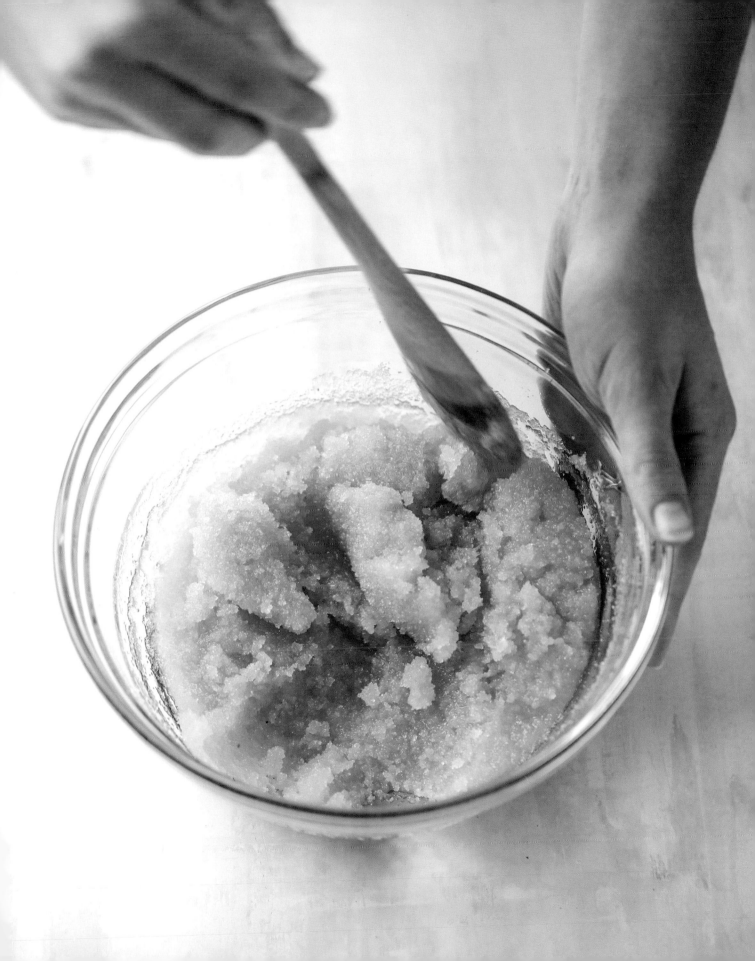

BIRTHDAY CAKE SCRUB

2 cups sugar

1 cup walnut or almond oil

8 drops vanilla essential oil

¾ cup dye-free sprinkles

Place the sugar in a bowl. Add the walnut or almond oil and the essential oil and stir together well, until the mixture is combined and fragrant. Fold in the sprinkles. Package in a jar with a seal-tight lid.

MAKES 2 CUPS

TIP: Make sure your sprinkles are dye-free so they don't color your tub or skin!

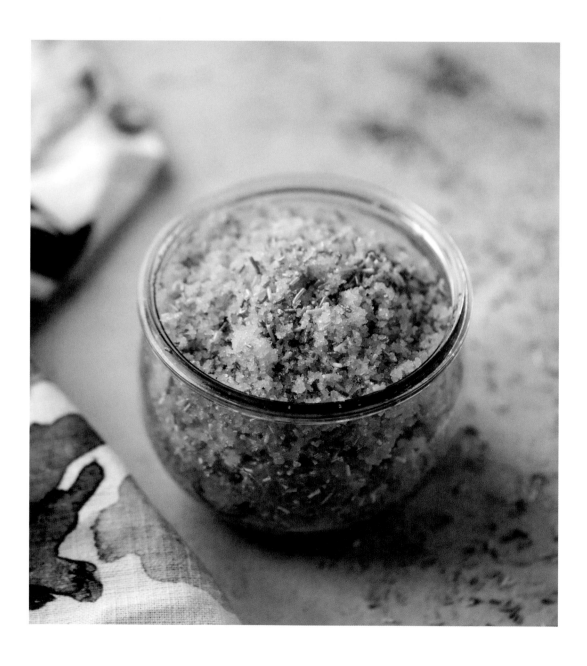

VANILLA BEAN ROSE SCRUB

2 cups sugar

1 cup walnut oil

1 vanilla bean, seeds scraped out

5 drops vanilla essential oil

½ cup crushed dried culinary rose petals

In a bowl, stir together the sugar and walnut oil. Add in the scraped vanilla seeds and essential oil and stir. Stir in the rose petals. Package in a jar with a seal-tight lid. MAKES 2 CUPS

TIP: For the "healthiest" skin scrub, make sure the dried rose petals are culinary grade, which ensures they weren't treated with chemicals.

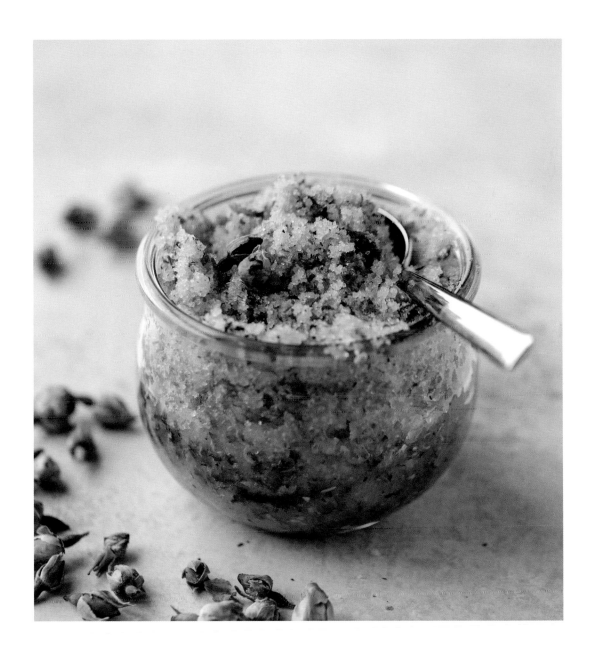

PEPPERMINT MOCHA SCRUB

2 cups sugar

½ cup fine coffee grounds

2 teaspoons unsweetened cocoa powder

1 cup walnut oil

5 drops peppermint essential oil

2 drops vanilla essential oil

In a bowl, stir together the sugar, coffee, and cocoa. Stir in the walnut oil until combined. Add in the essential oils and stir. Package in a jar with a seal-tight lid.   MAKES ABOUT 2 CUPS

TIP: I like to add a few pieces of chopped candy cane on top for gifting, but be sure to remove these before use! Do not mix them into the scrub, where they will get lost and possibly clog the drain. Tip: Make sure your sprinkles are dye-free so they don't color your tub or skin!

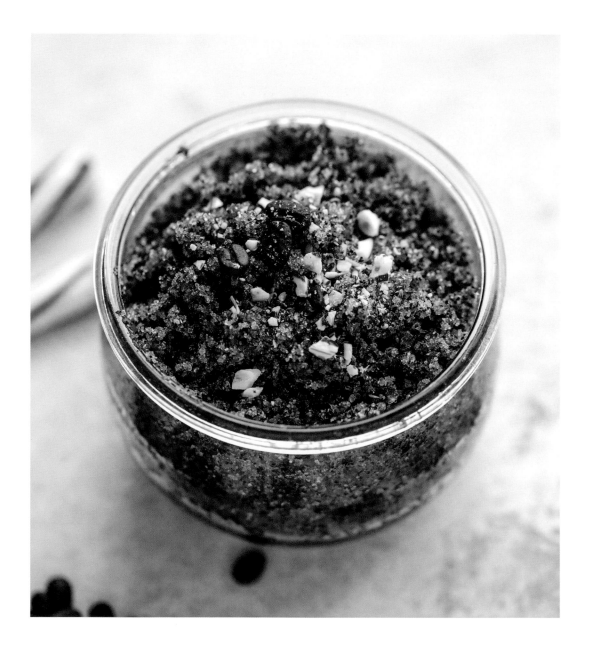

GRAPEFRUIT SCRUB

2   cups sugar
1   cup walnut oil
3   teaspoons grated grapefruit
    zest
4   drops grapefruit essential oil

In a bowl, stir together the sugar and walnut oil. Stir in the grapefruit zest and essential oil until combined. Package in a jar with a seal-tight lid. MAKES 2 CUPS

PUMPKIN CHAI SCRUB

1½ cups brown sugar
½   cup granulated sugar
3   tablespoons pumpkin pie spice
2   teaspoons allspice
2   teaspoons cardamom
2   drops cinnamon essential oil
4   drops vanilla essential oil
1   drop cardamom essential oil

In a bowl, stir together the sugars and spices. Add the essential oils and stir together well, until the mixture is combined and fragrant. Package in a jar with a seal-tight lid. MAKES ABOUT 2 CUPS

MORNING EUCALYPTUS SCRUB

2   cups sugar
1   cup walnut oil
5   drops eucalyptus essential oil
2   drops vanilla essential oil

In a bowl, stir together the sugar and walnut oil. Add in the essential oils and stir until combined. Package in a jar with a seal-tight lid. MAKES 2 CUPS

OATMEAL HONEY SCRUB

½   cup old-fashioned rolled oats
1   tablespoon brown sugar
3   tablespoons honey
3   tablespoons coconut oil, melted

Place the oats in a food processor and pulse until finely ground, but not a powder. MAKES ½ CUP

In a bowl, stir together the oats, sugar, honey, and coconut oil until it's a sugary paste. This scrub is best when used right away, so be sure to make it right before scrubbing! It's one of the few scrubs that I do use on my face occasionally because it's so gentle.

OATMEAL SUGAR SCRUB

½   cup old-fashioned rolled oats
3   tablespoons brown sugar
3   tablespoons coconut oil, melted
1   drop vanilla essential oil

Place the oats in a food processor and blend until finely ground, but not a powder.

In a bowl, stir together the oats, sugar, and coconut oil until it's a sugary paste. Stir in the essential oil. This scrub is best when used right away, so be sure to make it right before scrubbing! It's one of the few scrubs that I do use on my face since the oats and soft brown sugar are so gentle. MAKES ½ CUP

homemade sugar lip scrubs

In addition to my love for body scrubs, I've been a frequent lip scrub user as well. The first lip scrub I ever discovered was from The Body Shop while I was in high school, and it came in stick form—like a lipstick that was filled with sand. I thought this was the coolest idea—and never knew that I could easily remove dry skin flakes from my lips with a toothbrush or something similar.

As time went on, I fell prey to the multiple lip scrubs out there that had delicious flavors attached. Red velvet cake! Vanilla bean! Chocolate milkshake! I mean, of course I wanted a lip scrub that tasted like dessert. Hello.

The truth is, though, that those lip scrubs are purely sugar. Just sugar! You can easily grab a spoonful of sugar from your kitchen, mix it with a little coconut or olive oil, and rub it all over your lips each morning before your bright red lipstick goes on flawlessly. So easy, right?

If you'd like a slightly fancier option, or if you want a fun project to do on girls' night or an easy homemade holiday gift, these are some of my favorite homemade flavors below.

MOJITO LIP SCRUB

½   cup sugar
¼   cup walnut oil
1   drop spearmint essential oil
2   drops lime essential oil
4   drops vanilla essential oil

In a bowl, stir together the sugar and walnut oil until combined. Stir in the essential oils until combined. Package in a sealed jar. (I use ones made by Weck.) **MAKES ½ CUP**

LAVENDER VANILLA LIP SCRUB

½   cup sugar
¼   cup walnut oil
1   drop lavender essential oil
4   drops vanilla essential oil

In a bowl, stir together the sugar and walnut oil until combined. Stir in the essential oils until combined. Package in a sealed jar. **MAKES ½ CUP**

HONEY CREAMSICLE LIP SCRUB

½   cup sugar
¼   cup walnut oil
1   tablespoon honey
5   drops orange essential oil
2   drops vanilla essential oil

In a bowl, stir together the sugar, walnut oil, and honey until combined. Stir in the essential oils until combined. Package in a sealed jar. **MAKES ½ CUP**

LEMON VANILLA CAKE LIP SCRUB

½ cup sugar

¼ cup walnut oil

1 drop lemon essential oil

4 drops vanilla essential oil

In a bowl, stir together the sugar and walnut oil until combined. Stir in the essential oils until combined. Package in a sealed jar. MAKES ½ CUP

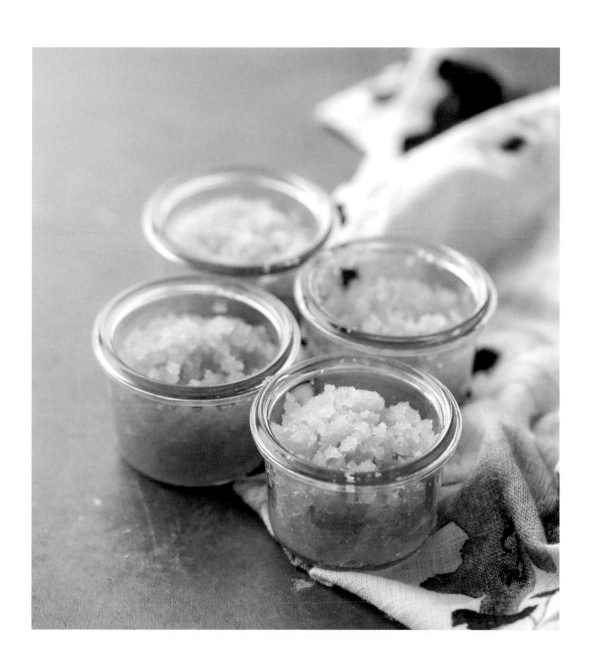

PEPPERMINT SEA SALT FOOT SCRUB

The one exception I make for coarse salt scrubs is on the feet. I'm going to be honest: I'm one of those weirdos who really hate feet, so to add something about feet in my cookbook took an itty-bitty leap of faith. And some caffeine.

I like using a coarse salt and peppermint oil in my foot scrub, mostly because the first foot scrub I ever tried way back in the day was made of something similar, and it stuck. It's a refreshing scent, and the coarse salt helps to slough off dry skin. This is also one area of the body where I think it's fine to exfoliate multiple times per week, even on consecutive days.

1 cup coarse sea salt

½ cup coconut oil, melted

5 drops peppermint essential oil

In a bowl, stir together the sea salt and coconut oil. Stir in the essential oil. Store in a sealed jar. The coconut oil will harden at room temperature, but running the jar under warm water will soften it again. I like to use it both ways! MAKES ABOUT 1 CUP

ROSEMARY SPEARMINT HAND SCRUB

My favorite hand soap in our kitchen is a rosemary mint scent, and we get a ridiculous number of compliments on it. Hand soap! It's crazy.

The scent of this hand scrub is so similar, and I love keeping a jar of this under the kitchen sink so I can easily grab it a few times per week, right as I finish cleaning up for the evening.

Rosemary oil might be a bit difficult to find, though I can occasionally find it at Whole Foods or specialty stores that carry essential oils. If you don't want to splurge on the oil, you can absolutely use dried rosemary instead. I would suggest crushing it down even more in a bowl or by using a mortar and pestle, so it's evenly distributed throughout the scrub.

Stick this in the powder room or on your kitchen counter the next time that you have friends over for a little extra pampering experience!

1 cup sugar

½ cup walnut oil

2 drops spearmint essential oil

1 drop rosemary essential oil

In a bowl, stir together the sugar and walnut oil until combined. Stir in the essential oils. Store in a sealed jar under the kitchen sink! MAKES 1 CUP

LEMON SUGAR HAND SCRUB

1 cup sugar

½ cup walnut oil

3 drops lemon essential oil

In a bowl, stir together the sugar and walnut oil until combined. Stir in the essential oil. Store in a sealed jar under the kitchen sink! MAKES 1 CUP

homemade bath soaks

I was never a bath person until after I had my son. Before that, I thought that baths were the equivalent to sitting in a tub of dirty water (sort of?), but I soon realized just how wonderful and relaxing they could be.

Super-hot baths aren't great for my dry skin, but sometimes I just can't resist. When we were kids, my mom would throw us in oatmeal baths if we had the chicken pox or when my brothers would be covered in poison ivy. Not exactly the most relaxing memories, but these baths are still a weirdly nostalgic thing for me. These are some of my favorite homemade add-ins that I love to drop in the tub for an at-home spa-like experience.

LAVENDER OATMEAL BATH SOAK

½ cup finely ground old-
   fashioned rolled oats

2 drops lavender essential oil

Once the tub is filled with warm bathwater, drop in the oats and the essential oil. Get in there and soak! MAKES 1 SOAK, IS EASILY MULTIPLIED

TIP: To grind the oats, I place them in a food processor and blend until fine crumbs remain.

ROSE WATER OATMEAL BATH SOAK

½ cup finely ground old-
   fashioned rolled oats

½ cup rose water

Fresh, untreated rose petals,
   for sprinkling (optional)

Once the tub is filled with warm bathwater, drop in the oats and rose water. If desired, sprinkle some rose petals in the tub! Get in there and soak! MAKES 1 SOAK, IS EASILY MULTIPLIED

LEMON PEPPERMINT BATH SOAK

½ cup Epsom salts

1 drop lemon essential oil

1 drop peppermint essential oil

Pour the Epsom salts into the tub while the warm water is running. Drop in the essential oils and soak! MAKES 1 SOAK, IS EASILY MULTIPLIED

ALMOND OATMEAL BATH SOAK

½ cup finely ground old-
   fashioned rolled oats

½ cup almond oil

Once the tub is filled with warm bathwater, drop in the oats and almond oil. Soak it up! MAKES 1 SOAK, IS EASILY MULTIPLIED

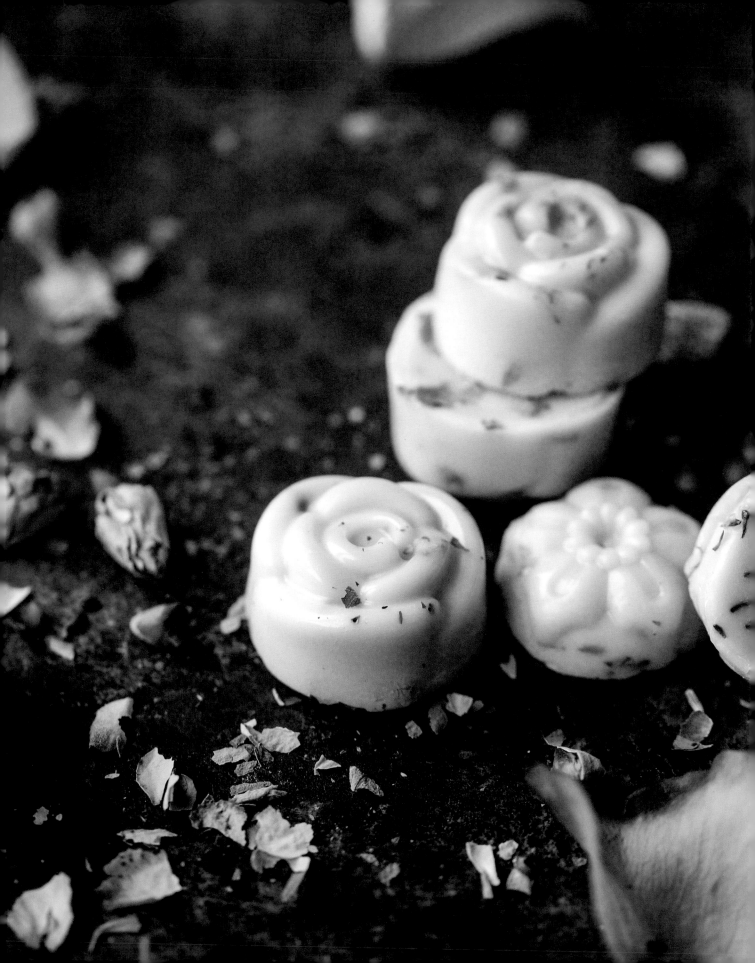

homemade bath melts

Bath melts are a luxurious scented way of adding moisture to your bath! I love how silky they make the water feel, because it leaves your skin feeling soft and just lightly delicious.

Making bath melts at home is similar to making lip balm—they need a touch of beeswax so they firm up. This makes them portable and, better yet, so giftable! You can find a ton of cute molds on Amazon on in craft stores, but an ice cube tray (kept solely for making melts!) does great in a pinch. Make these as party favors or as Mother's Day or holiday gifts. Or just for yourself because you're oh-so special!

CHOCOLATE ICE CREAM BATH MELT

½ cup cocoa butter

1 teaspoon beeswax

4 drops vanilla essential oil

1 teaspoon unsweetened cocoa powder

In a double boiler, heat the cocoa butter and beeswax over medium-low heat until they melt. Stir in the essential oil. Let cool slightly. Once cool, stir in the cocoa. Gently pour the mixture into 2 molds and let firm up overnight. Once the molds are set, package them in cute containers or jars. MAKES 2

MINTED CITRUS BATH MELT

½ cup shea butter

1 teaspoon beeswax

3 drops orange essential oil

1 drop peppermint essential oil

½ teaspoon grated orange zest

In a double boiler, heat the shea butter and beeswax over medium-low heat until they melt. Stir in the essential oils. Let cool slightly. Once cool, stir in the orange zest. Gently pour the mixture into 2 molds and let firm up overnight. Once the molds are set, package them in cute containers or jars. MAKES 2

VANILLA ROSE BATH MELT

½ cup shea butter

1 teaspoon beeswax

4 drops vanilla essential oil

1 drop rose essential oil

2 teaspoons dried untreated rose petals

In a double boiler, heat the shea butter and beeswax over medium-low heat until they melt. Stir in the essential oils. Let cool slightly. Once cool, stir in the rose petals. Gently pour the mixture into 2 molds and let firm up overnight. Once the molds are set, package them in cute containers or jars. MAKES 2

CAKE BATTER BATH MELT

½ cup cocoa butter

1 teaspoon beeswax

6 drops vanilla essential oil

Assorted dye-free sprinkles

In a double boiler, heat the cocoa butter and beeswax over medium-low heat until they melt. Stir in the essential oil. Let cool slightly. Once cool, stir in the sprinkles. Gently pour the mixture into 2 molds and let firm up overnight. Once the molds are set, package them in cute containers or jars. **MAKES 2**

LAVENDER HONEY BATH MELT

¼ cup shea butter

¼ cup cocoa butter

2 teaspoons honey

1 teaspoon beeswax

4 drops lavender essential oil

1 teaspoon dried lavender flowers

In a double boiler, heat the shea butter, cocoa butter, honey, and beeswax over medium-low heat until they melt. Stir in the essential oil. Let cool slightly. Once cool, stir in the dried lavender. Gently pour the mixture into 2 molds and let firm up overnight. Once the molds are set, package them in cute containers or jars. **MAKES 2**

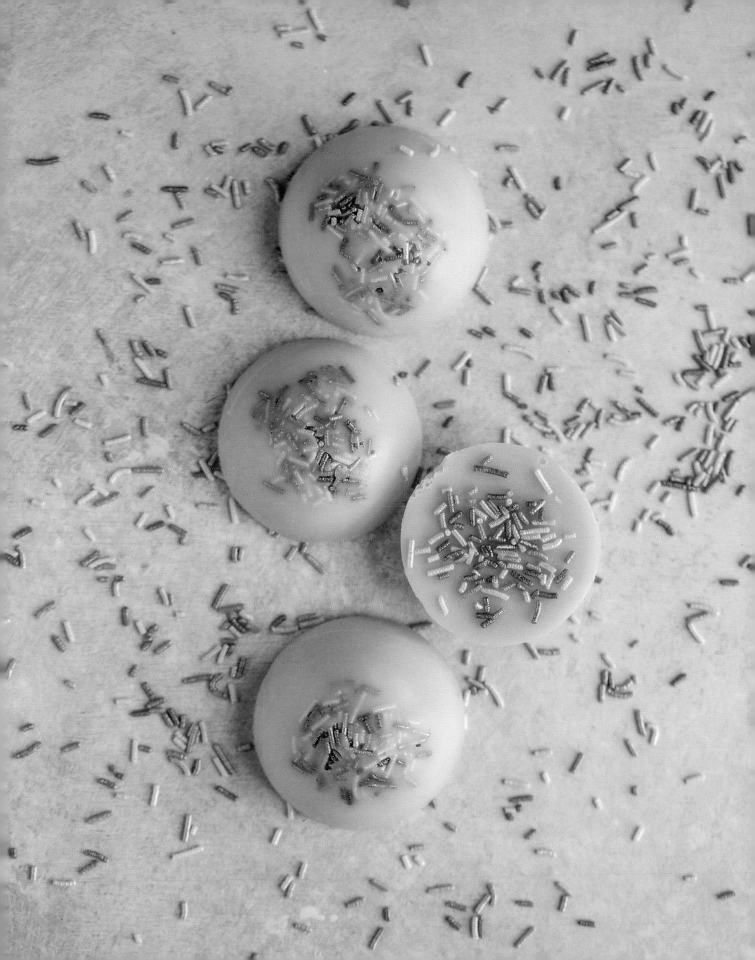

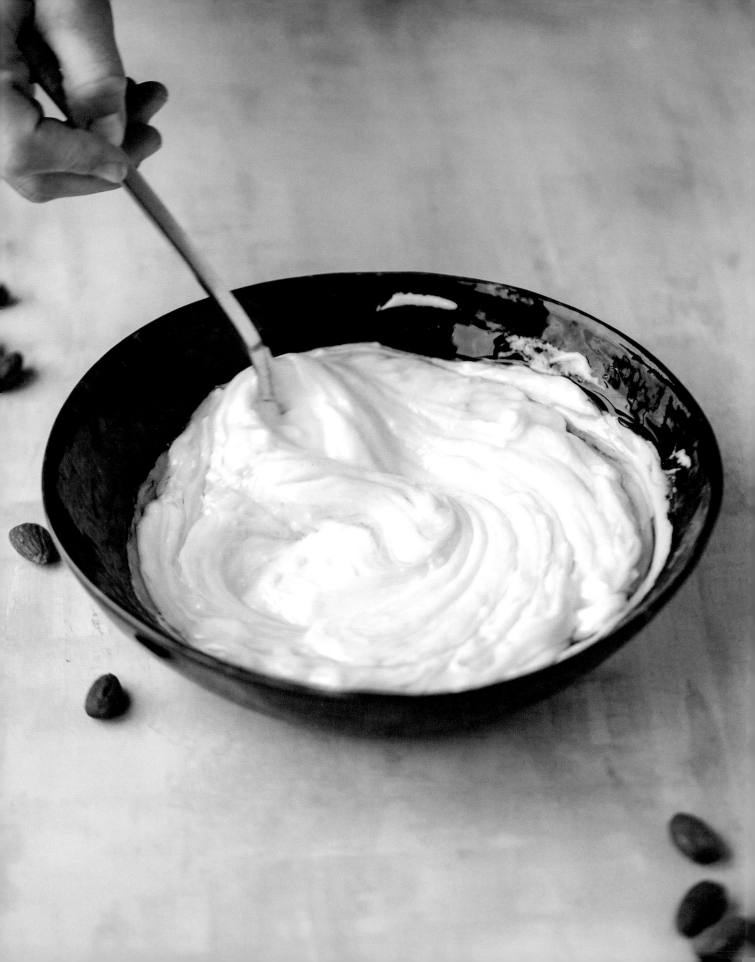

homemade face masks

As a child of the Internet generation, I have a difficult time disconnecting and slowing down. I also work from home, so since work is always with me, it can be challenging to turn off my computer and my brain.

I've done face masks with friends since my early tween years—those cheap ones in the drugstore were one of the first purchases we would make together for a sleepover. It was the cliché sleepover photo, too, what with our hair out of our faces with funny headbands, our faces slathered with mint green–colored clay, and cray pajamas. We'd also do things like prank call friends and boys, which probably doesn't even exist anymore since everyone has their own cell phone these days.

Now that I'm older, I use face masks (and especially sheet masks) to decompress, relax, and rehydrate my skin when I just need to take a "moment." You'll notice that most of my beauty DIYs lend themselves to moisturizing the skin, because not only is that my biggest challenge, but it's also a challenge we face as we grow older. However, my husband has oilier skin than I do, and he still loves a good drying, clay face mask every now and then. I've included a few fun options below (that smell like dessert, of course) to make at home, ranging from light exfoliation to extra hydration!

It should be noted that these are one-time-use masks that should be prepped right before using!

OATMEAL FACE MASK
SLIGHTLY EXFOLIATING, MOISTURIZING

¼ cup plain Greek yogurt

2 tablespoons finely ground old-fashioned rolled oats

2 teaspoons honey

In a bowl, stir together the yogurt, oats, and honey. Rub the mixture on your clean face and let it soak in for 20 minutes. Remove with warm water and a soft washcloth.

COCONUT YOGURT FACE MASK
MOISTURIZING

¼ cup plain Greek yogurt

2 tablespoons coconut oil, melted and cooled

1 tablespoon full-fat coconut milk

In a bowl, stir together the yogurt, cooled coconut oil, and coconut milk. Rub the mixture on your clean face and let it soak in for 20 minutes. Remove with warm water and a soft washcloth.

CHOCOLATE COFFEE FACE MASK
EXFOLIATING AND MOISTURIZING

¼ cup plain Greek yogurt

1 teaspoon unsweetened cocoa
powder

1 teaspoon finely ground coffee
grounds

In a bowl, stir together the yogurt, cocoa, and coffee grounds. Rub the mixture gently on your clean face (rubbing will give it a bit of exfoliating action!) and let it soak in for 20 minutes. Remove with warm water and a soft washcloth.

CHOCOLATE CAKE FACE MASK
MOISTURIZING

¼ cup plain Greek yogurt

1 teaspoon unsweetened cocoa
powder

1 teaspoon almond oil

In a bowl, stir together the yogurt, cocoa, and almond oil. Rub the mixture on your clean face and let it soak in for 20 minutes. Remove with warm water and a soft washcloth.

HONEY ALMOND FACE MASK
MOISTURIZING, ANTI-AGING

¼ cup plain Greek yogurt

3 tablespoons honey

2 teaspoons almond oil

In a bowl, stir together the yogurt, honey, and almond oil. Rub it on your clean face and let it soak in for 20 minutes. Remove with warm water and a soft washcloth.

ACAI FACE MASK
MOISTURIZING, ANTI-AGING

¼ cup plain Greek yogurt

3 tablespoons honey

½ teaspoon acai powder

In a bowl, stir together the yogurt, honey, and acai powder. Rub the mixture on your clean face and let it soak in for 20 minutes. Remove with warm water and a soft washcloth.

AVOCADO BANANA FACE MASK
MOISTURIZING

½ avocado, peeled and mashed

½ banana, mashed

2 teaspoons avocado oil

In a bowl, stir together the avocado, banana, and avocado oil until combined. Slather the mixture on your clean face and let it soak in for 20 minutes. Remove with warm water and a soft washcloth.

COCONANA FACE MASK
MOISTURIZING

½ banana, mashed

1 teaspoon coconut oil, melted

½ teaspoon unsweetened
shredded coconut

In a bowl, stir together the banana, coconut oil, and shredded coconut. Rub the mixture gently on your clean face and let it soak in for 20 minutes. Remove with warm water and a soft washcloth.

hair masks

With the plight of having drier skin also comes drier hair. I am lucky to have a lot of hair that is fairly thick, but with the regular use of products and heat, it can really dry out. Occasionally I'll also have dry scalp issues since the rest of my skin is dry, and that is nothing short of humiliating. I also went through a good decade when I was into dying my very dark brown hair blonde, which did nothing but destroy the texture of my hair and make it feel like straw.

In the '90s, I was so desperate for my mom to buy me one of those old-school V8 hot oil hair packets. I have no idea why. The magazine advertisements and commercials sold me like the market-ers' dream that I am. It just seems so luxurious. So lovely to have warm oil in your hair, resulting in this super-shiny mane.

She never bit, and I never got to try the hot oil hair treatment. So here I am, 20 years later, still feeling deprived, but not foolish enough to go to the drugstore and buy the product that I believe is still around, so I made my own with avocado oil. Mmmmmm.

Below you can find some of my favorite hair treatments that can easily be whipped up in the kitchen. While I use a natural, store-bought shampoo and conditioner, I don't use any other treat-ments on my hair (aside from the occasional leave-in conditioner for tangles, or blow-dry spray to dry my hair quickly) for moisturizing than these ones straight out of my kitchen!

HOT AVOCADO OIL
FOR DEEP CONDITIONING

¼ cup avocado oil, warmed slightly

Use the oil on damp or dry hair, working it from the middle of the head down to the ends and avoiding the roots. Leave it on for 1 hour and then rinse out.

GREEK YOGURT
FOR DEEP CONDITIONING

⅓ cup plain Greek yogurt

Coat damp or dry hair with the yogurt from the middle of the head down to the ends, avoiding the roots. Leave it on for 1 hour and then rinse out.

BANANA BREAD

1   banana, mashed

2   tablespoons coconut oil, melted

In a bowl, combine the banana and coconut oil. Coat damp or dry hair with the mixture from the middle of the head down to the ends, avoiding the roots. Leave it on for 1 hour and then rinse out.

AVOCADO HONEY
TO MOISTURIZE AND STRENGTHEN

1   avocado, pitted, peeled, and mashed

2   tablespoons honey

In a bowl, combine the avocado and honey. Coat damp or dry hair with the mixture from the middle of the head down to the ends, avoiding the roots. Leave it on for 1 hour and then rinse out.

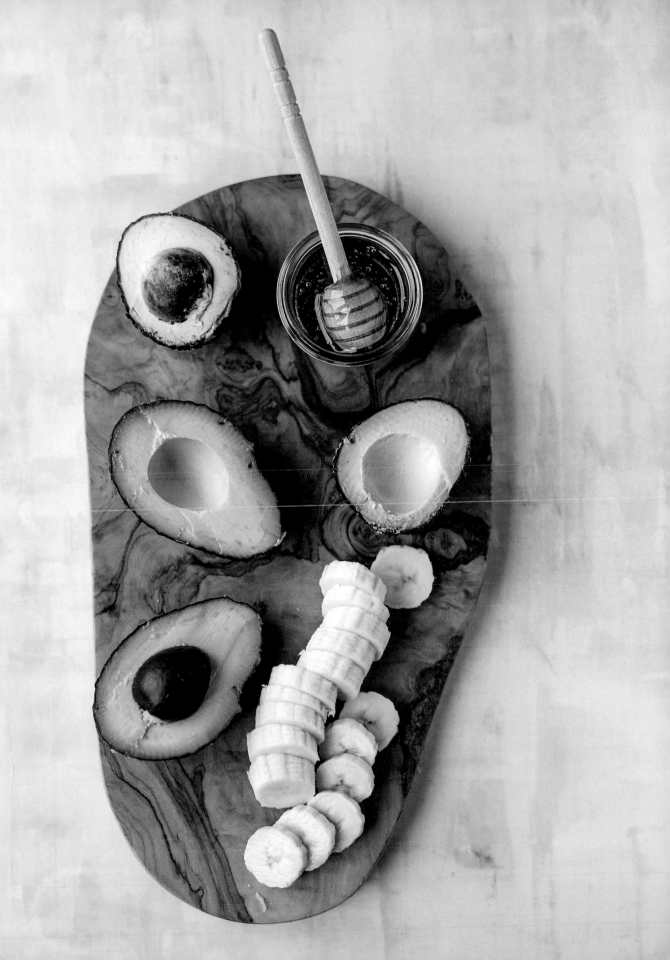

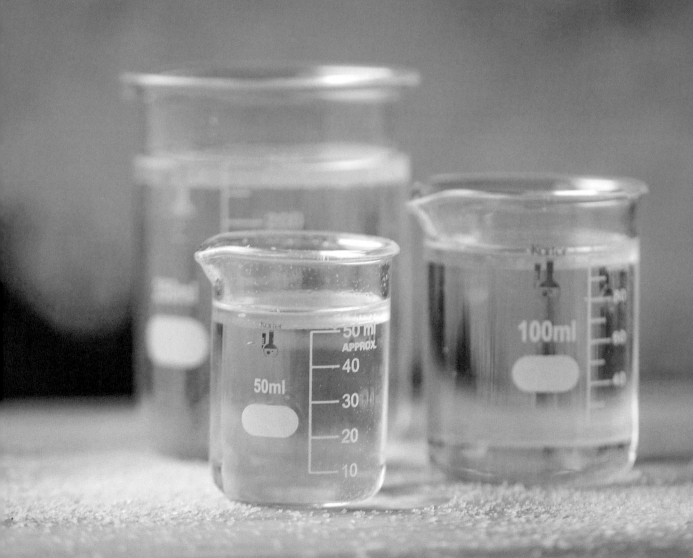

beachy waves sea salt spray

So, now that I've ranted on about how incredibly dry my skin and hair usually are, I'm going to go ahead and tell you a way to make it drier.

I know. It seems a bit hypocritical, and it very much is. But if you have longer hair and crave the beachy waves look? Homemade texture spray is one way to go. And as long as you don't use it every single day, it won't dry out your hair to the point of exhaustion.

I feel like the beachy waves look has been "in" for more than 20 years. Easily since I was 10 or 11 years old, when I would purchase the aqua bottle of John Frieda beach waves sea salt spray and use it daily for three months straight to pretend I was always at the beach.

This is just like that! While the sea salt can be drying, it helps to give your hair texture and really promote that effortless wavy look. My hair has a weird natural wave to it, but I like to throw a few waves into it with a curling wand or straightener before using this spray, because I find it's a way to use less spray.

Also! You can totally make this beach-scented with a few drops of coconut extract. It is alcohol based, which is also drying, but it's not enough to damage your hair with occasional use, and as long as you are conditioning, it should be all good!

1½ cups warm water

1½ teaspoons sea salt

1½ teaspoons avocado oil or fractionated coconut oil

2 teaspoons vanilla essential oil

¼ teaspoon coconut extract (optional)

In a bowl, whisk together the warm water and sea salt until the salt dissolves. Stir in the oils and coconut extract (if using). Pour the mixture into a spray container (preferably glass). Shake before using!

homemade lip balms

My collection of lip balms and glosses could be considered something out of the show Hoarders.

Okay, okay, it might not be that bad, but I certainly love to "collect" these gems of scent, flavor, and color.

Coconut oil on its own is an amazing lip moisturizer, but it's not the most easily transportable. If you mix just a touch of beeswax with the coconut oil, it will help it remain firm so you can throw it in your purse on the go!

And now, for my favorite scents . . .

VANILLA LIP BALM

1½ tablespoons coconut oil

1 tablespoon beeswax

3 drops vanilla essential oil

In a double boiler, heat the coconut oil and beeswax over medium-low heat until just melted. Remove from the heat and stir in the essential oil. Very gently pour the mixture into a container with a lid and let it firm up. Use as desired.

LAVENDER MINT LIP BALM

1½ tablespoons coconut oil

1 tablespoon beeswax

2 drops lavender essential oil

1 drop peppermint essential oil

In a double boiler, heat the coconut oil and beeswax over medium-low heat until just melted. Remove from the heat and stir in the essential oils. Very gently pour the mixture into a container with a lid and let it firm up. Use as desired.

MACAROON LIP BALM

1½ tablespoons coconut oil

1 tablespoon beeswax

1 teaspoon almond oil

4 drops vanilla essential oil

In a double boiler, heat the coconut oil, beeswax, and almond oil over medium-low heat until just melted. Remove from the heat and stir in the essential oil. Very gently pour the mixture into a container with a lid and let it firm up. Use as desired.

ACAI LIP BALM

1½ tablespoons coconut oil

1 tablespoon beeswax

2 drops vanilla essential oil

¼ teaspoon acai powder

In a double boiler, heat the coconut oil and beeswax over medium-low heat until just melted. Remove from the heat and stir in the essential oil and acai powder. Very gently pour the mixture into a container with a lid and let it firm up.

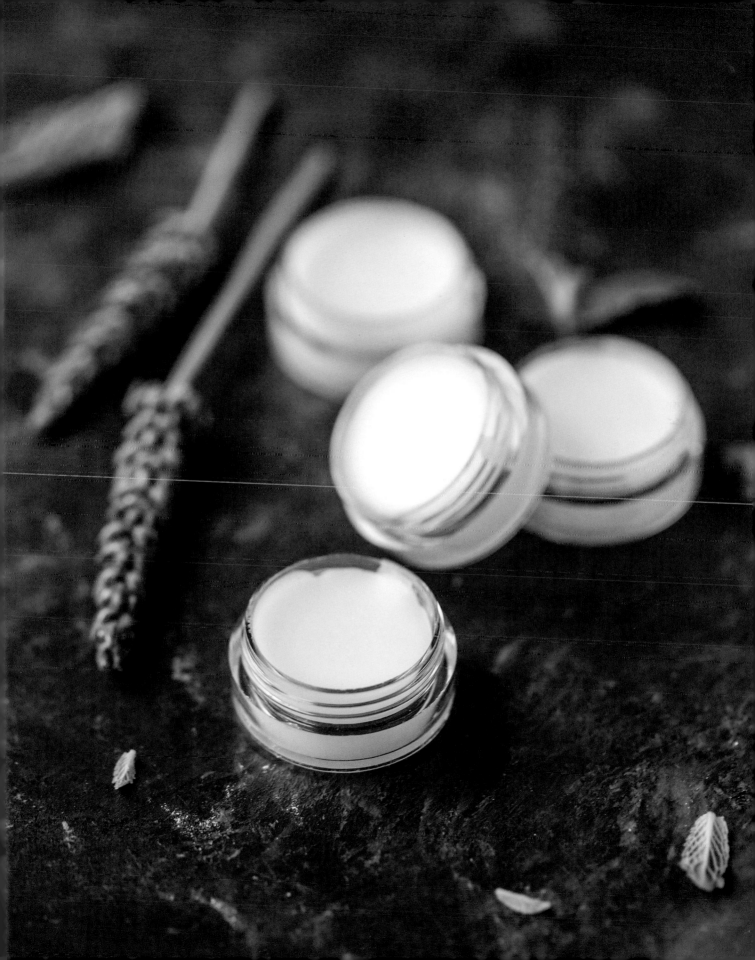

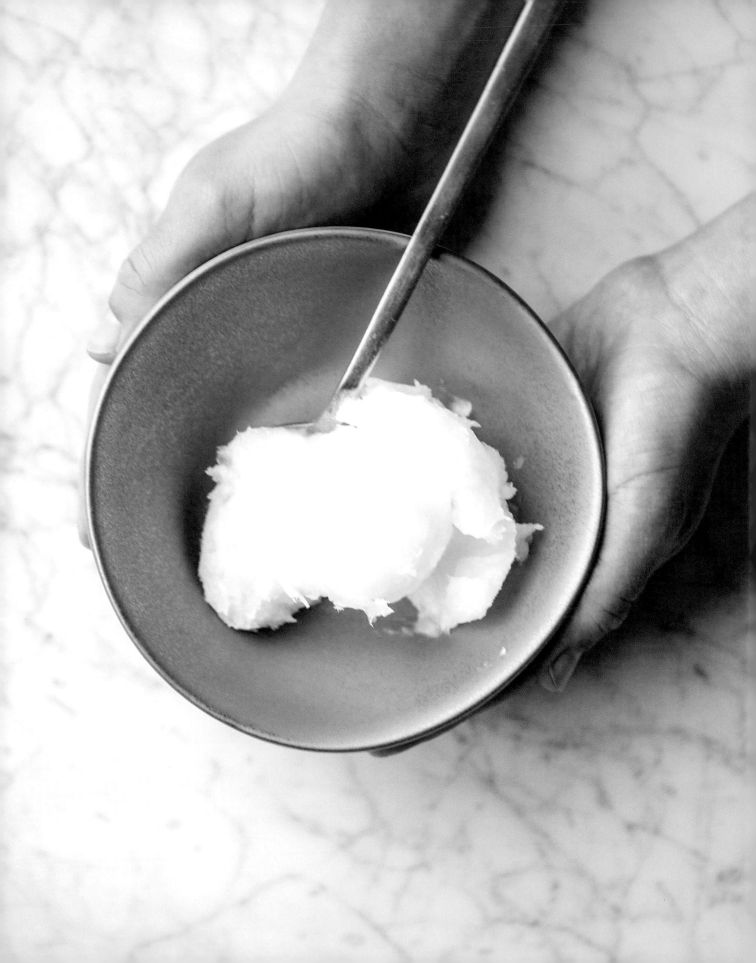

COCONUT OIL MAGIC!
MY FAVORITE USES FOR COCONUT OIL

Coconut oil *is* magic. I swear it is. I've said it before, and I'll say it again: I was using coconut oil before coconut oil was cool.

These are my favorite ways to use it in my everyday beauty routine.

Easy eye makeup remover.
I've used coconut oil on my eyelids to remove makeup off and on for at least 6 years. While I do prefer some oil makeup removers that are in a pump (for hygiene and convenience purposes), if I'm in a pinch and have only coconut oil, massaging it into the eyelids for a few seconds removes all mascara and eyeliner! It's wonderful and, of course, not drying whatsoever.

Homemade body cream.
If you throw coconut oil in solid form in your stand mixer and whip it with the whisk attachment, it becomes nice and creamy, like actual body cream. This is an awesome way to use coconut oil if the oil form freaks you out or feels too greasy! Of course, you can always add a drop of essential oil in there, too, for scent.

Cuticle cream.
I love mixing 1 or 2 tablespoons of coconut oil with ½ teaspoon almond oil and storing it in a jar for a nighttime cuticle cream.

Deep conditioner for hair ends.
Most often, I use coconut oil to moisturize the ends of my hair. Occasionally, I even sleep with it in my hair! I will massage 2 tablespoons into the ends of my hair and wrap it in a soft jersey towel. I rinse it out after a few hours or first thing in the morning.

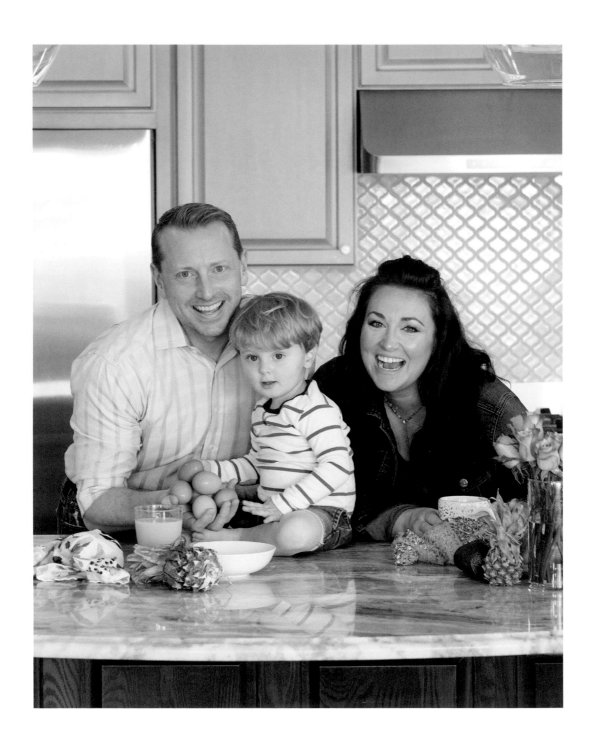

acknowledgments

To Eddie, for not only unloading the dishwasher at 4am on long recipe days and for not only dealing with eleven unfolded baskets of laundry around our house for two weeks, for living amongst a pile of bowls and plates and fridges so stuffed to the brim that they can barely be opened without ingredients falling to the floor, thank you for your constant support for my passion and everything you do to help bring this dream alive. You and Max and this babe on the way are on my life.

To my mom, who never walks into my house on a recipe testing day and loses her mind or asks me "how we live in this disaster" even though she surely must think it. You are the best!

To all of my family and friends, who constantly inspire me and taste my creations. I love you so much!

To Dervla Kelly, who is not only my dream editor but also my good friend. Thank you so much for your constant dedication to making sure this book was the absolute best it could be!

To Yeon, Anna, Amy and the entire Rodale team. Thank you so much for making this one of the most gorgeous books I have ever laid eyes on! I cannot even begin to explain how much I love it.

To Stacey Glick, who somehow constantly always believes in me and graciously answers my wordy, neurotic emails and texts with even more encouragement than I deserve. I will forever thank you for my very first pretzel croissant!

To Erin Alvarez, who seriously saved my soul in the year of 2017 with all of her incredible food styling help. You make even the ugliest of dishes (hello, orange everything!) look gorgeous and I can't thank you enough for helping me to not hate every photo I take.

To everyone that helped bring this cookbook alive in the testing and photography process, especially Alex, Colleen and Katy. I couldn't have done it without you!

Finally, to all the amazing readers of How Sweet Eats, who are the only reason that this book exists. Thank you so much for sharing daily rambles with me and building our community and existing in this invisible internet world. And for allowing me to have my dream job.

ACKNOWLEDGMENTS |

index

Underscored page references indicate boxed text. **Boldfaced** page references indicate photographs.